LEARN TO CUT

A structured program of cutting tasks with reproducible patterns

by Robin R. Wolfe

Communication Skill Builders®
3830 E. Bellevue/P.O. Box 42050
Tucson, Arizona 85733
(602) 323-7500

Duplicating

You may prefer to copy the designated reproducible materials by using stencils or spirit masters. It is not necessary to tear pages out of this book. Make a single photocopy of the desired page. Use that photocopy to make a stencil or spirit master on a thermal copier.

Communication Skill Builders, Inc.®
3830 E. Bellevue/P.O. Box 42050
Tucson, Arizona 85733
(602) 323-7500

ISBN 0-88450-994-X Catalog No. 7401

10 9 8 7 6 5
Printed in the United States of America

Contents

Part 2—Art Projects

Holiday Art Projects

Introduction

Learn to Cut is a structured program designed to teach the skill of cutting and shape recognition simultaneously. Suggestions are given for enhancing language skills while teaching cutting techniques.

In Part 1 of the *Learn to Cut* program, the fine motor task of cutting is broken down into eight major Skills structured in a hierarchy of Steps. The eight Skills are:

Skill 1—Snipping lines of varying lengths
Skill 2—Cutting lines of varying widths
Skill 3—Cutting a simple shape with a ¼" line
Skill 4—Cutting a simple shape with a ⅛" line
Skill 5—Cutting two simple shapes with a ⅛" line
Skill 6—Cutting a complex shape with a ¼" line
Skill 7—Cutting a complex shape with a ⅛" line
Skill 8—Cutting two complex shapes with a ⅛" line

Objectives for each Skill are clearly stated for meeting IEP goals.

A detailed task analysis of Steps is described for each Skill.

Pre- and Posttests measure achievement for each Skill. The tests serve as both an indicator of mastery and as a tool in placing the student at the correct Skill level. Students begin the *Learn to Cut* program on the Skill level indicated by the first pretest error.

Each pretest item is paralleled by a structured worksheet. The worksheets are designed to teach each Step that leads to Skill mastery. They are used for daily practice.

A recording sheet is included for tracking each student's tests and daily progress.

All materials may be reproduced.

At Skills 1 and 2, the teacher works individually with each student, offering assistance in correct scissors manipulation. At the higher Skills, the teacher may choose to work with individual students or with small groups, encouraging independence in accomplishing the task.

Part 2 of the *Learn to Cut* program contains 61 individual art projects, including 25 holiday cutting activities. Patterns are given for each project. All patterns may be reproduced. Students are encouraged to start and complete each cutting project independently.

Suggestions for Language Enhancement

Language skills may be enriched while teaching cutting skills. The following example may be adapted to each task in the *Learn to Cut* program.

The teacher places a picture in front of the student.

Teacher: What is this picture?
Student: An elephant.
Teacher: Good! This is a picture of an elephant!

Or: Teacher: What is this picture?
(The student does not respond.)
Teacher: This is a picture of an elephant. What is this picture?
Student: Elephant.
Teacher: Good! This is a picture of an elephant.

The teacher places a cutting shape in front of the student.

Teacher: What do we call this shape?
Student: A square.
Teacher: Good! This is a square.

Or: Teacher: What do we call this shape?
(The student does not respond.)
Teacher: This shape is a square. What do we call this shape?
Student: A square.
Teacher: Good! Now you are going to cut out the square.

The teacher hands the student a pair of scissors. The student begins to cut.

Teacher: What are you doing?
Student: Cutting.
Teacher: Good! You are cutting out a square.

Or: Teacher: What are you doing?
(The student does not respond.)
Teacher: You are cutting out a square. What are you doing?
Student: Cutting out a square.
Teacher: Good!

Continue to question and extend the student's vocabulary throughout the cutting process. The number and kinds of questions you ask will depend on the individual student and the project being cut. Other questions might be, "Where does the square go? Have you ever seen an elephant? Where did you see the elephant?"

You may want to record the student's verbal responses, particularly if increasing responses is an IEP objective.

Be creative—and have fun! Having a pleasant, fun conversation tends to trigger responses. Don't make the session threatening; the student should look forward to this special individual time! Conclude each session on a positive note, with a smile and a word of encouragement!

Goals and Objectives

SKILL 1—SNIPPING

Objective: Student cuts a line ¼" wide, stopping at the designated length, with 80% accuracy.

Step 1—Student cuts a line ¼" wide, 1" long.

Step 2—Student cuts a line ¼" wide, 2" long.

Step 3—Student cuts a line ¼" wide, in varying lengths.

SKILL 2—CUTTING A LINE

Objective: Student cuts a picture in half, staying on the line, 80% of the time.

Step 1—Student cuts a line ½" wide.

Step 2—Student cuts a line ¼" wide.

Step 3—Student cuts a line ⅛" wide.

SKILL 3—CUTTING A SIMPLE SHAPE—¼" LINE

Objective: Student cuts out a simple shape with a line ¼" wide, and pastes it on a fixed outline, with 80% accuracy.

Step 1—Strips

Step 2—Squares

Step 3—Rectangles

Step 4—Triangles

Step 5—Diamonds

SKILL 4—CUTTING A SIMPLE SHAPE—⅛" LINE

Objective: Student cuts out a simple shape with a line ⅛" wide, and pastes it on a fixed outline, with 80% accuracy.

Step 1—Strips

Step 2—Squares

Step 3—Rectangles

Step 4—Triangles

Step 5—Diamonds

SKILL 5—CUTTING COMBINED SIMPLE SHAPES—⅛" LINE

Objective: Student cuts out two familiar shapes with a line ⅛" wide, and pastes them on the corresponding fixed outlines, with 80% accuracy.

Step 1—Combined Shapes

Step 2—Smaller Combined Shapes

SKILL 6—CUTTING CIRCLES AND COMPLEX SHAPES—¼" LINE

Objective: Student cuts out circles and complex shapes of varying sizes with a line ¼" wide, and pastes them on the corresponding fixed outlines, with 80% accuracy.

Step 1—Circles

Step 2—Ovals

Step 3—Crescents

Step 4—Hearts

Step 5—Stars

SKILL 7—CUTTING CIRCLES AND COMPLEX SHAPES—⅛" LINE

Objective: Student cuts out circles and complex shapes of varying sizes with a line ⅛" wide, and pastes them on the corresponding fixed outlines, with 80% accuracy.

Step 1—Circles

Step 2—Ovals

Step 3—Crescents

Step 4—Hearts

Step 5—Stars

SKILL 8—CUTTING COMBINED CIRCLES AND COMPLEX SHAPES—⅛" LINE

Objective: Student cuts out two familiar shapes with a line ⅛" wide, and pastes them on the corresponding fixed outlines, with 80% accuracy.

Step 1—Combined Shapes

Step 2—Smaller Combined Shapes

Learn to Cut

Recording Sheet

Name ____ Page ____

Date	Skill	Step	Pretest Passed	Worksheet	Posttest Passed	Comments

Criterion: 80% accuracy cutting on line

PART 1
Skills and Steps

Skill 1—Snipping

Objective: Student cuts a line ¼" wide, stopping at the designated length, with 80% accuracy.

Procedure

Pretest: Student takes Skill 1 Pretest.

If criterion met: Student advances to Skill 2.

If criterion not met:

1. Student cuts Skill 1 worksheets:
   - Step 1—Student cuts a line ¼" wide, 1" long.
   - Step 2—Student cuts a line ¼" wide, 2" long.
   - Step 3—Student cuts a line ¼" wide, in varying lengths.
2. Student takes Skill 1 Posttest.

   If criterion met: Student advances to Skill 2.

   If criterion not met: Student repeats Skill 1 worksheets and Posttest.

Skill 1—Snipping
Pre/Posttest

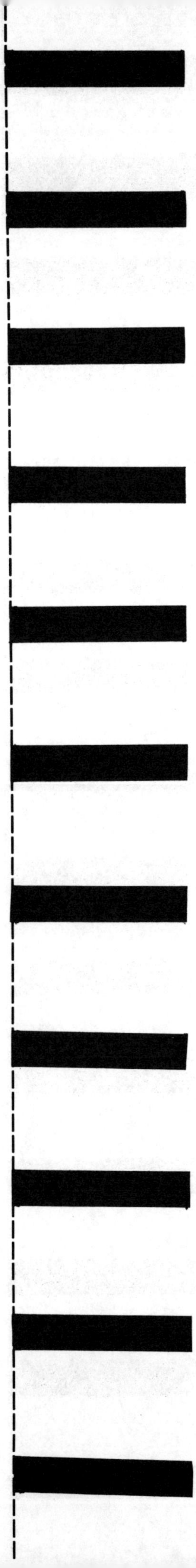

Skill 1—Snipping
Step 2 Worksheet

Skill 1—Snipping
Step 3 Worksheet

Skill 2—Cutting a Line

Objective: Student cuts a picture in half, staying on the line, 80% of the time.

Procedure
Pretest: Student takes Skill 2 Pretest.

If criterion met: Student advances to Skill 3.

If criterion not met:
1. Student cuts Skill 2 worksheets:
   Step 1—Student cuts a line ½" wide (4 worksheets).
   Step 2—Student cuts a line ¼" wide (4 worksheets).
   Step 3—Student cuts a line ⅛" wide (3 worksheets).
2. Student takes Skill 2 Posttest.
   If criterion met: Student advances to Skill 3.
   If criterion not met: Student repeats Skill 2 worksheets and Posttest.

Skill 2—Cutting a Line
Pre/Posttest

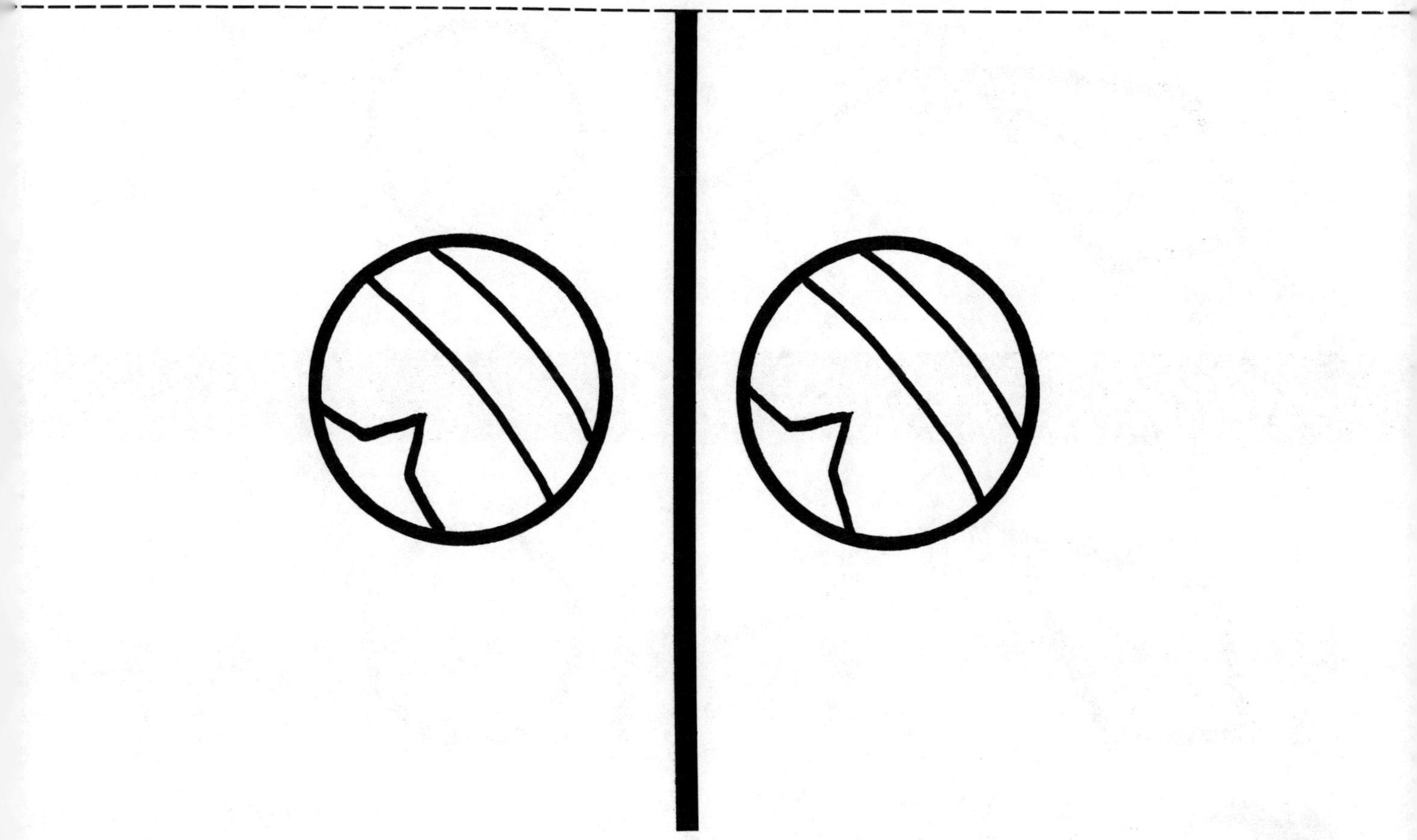

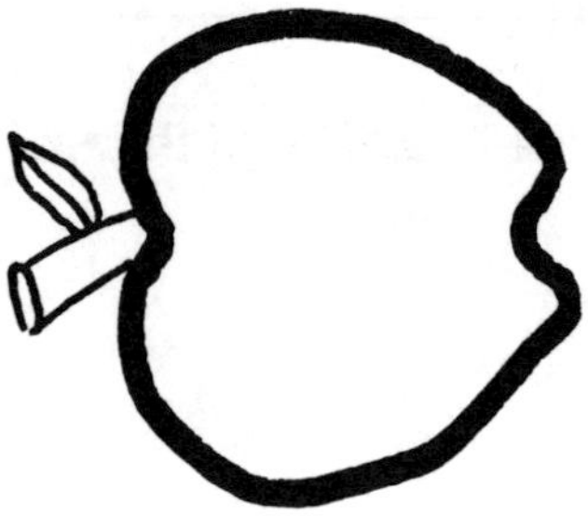

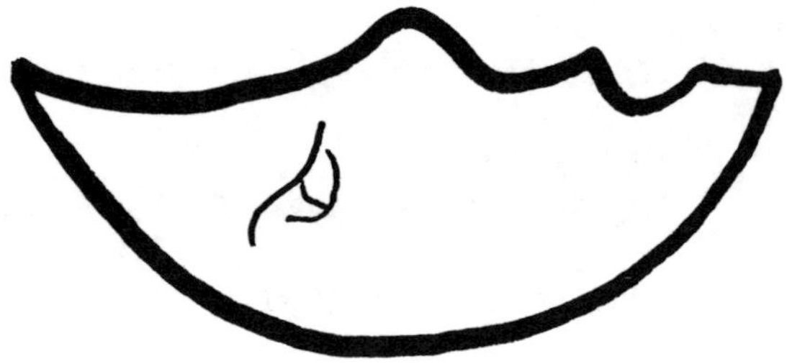

Skill 2
Step 1 Worksheet

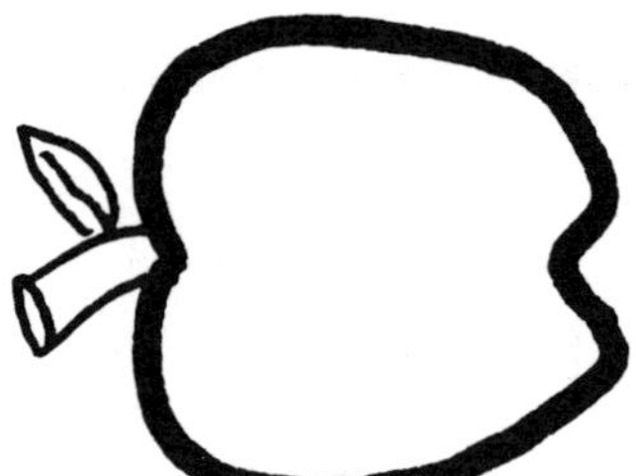

Skill 2
Step 1 Worksheet

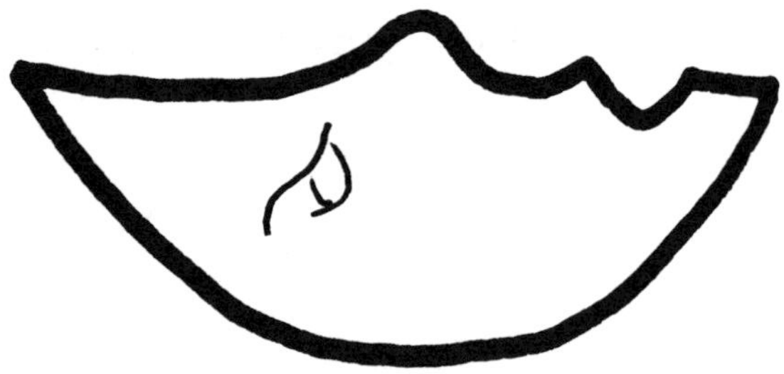

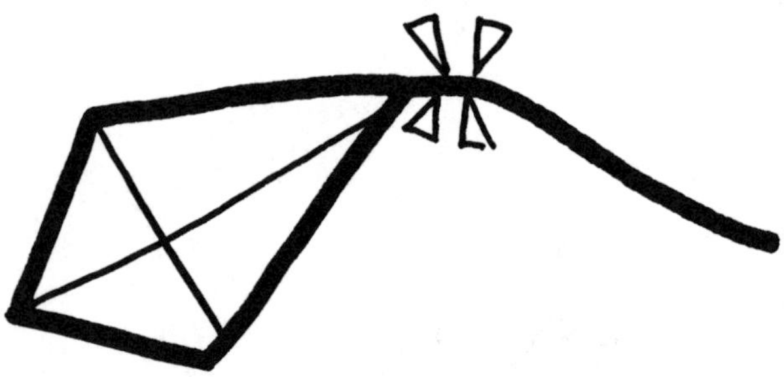

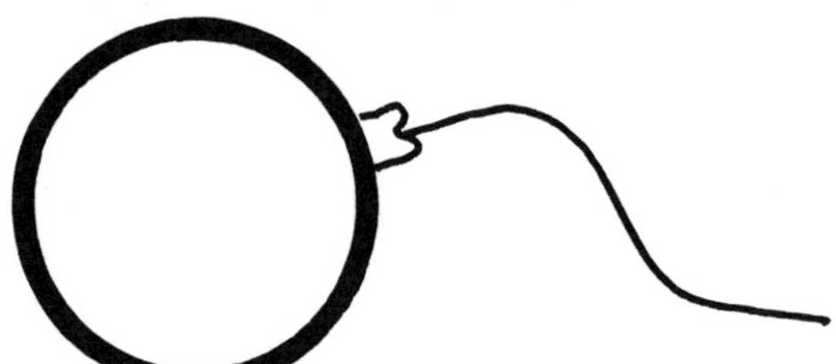

Skill 2
Step 1 Worksheet

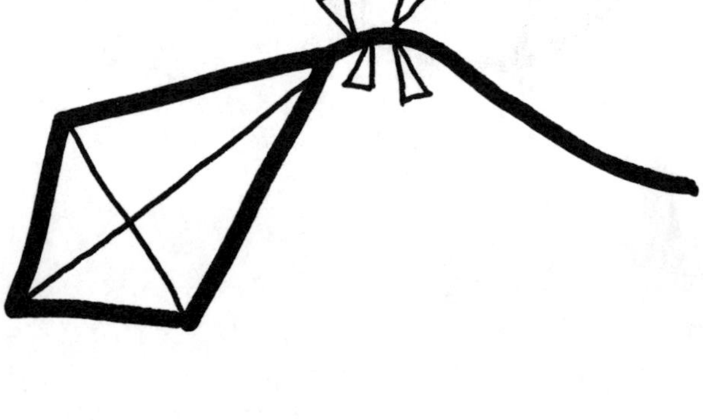

Skill 2
Step 1 Worksheet

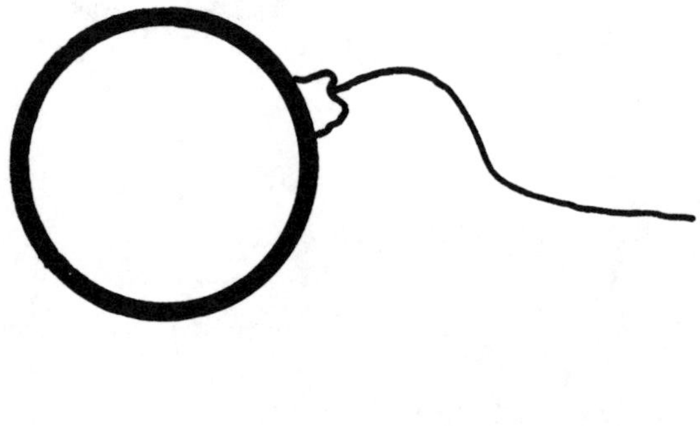

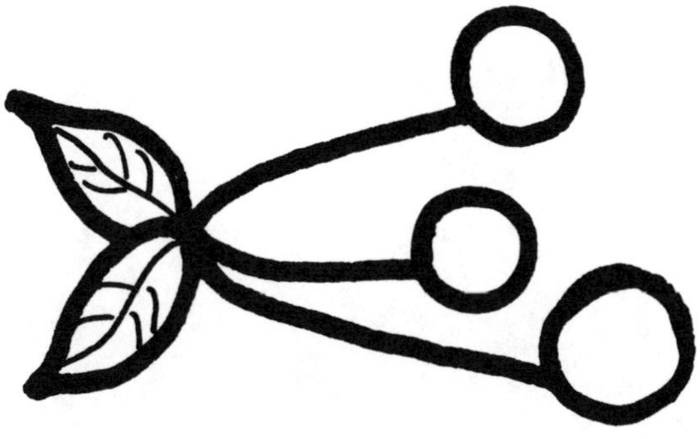

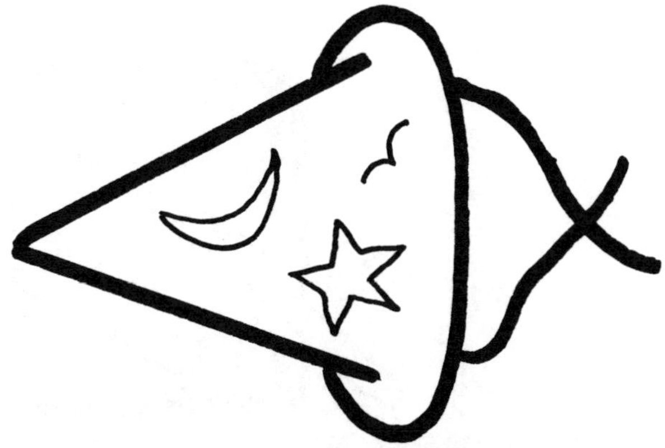

Skill 2
Step 2 Worksheet

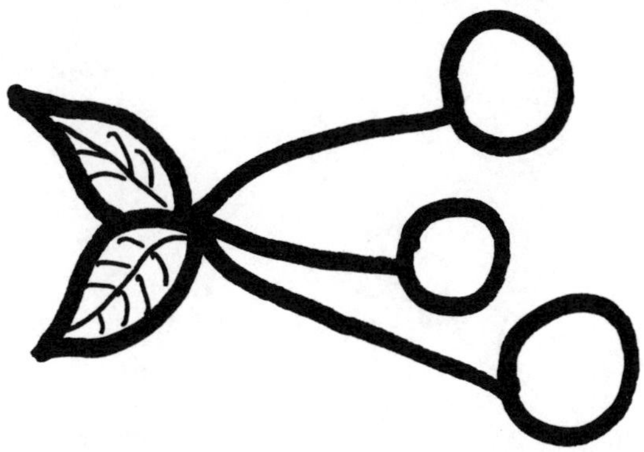

Skill 2
Step 2 Worksheet

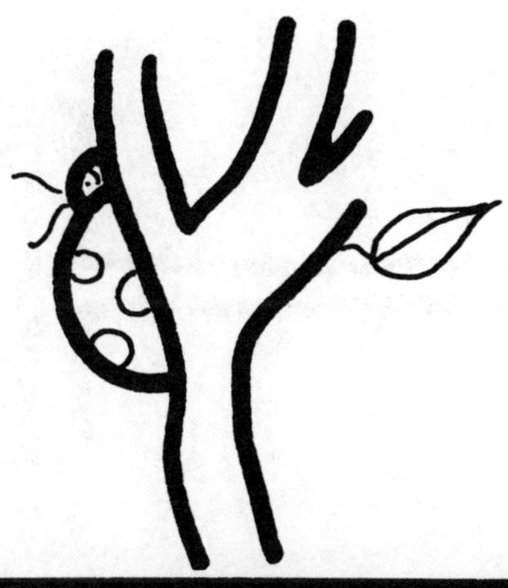

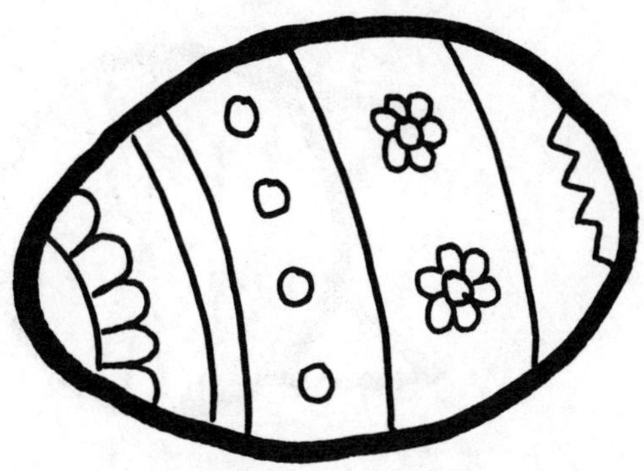

Skill 2
Step 2 Worksheet

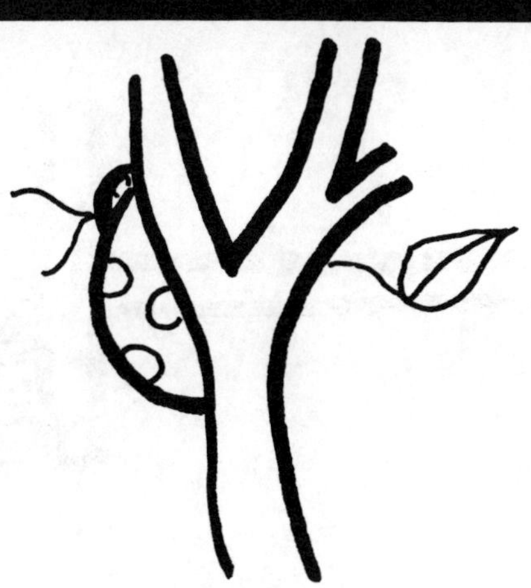

Skill 2
Step 2 Worksheet

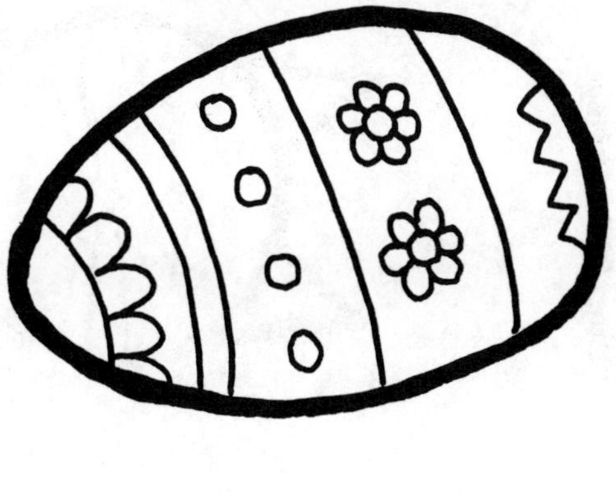

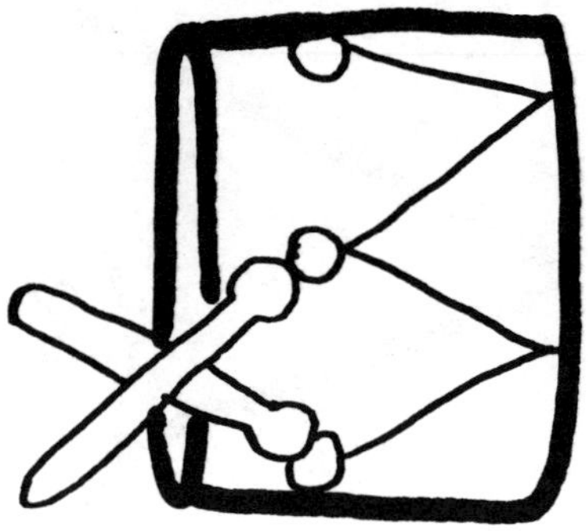

Skill 2
Step 3 Worksheet

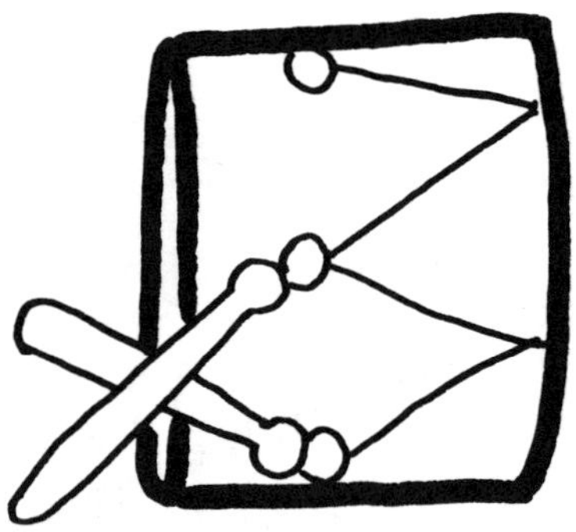

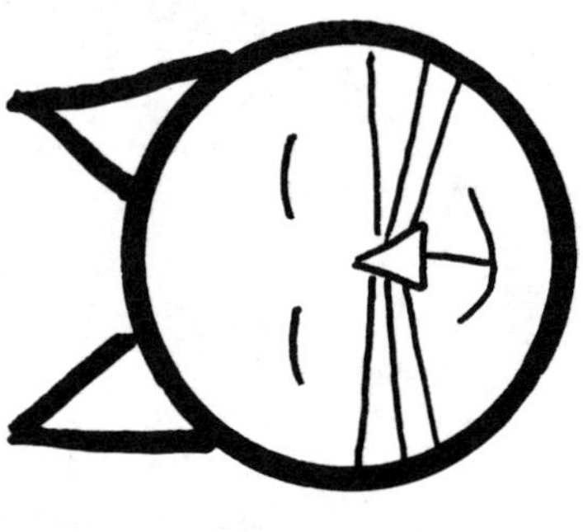

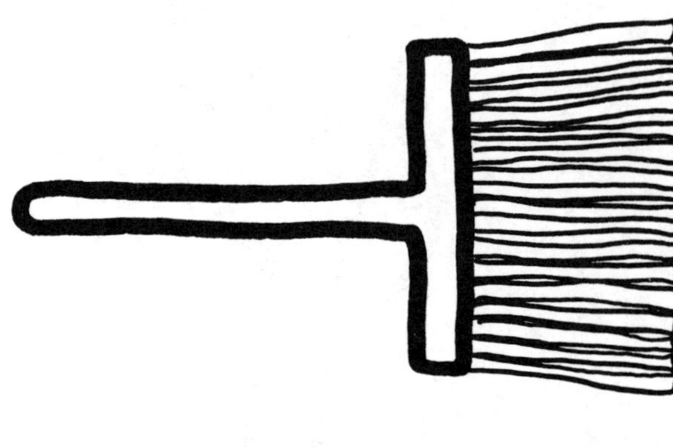

Skill 2
Step 3 Worksheet

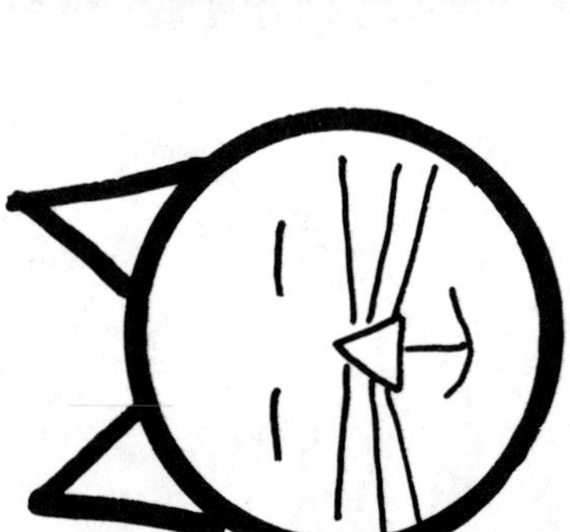

Skill 2
Step 3 Worksheet

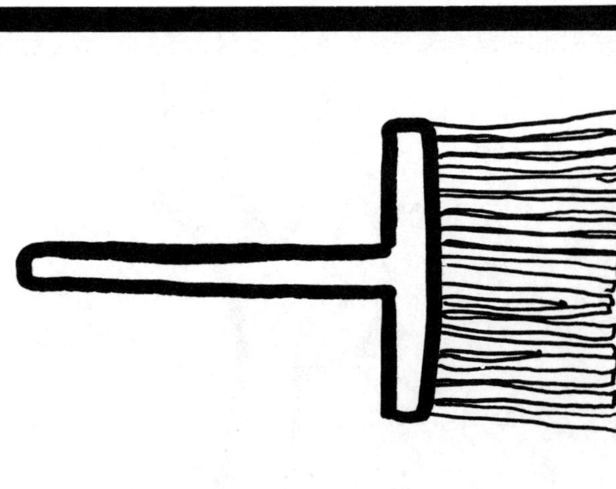

Skill 3—Cutting a Simple Shape—¼" Line

Objective: Student cuts out a simple shape with a line ¼" wide, and pastes it on a fixed outline, with 80% accuracy.

SKILL 3—STEP 1—STRIPS

Level #1—Strips 1" thick, ¼" wide line
Pretest: Student takes Level #1 Pretest (picture frame—10" strips).

If criterion met: Student advances to Level #2.

If criterion not met:
1. Student cuts Level #1 worksheets:
   window—7"
   crayons—6"
   knife, fork, spoon—6½"
2. Student takes Level #1 Posttest (picture frame).
   If criterion met: Student advances to Level #2.
   If criterion not met: Student repeats Level #1 worksheets and Posttest.

Level #2—Short Strips ½" thick,—¼" wide line
Pretest: Student takes Level #2 Pretest (bird in cage —6" strips).

If criterion met: Student advances to Level #3.

If criterion not met:
1. Student cuts Level #2 worksheets:
   broom—3¾"
   helicopter—4"
   sunburst—4"
   tiger in cage—4½"
2. Student takes Level #2 Posttest (bird in cage).
   If criterion met: Student advances to Level #3.
   If criterion not met: Student repeats Level #2 worksheets and Posttest.

Level #3—Longer Strips ½" thick—¼" wide line
Pretest: Student takes Level #3 Pretest (guitar, 8" strips).

If criterion met: Student advances to Level #4

If criterion not met:
1. Student cuts Level #3 worksheets:
   house—8"
   swing—6½"
   fence—7"
2. Student takes Level #3 Posttest (guitar).
   If criterion met: Student advances to Level #4.
   If criterion not met: Student repeats Level #3 worksheets and Posttest.

Level #4—Combined Strips ½" thick—¼" wide line
Pretest: Student takes Level #4 Pretest (spider—8 strips).

If criterion met: Student advances to Step 2—Squares.

If criterion not met:
1. Student cuts Level #4 worksheet (flowers—3 strips).
2. Student takes Level #4 Posttest (spider).
   If criterion met: Student advances to Step 2—Squares.
   If criterion not met: Student repeats Level #4 worksheet and Posttest.

Step 1—Level #1 Pre/Posttest

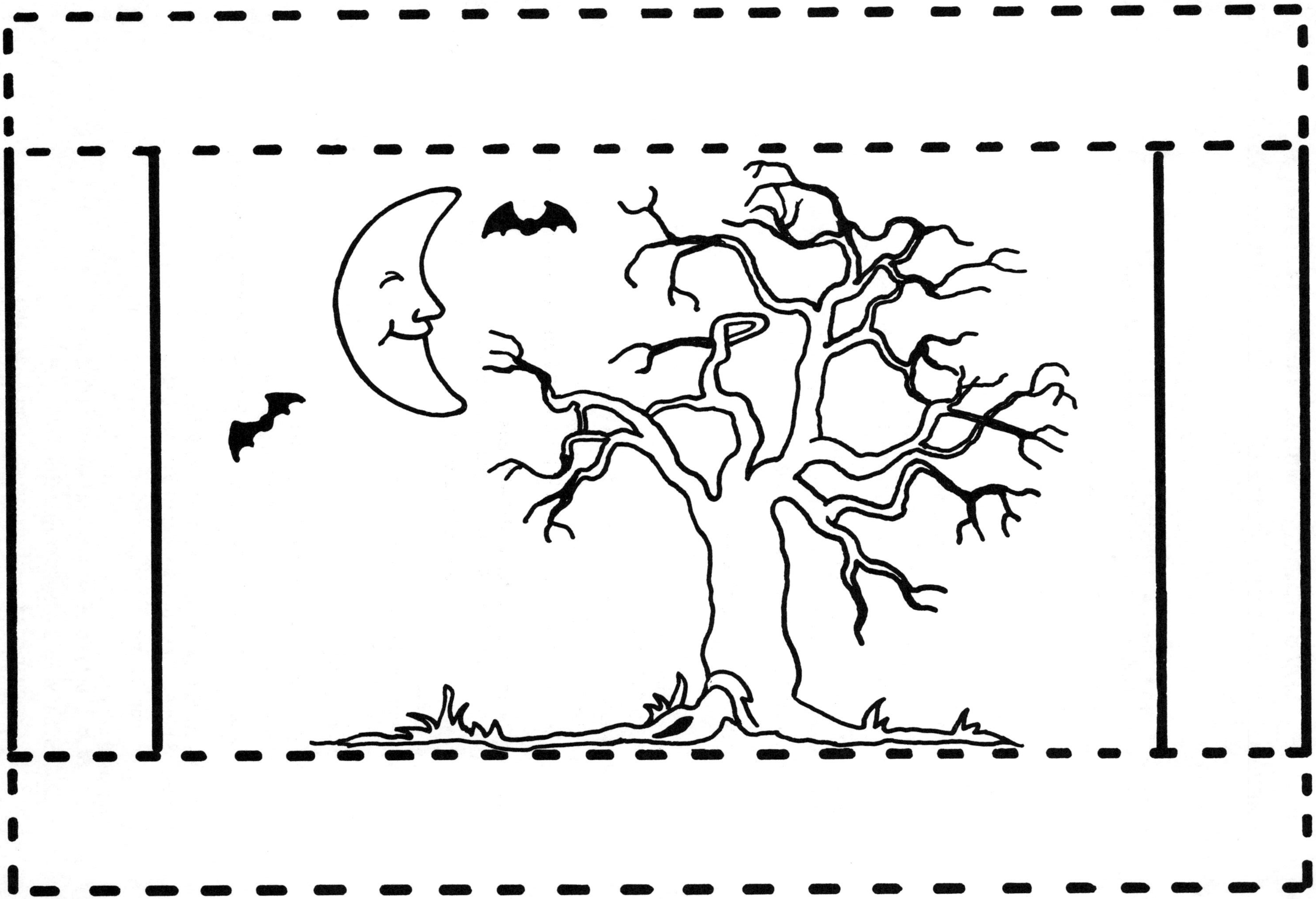

Step 1—Level #1 Worksheet

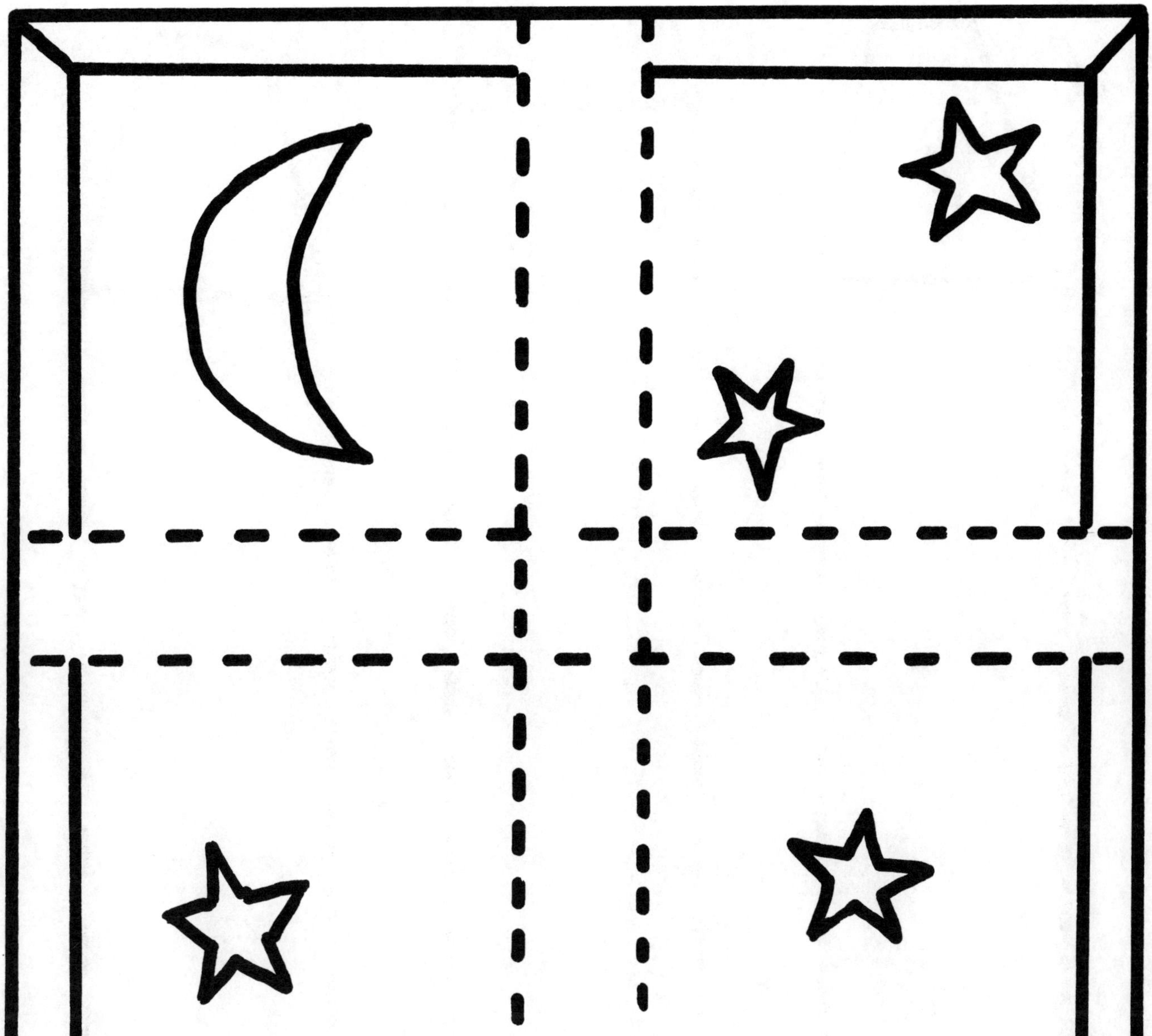

Step 1—Level #1 Worksheet

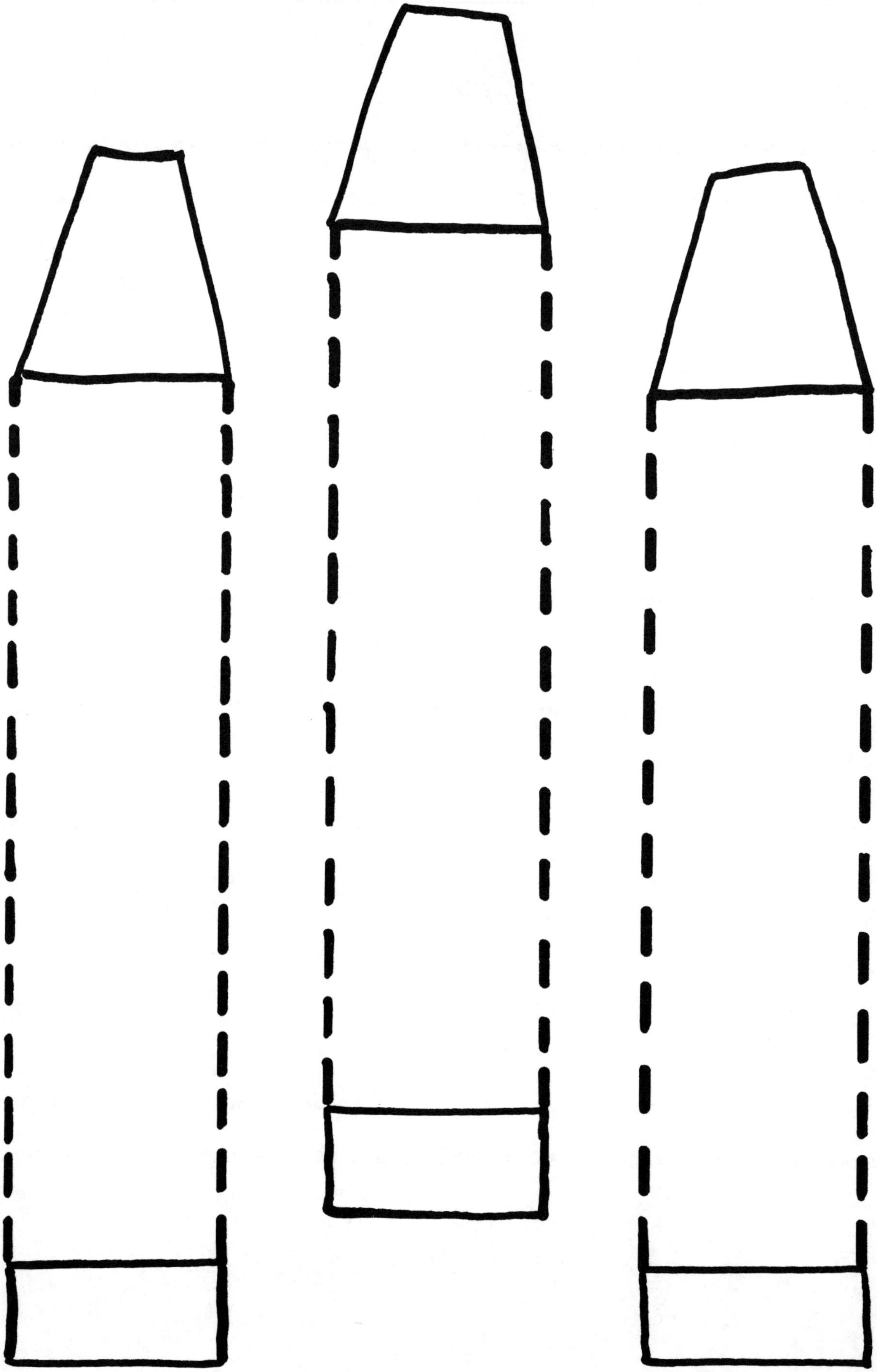

Step 1—Level #1 Worksheet

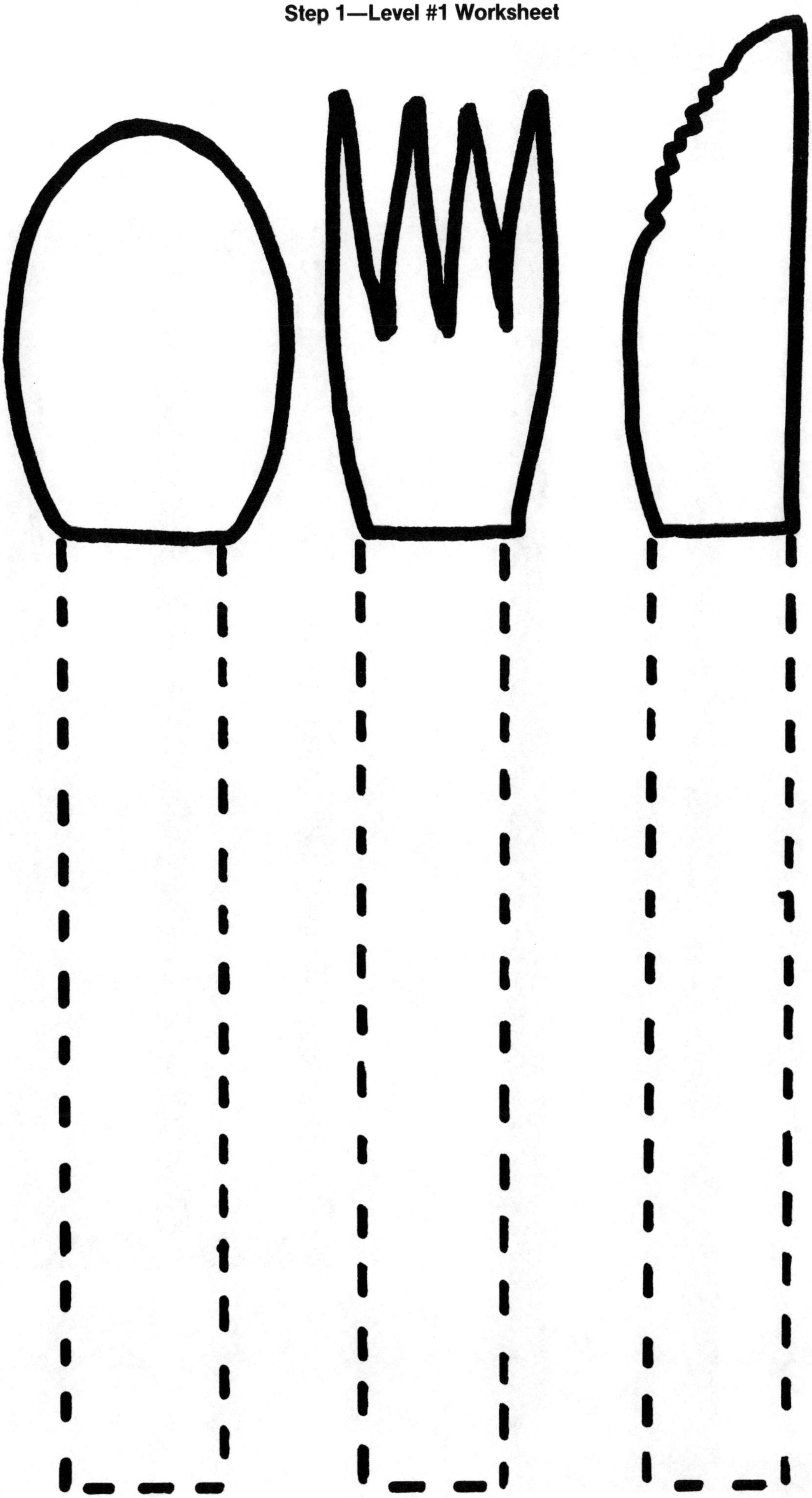

Skill 3
Step 1—Level #1 Pre/Posttest (picture frame)

Skill 3
Step 1—Level #1 Worksheet (window)

Skill 3
Step 1—Level #1 Worksheet (crayons)

Skill 3
Step 1—Level #1 Worksheet (knife, fork, spoon)

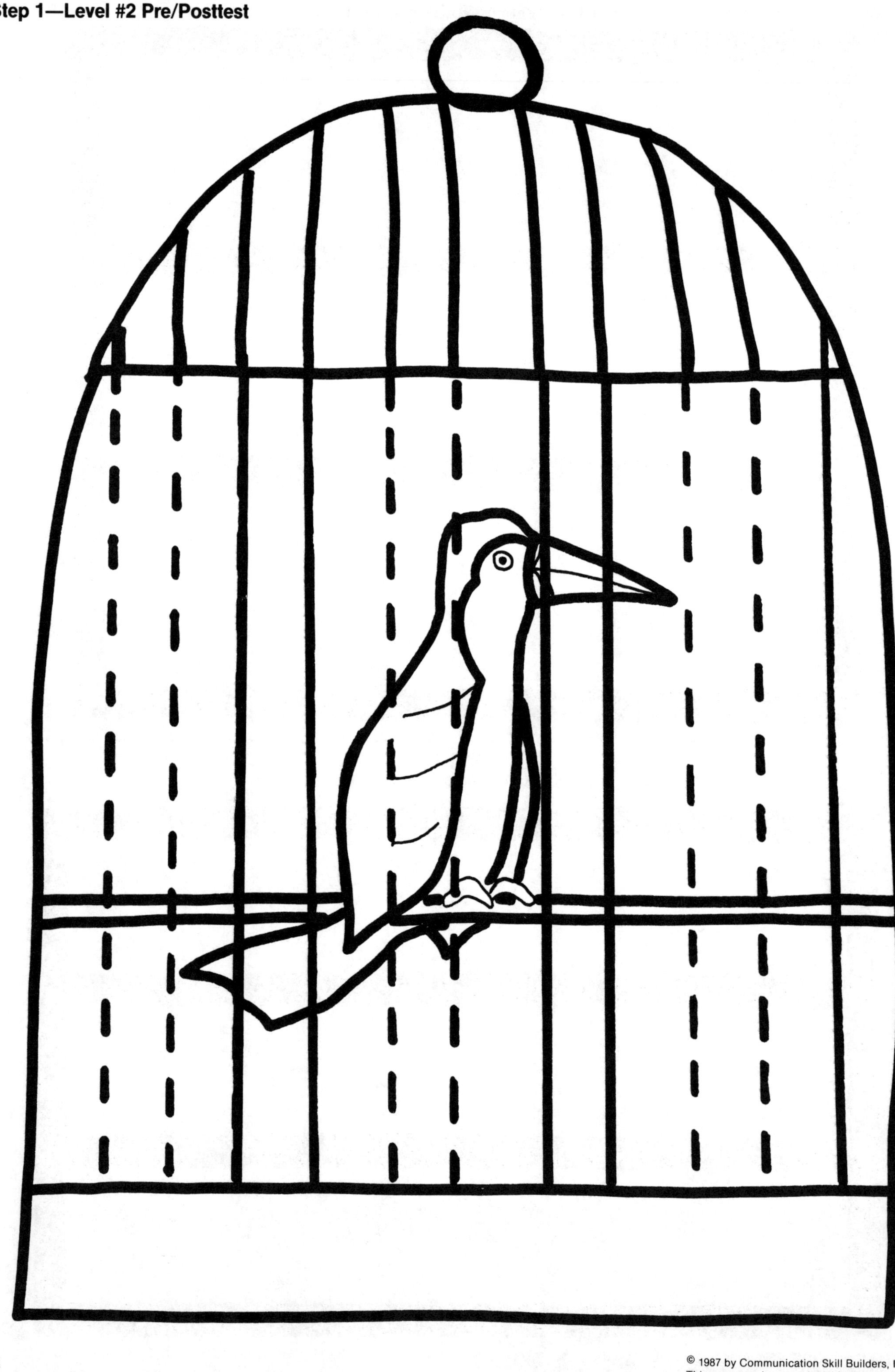

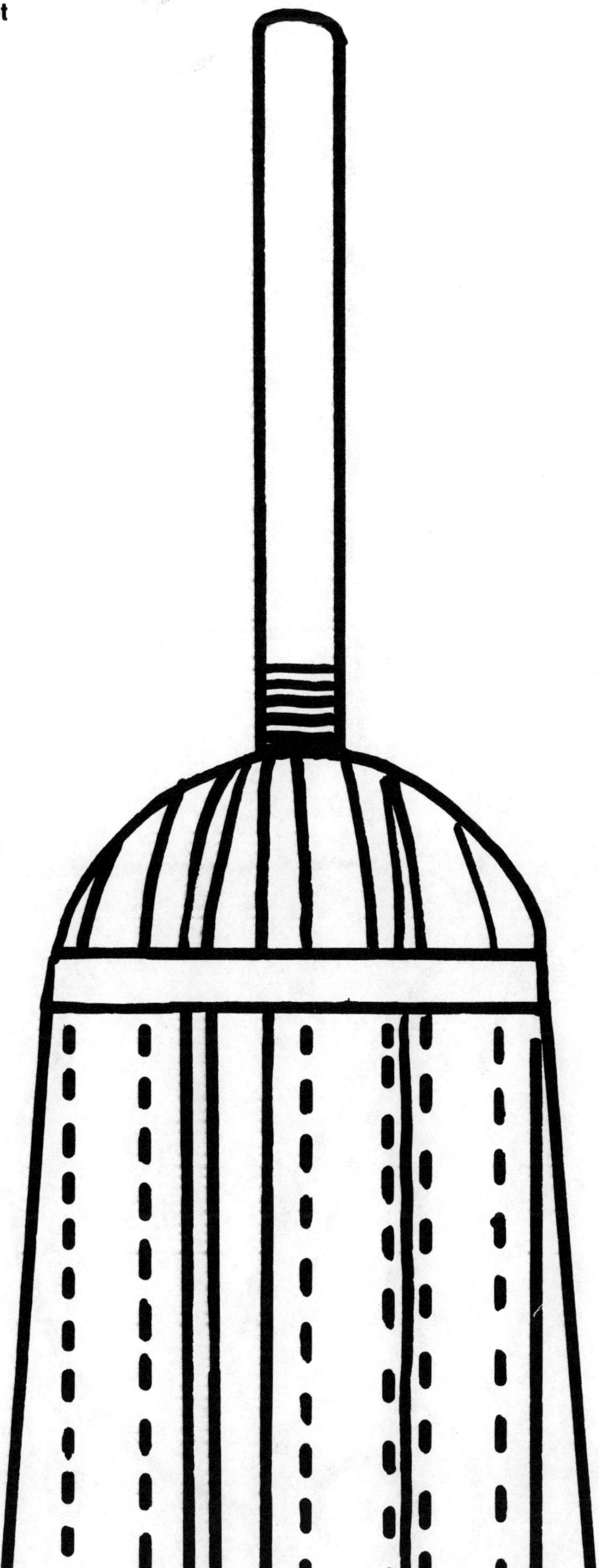

Step 1—Level #2 Worksheet

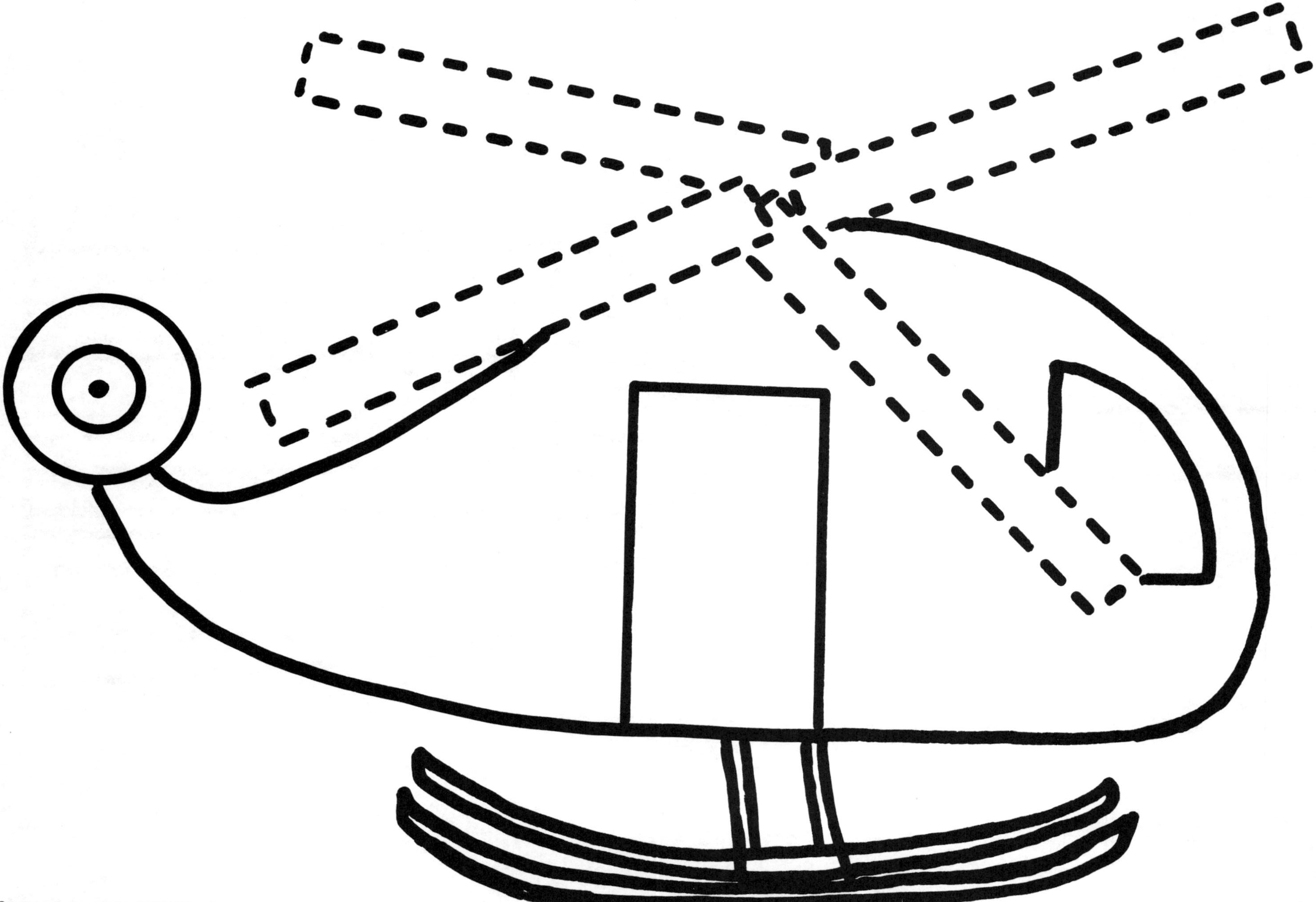

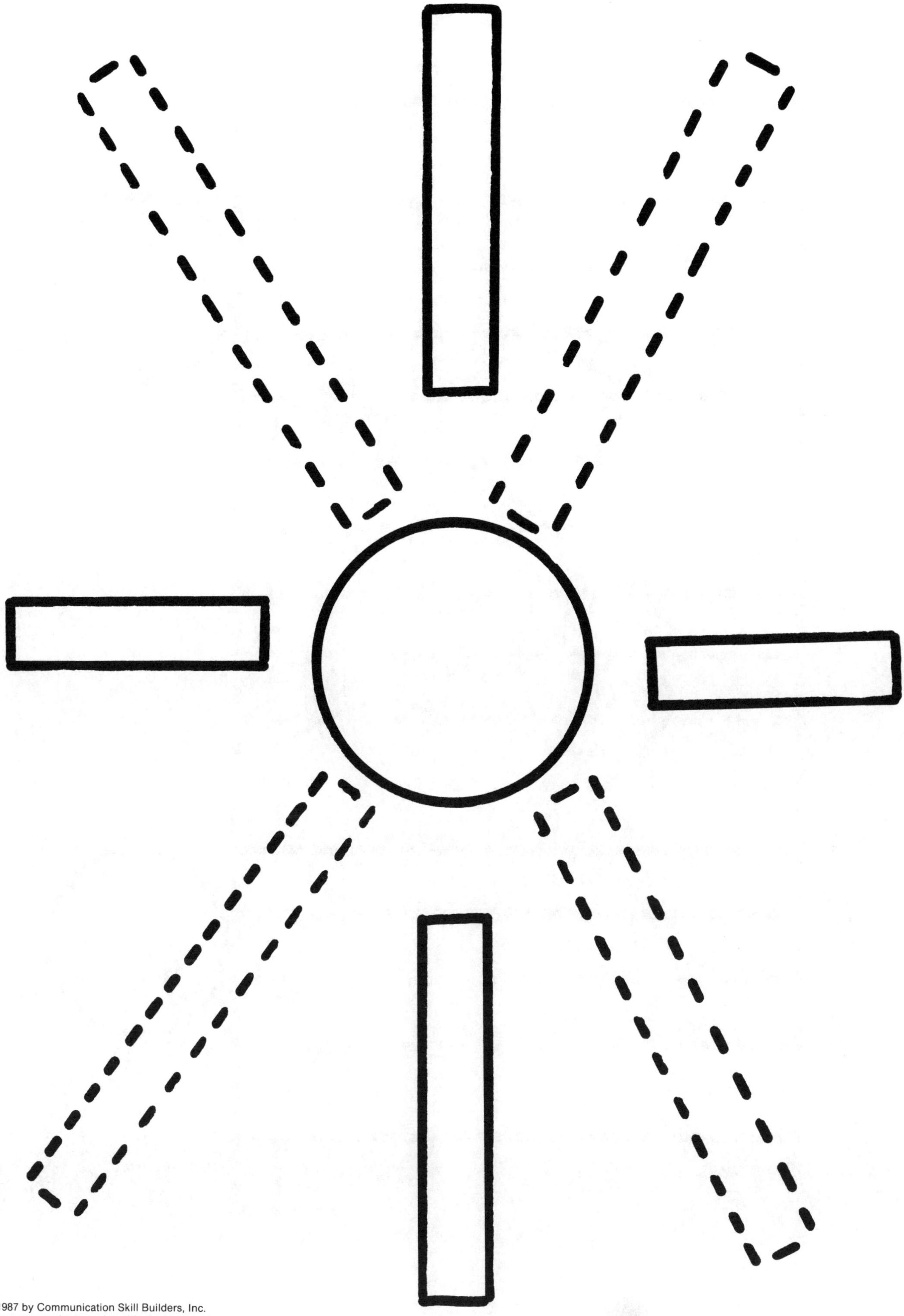

Step 1—Level #2 Worksheet

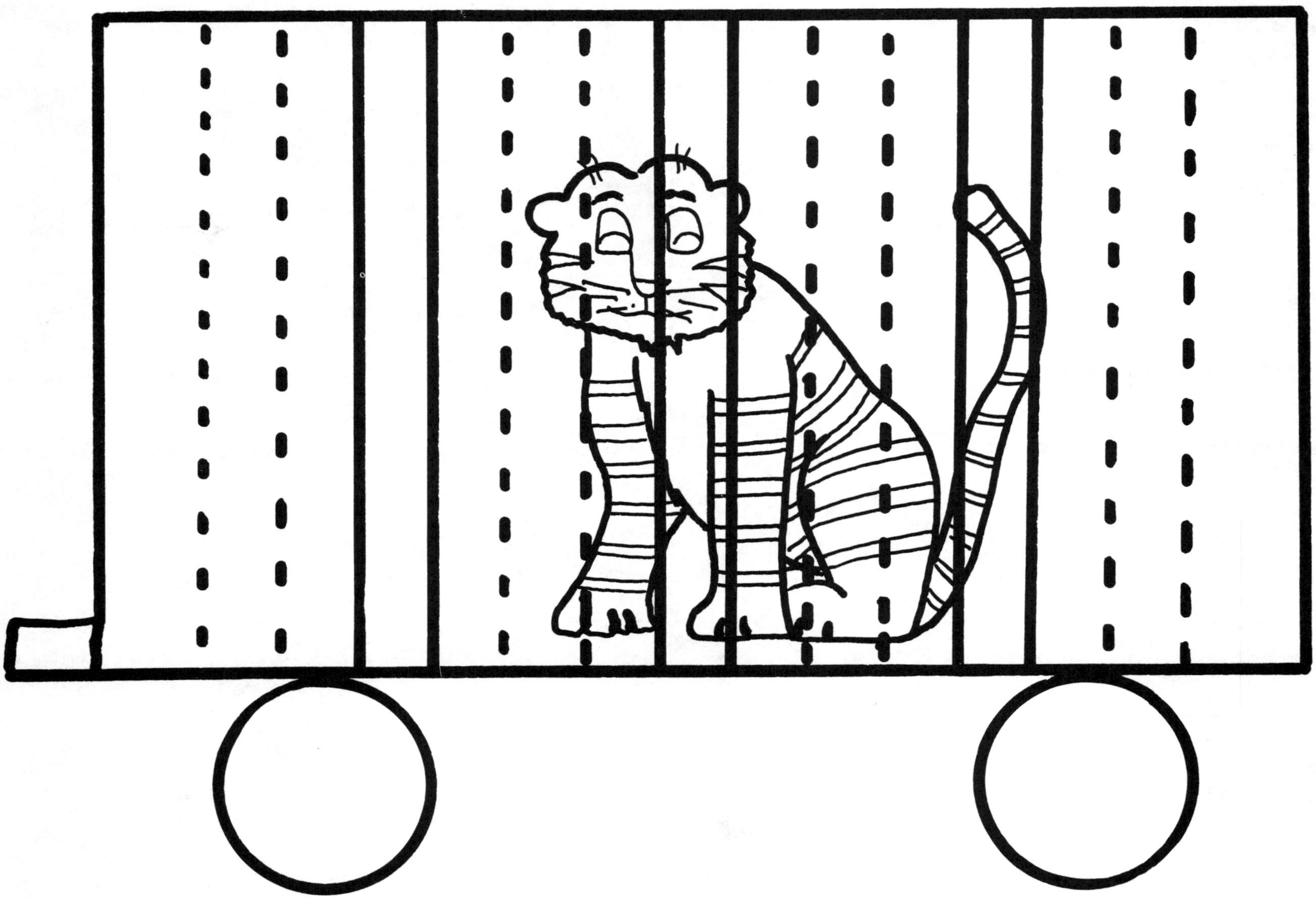

Skill 3
Step 1—Level #2 Pre/Posttest (bird in cage)

Skill 3
Step 1—Level #2 Worksheet (broom)

Skill 3
Step 1—Level #2 Worksheet (helicopter)

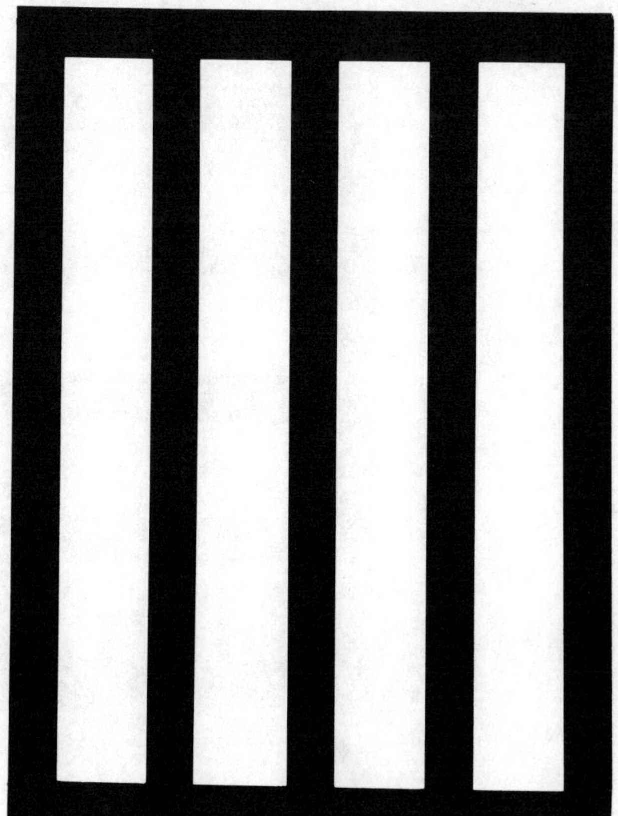

Skill 3
Step 1—Level #2 Worksheet (sunburst)

Skill 3
Step 1—Level #2 Worksheet (tiger in cage)

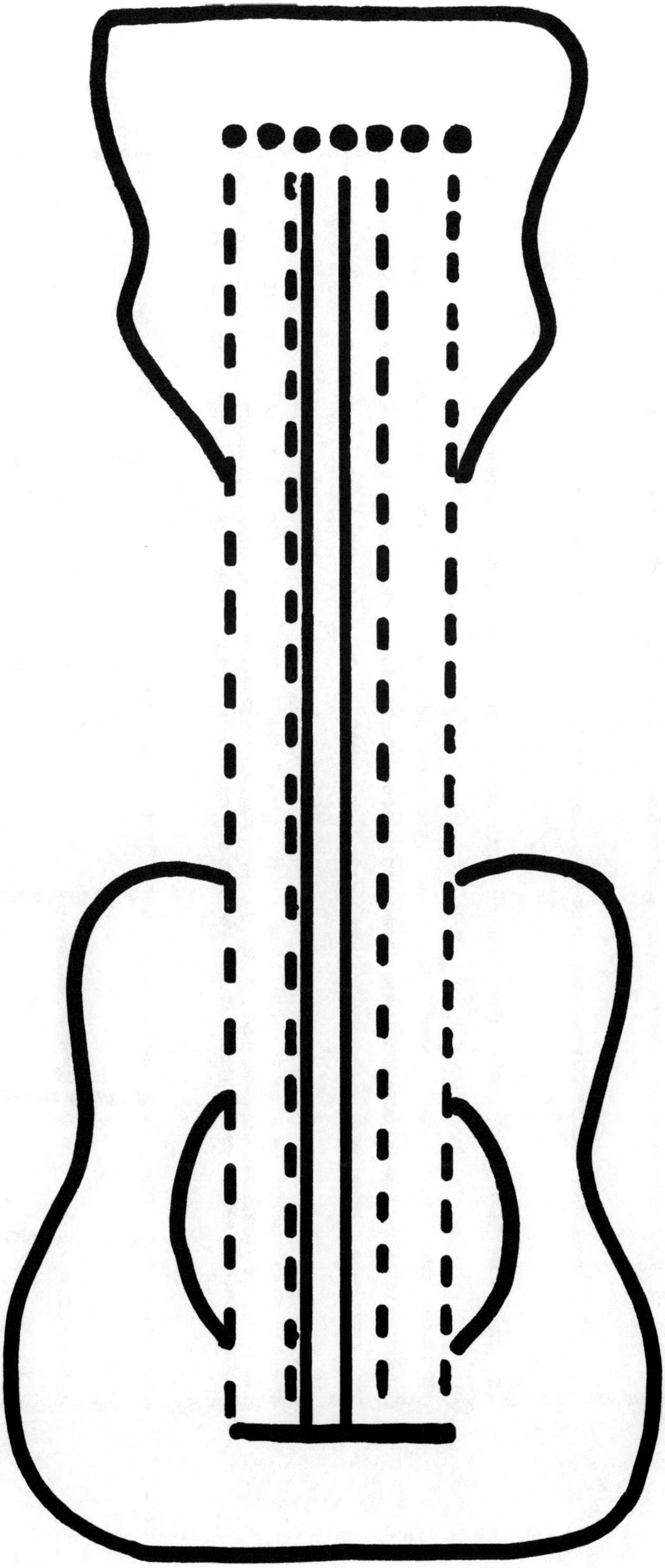

Step 1—Level #3 Worksheet

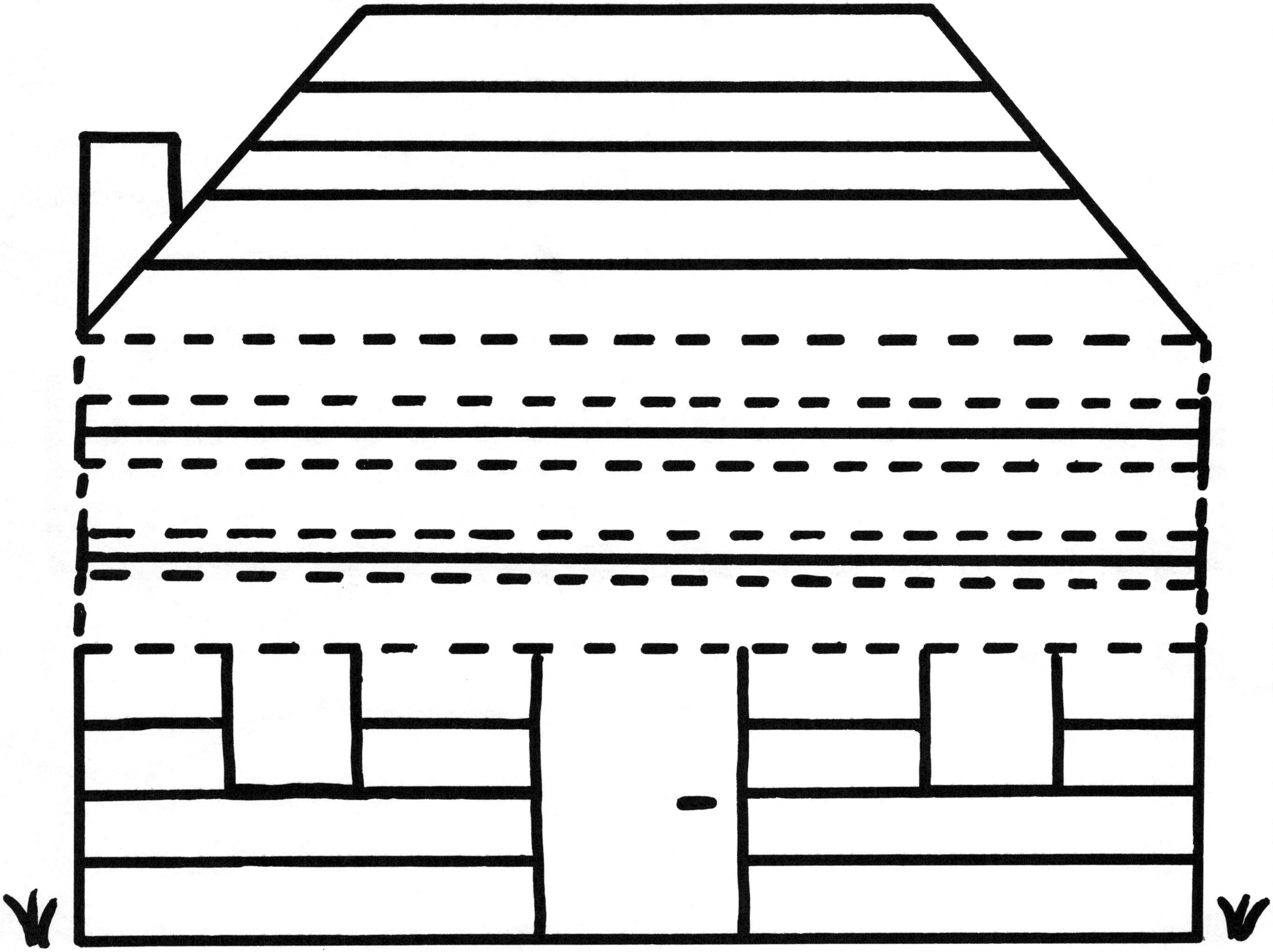

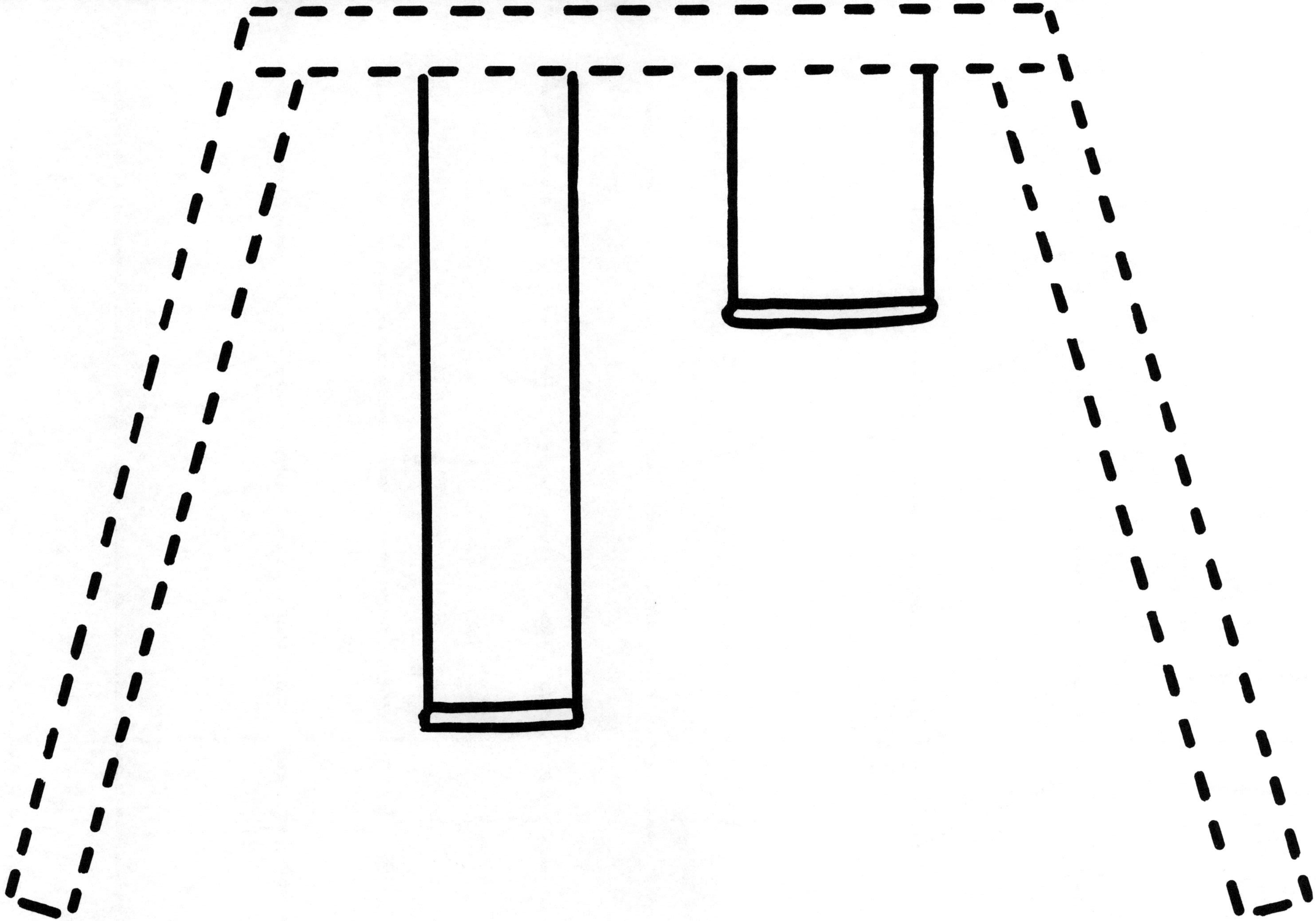

Step 1—Level #3 Worksheet

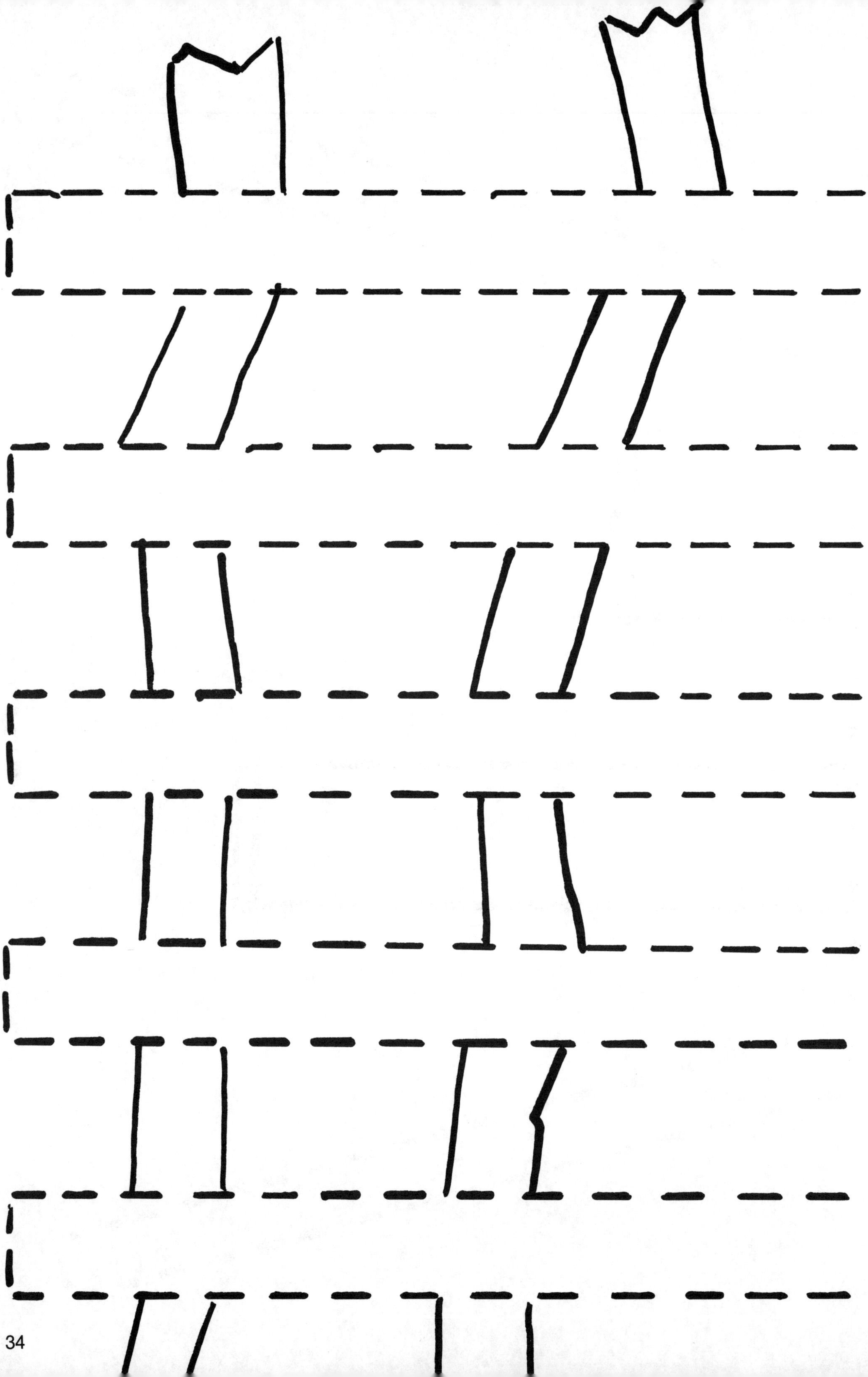

Step 1—Level #3 Worksheet

Skill 3
Step 1—Level #3 Pre/Posttest (guitar)

Skill 3
Step 1—Level #3 Worksheet (house)

Skill 3
Step 1—Level #3 Worksheet (swing)

Skill 3
Step 1—Level #3 Worksheet (fence)

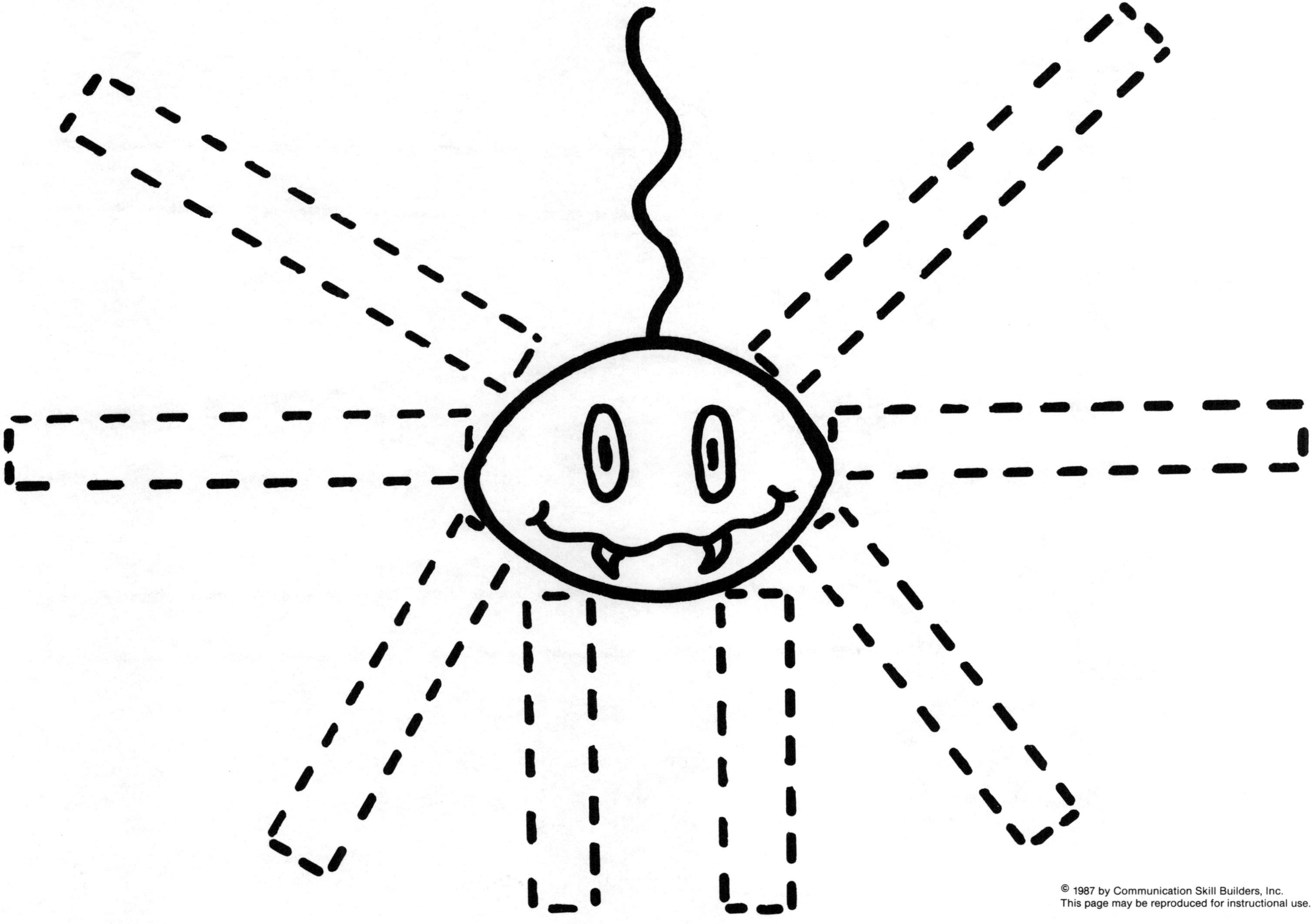

Step 1—Level #4 Worksheet

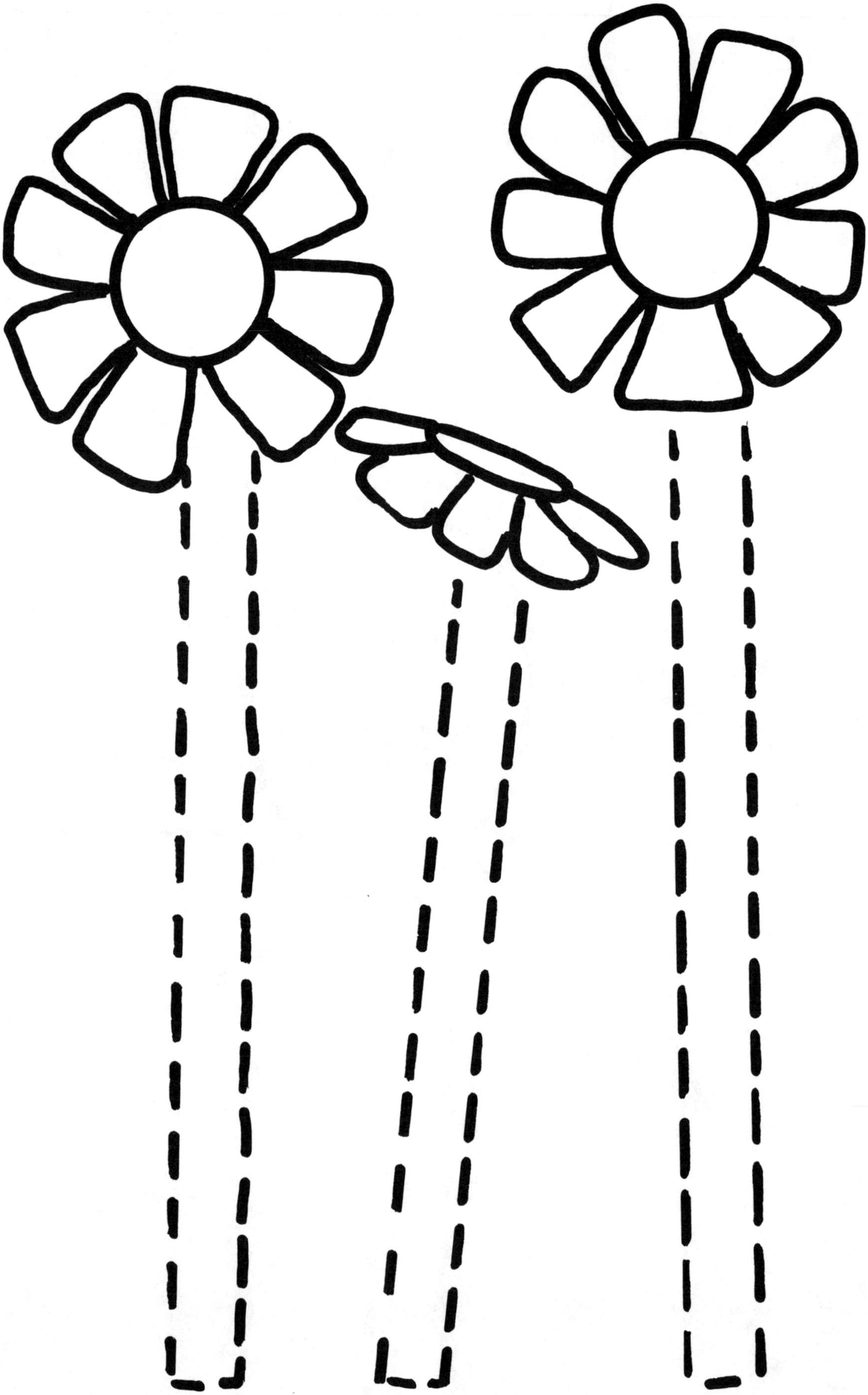

Skill 3
Step 1—Level #4 Pre/Posttest (spider)

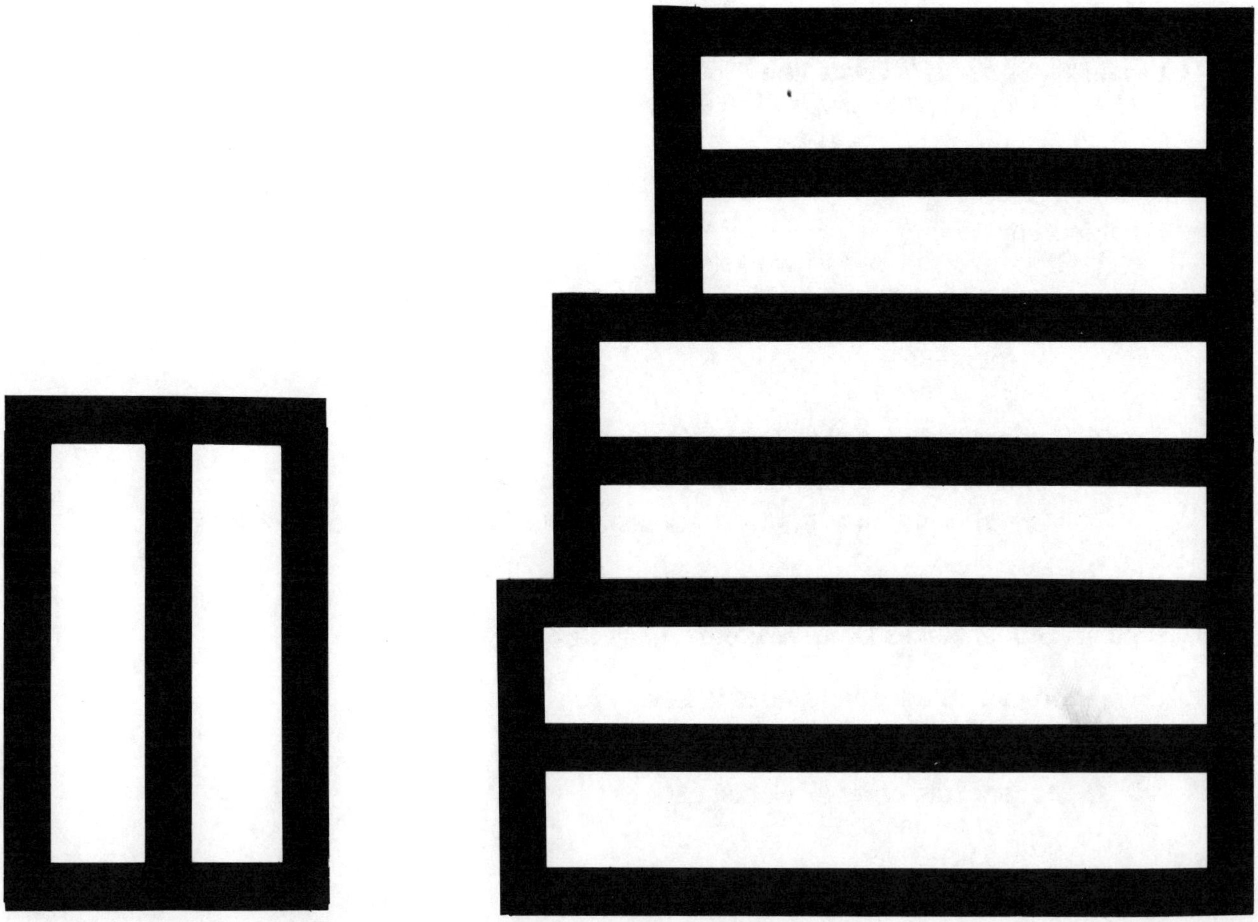

Skill 3
Step 1—Level #4 Worksheet (flowers)

SKILL 3—STEP 2—SQUARES

Level #1—Squares, 1/4" wide line
Pretest: Student takes Level #1 Pretest (shape man—3" square).

If criterion met: Student advances to Level #2.

If criterion not met:
1. Student cuts Level #1 worksheets:
   house—5"
   rabbit in hat—4"
   robot—3-1/4"
   TV screen—3"
2. Student takes Level #1 Posttest (shape man).
   If criterion met: Student advances to Level #2.
   If criterion not met: Student repeats Level #1 worksheets and Posttest.

Level #2—Smaller Squares, 1/4" wide line
Pretest: Student takes Level #2 Pretest (jack-in-the-box, 2½" square).

If criterion met: Student advances to Level #3.

If criterion not met:
1. Student cuts Level #2 worksheets:
   hot air balloon—3"
   book—3"
   clown's hat—3"
2. Student takes Level #2 Posttest (jack-in-the-box).
   If criterion met: Student advances to Level #3.
   If criterion not met: Student repeats Level #2 worksheets and Posttest.

Level #3—Combined Squares, 1/4" wide line
Pretest: Student takes Level #3 Pretest (school bus, three 1½" squares).

If criterion met: Student advances to Step 3—Rectangles.

If criterion not met:
1. Student cuts worksheet (blocks, two 2½" squares).
2. Student takes Level #3 Posttest (school bus).
   If criterion met: Student advances to Step 3—Rectangles.
   If criterion not met: Student repeats Level #3 worksheet and Posttest.

Step 2—Level #1 Pre/Posttest

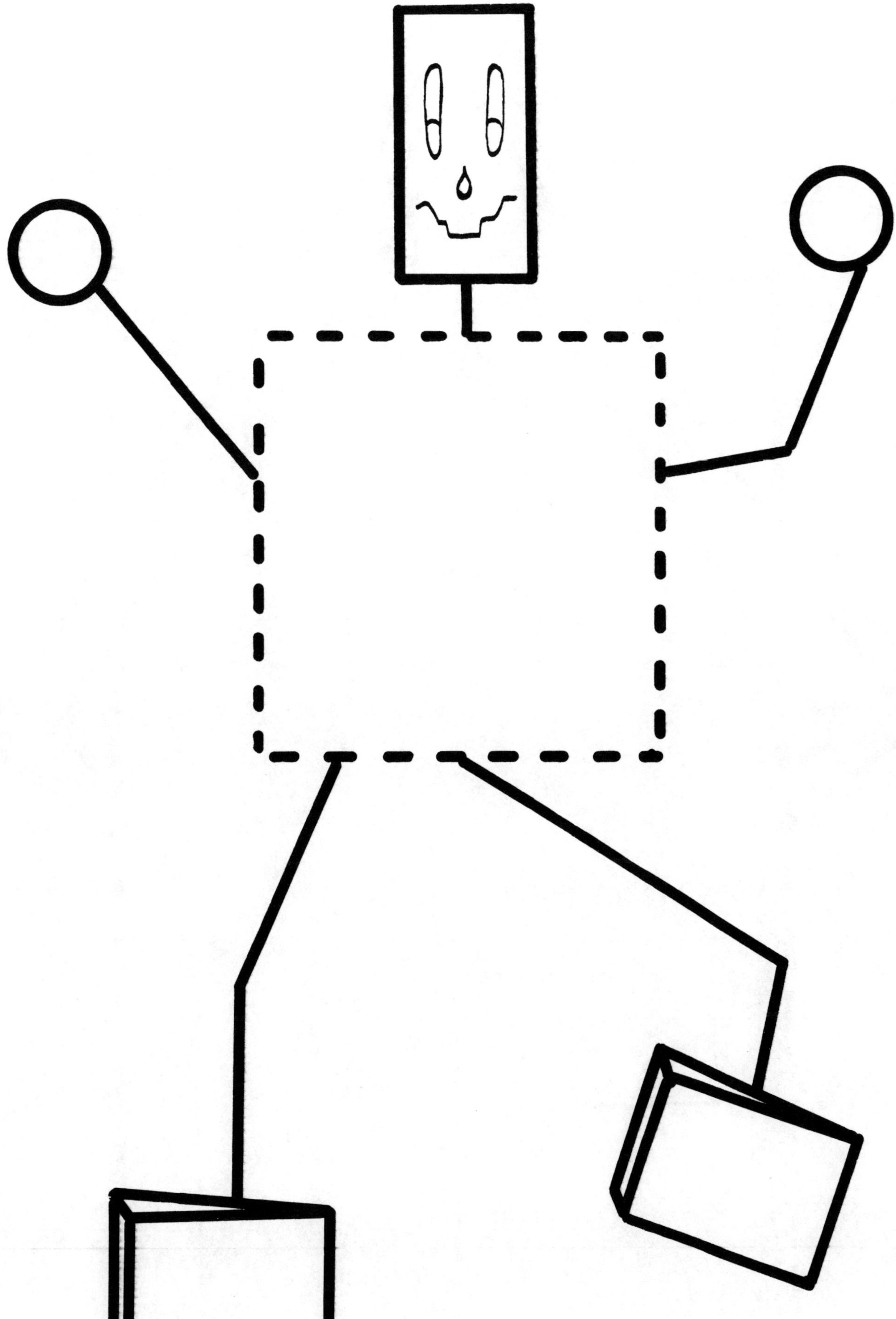

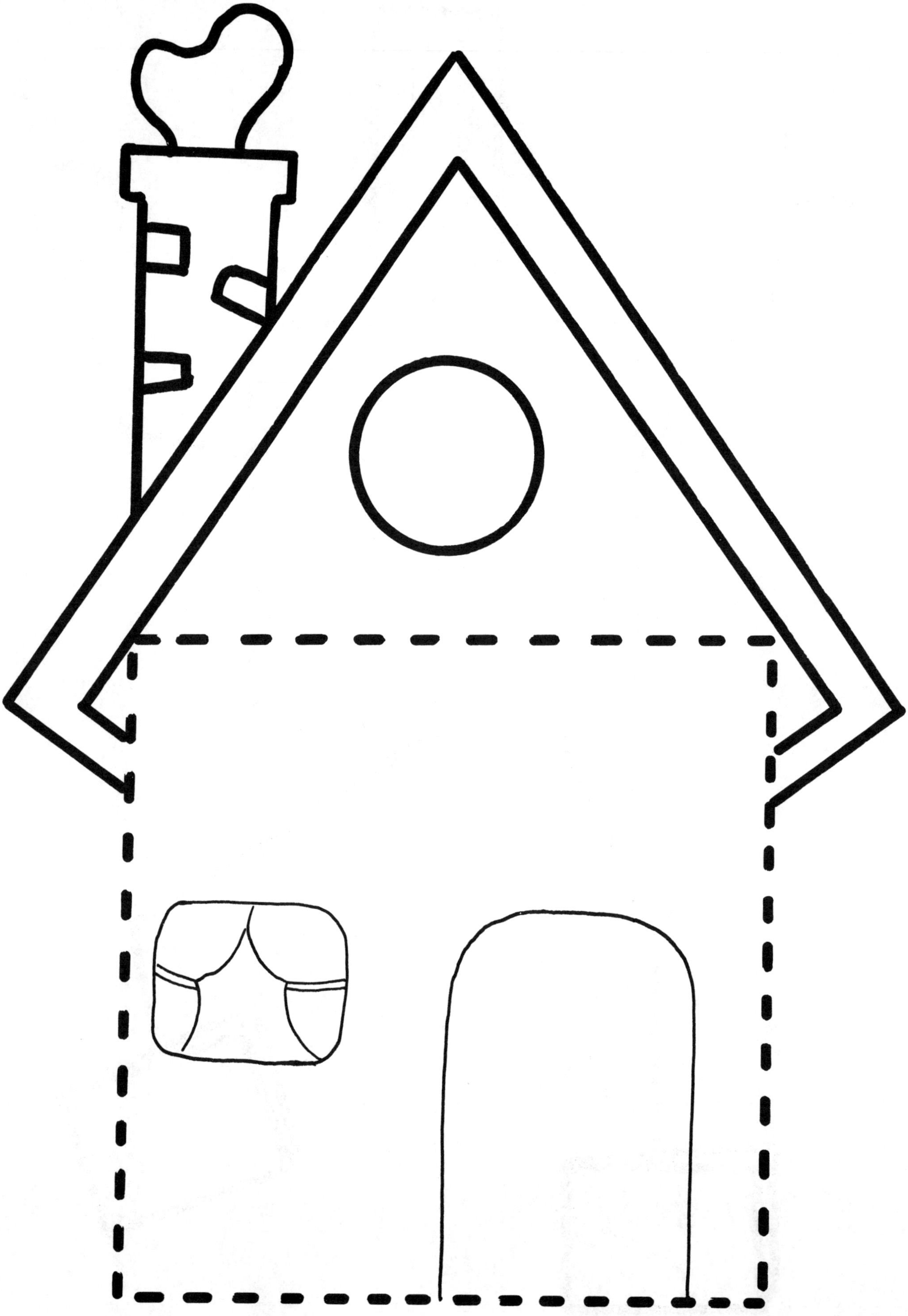

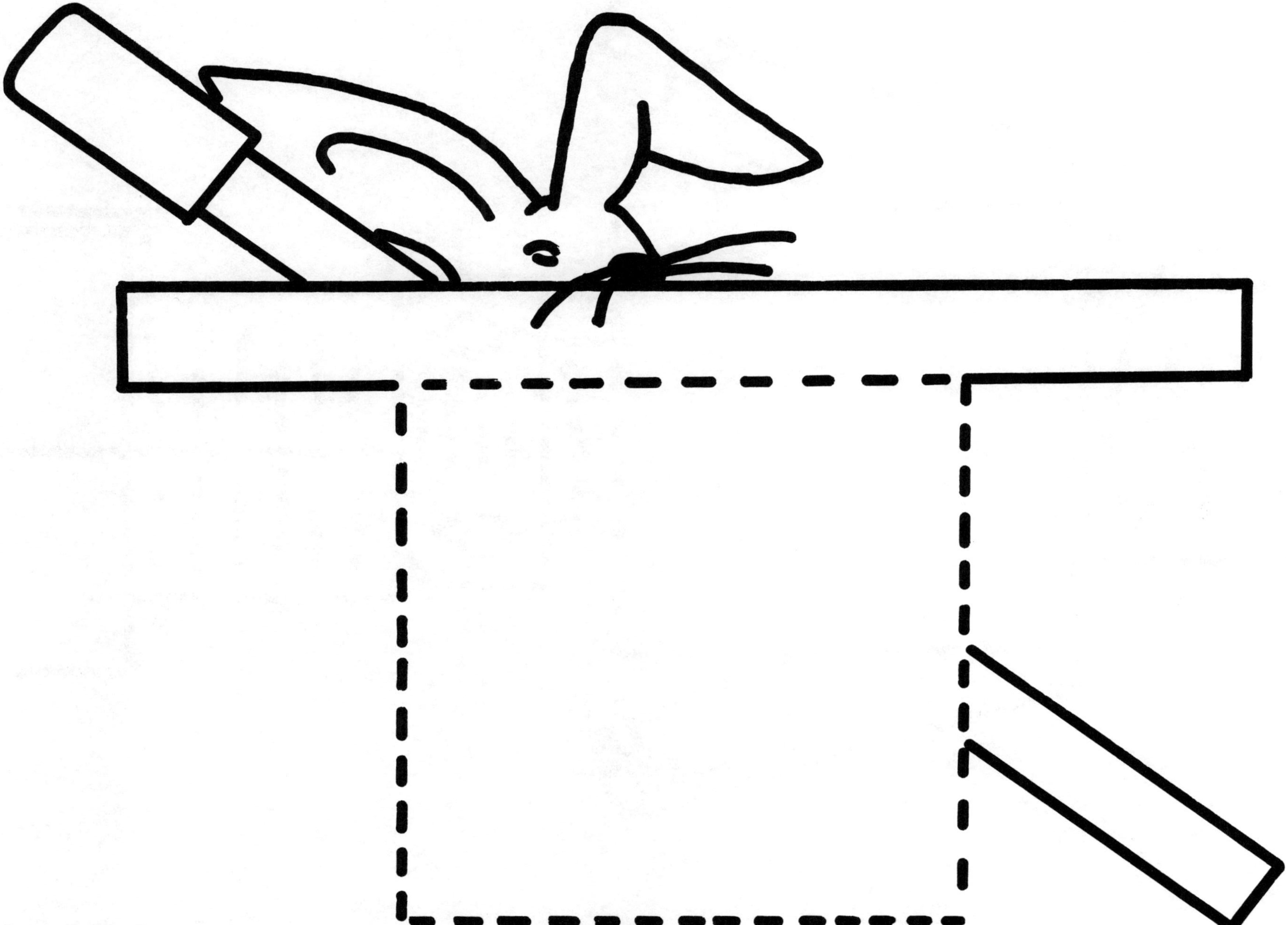

Step 2—Level #1 Worksheet

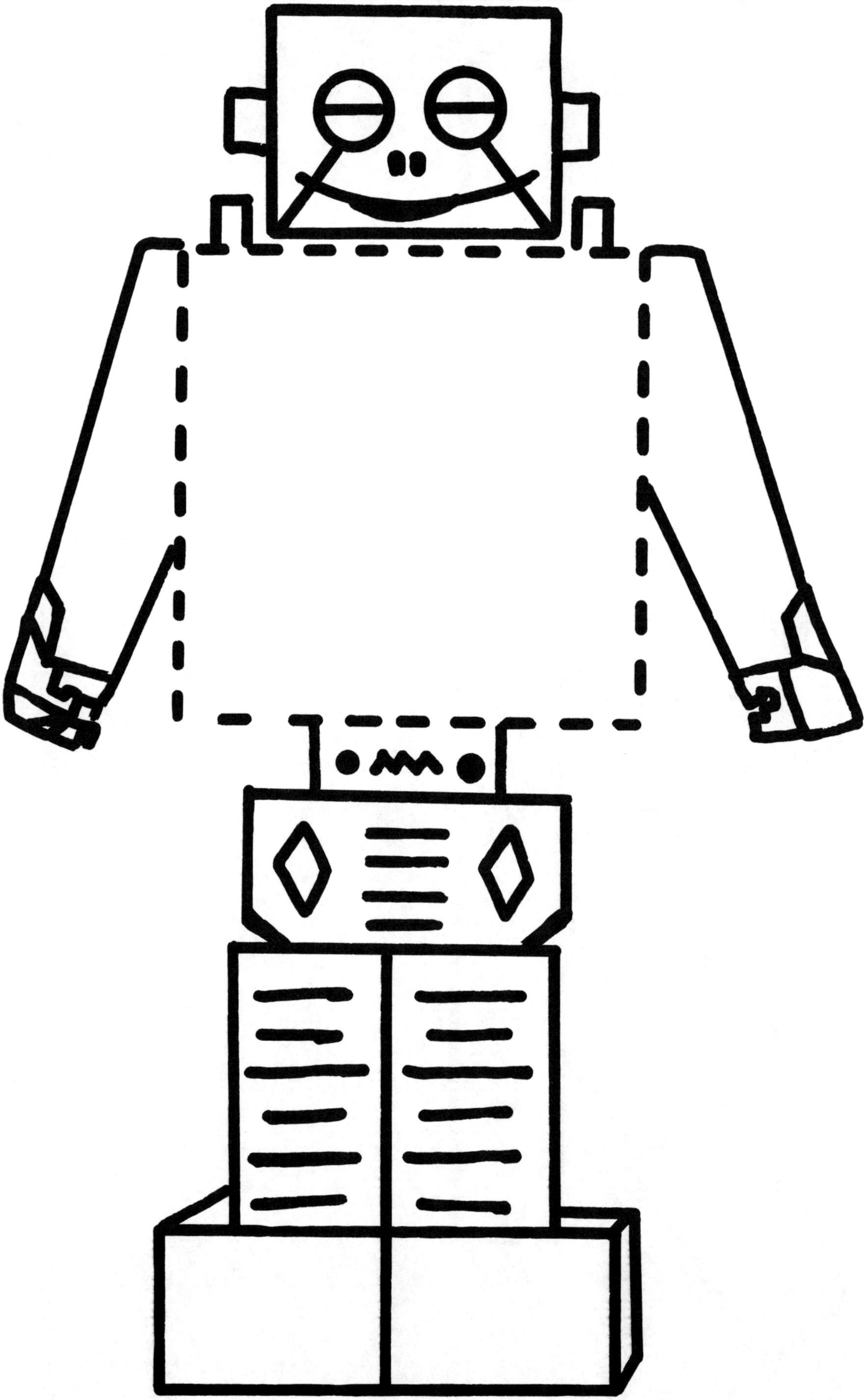

Step 2—Level #1 Worksheet

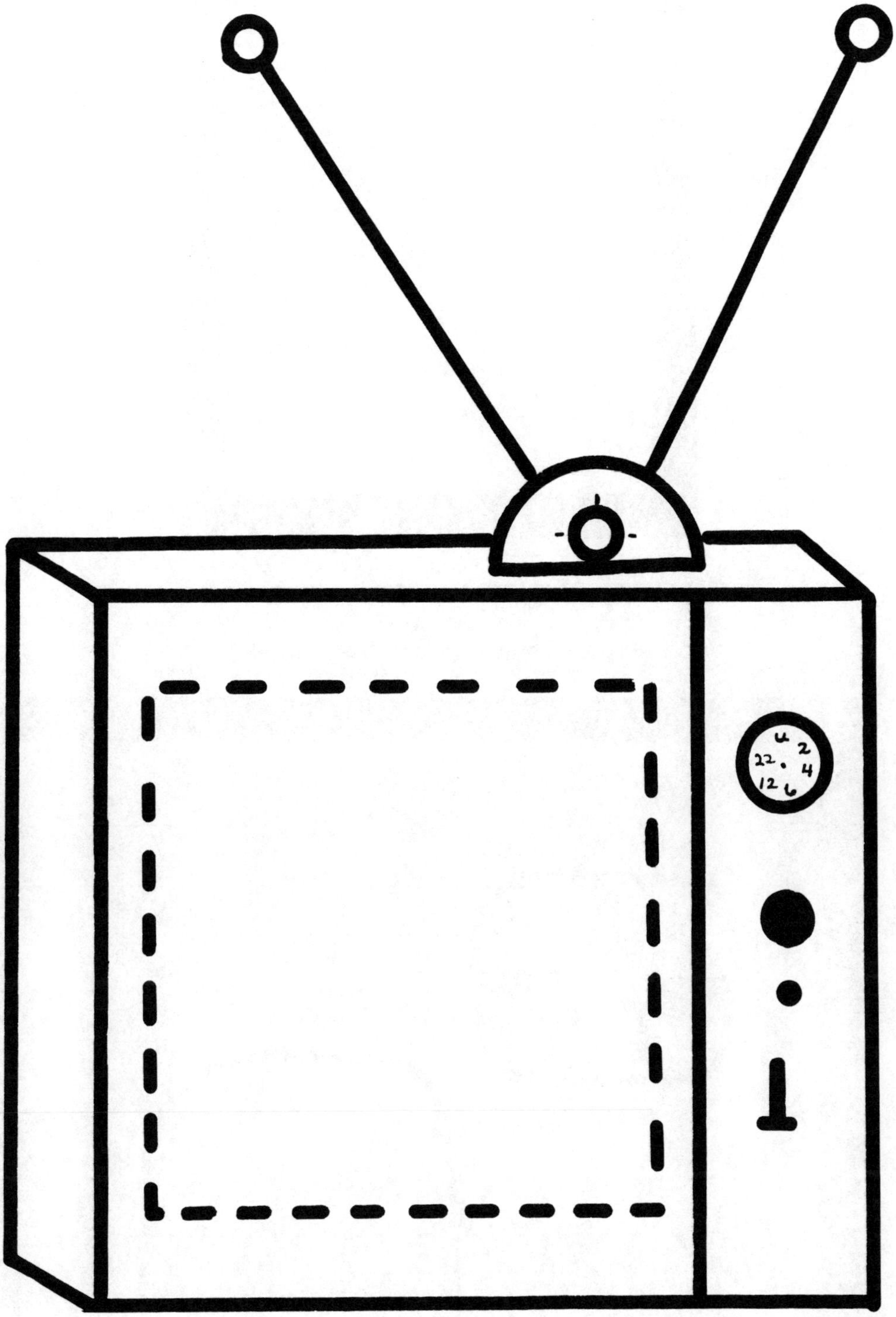

Skill 3
Step 2—Level #1 Pre/Posttest (shape man)

Skill 3
Step 2—Level #1 Worksheet (house)

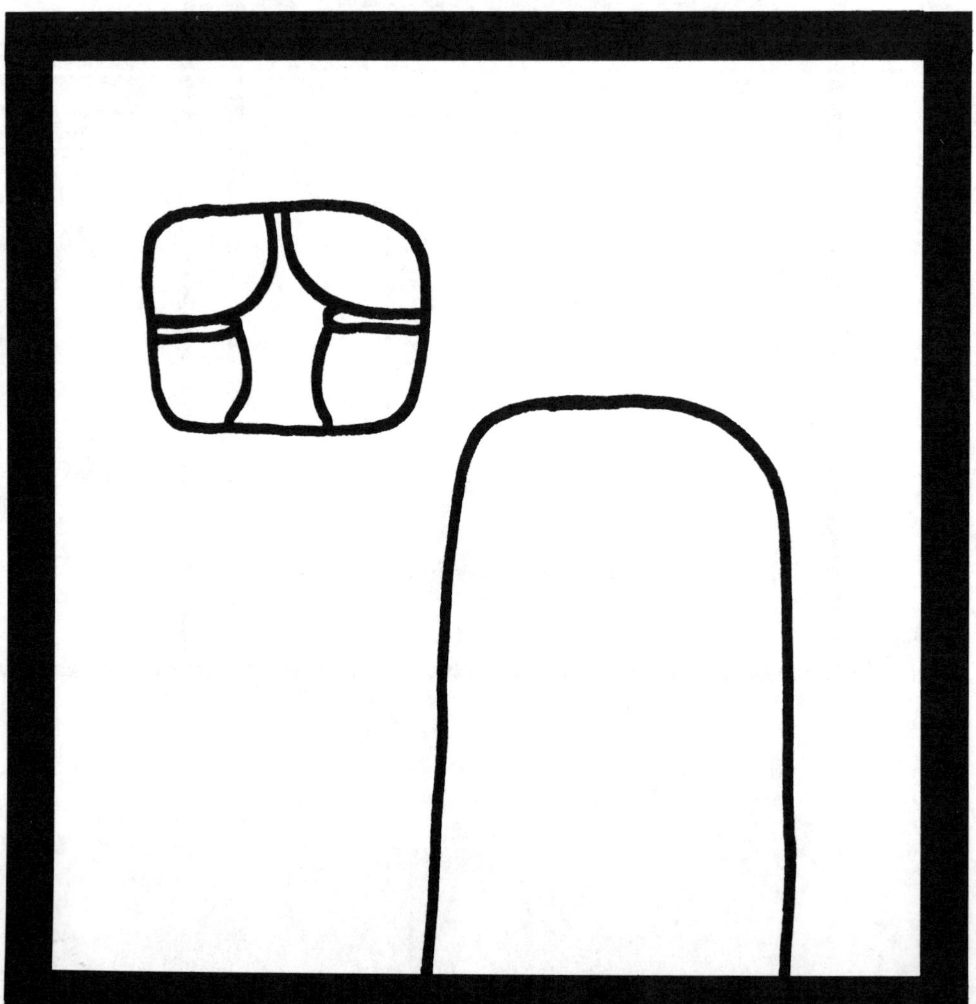

Skill 3
Step 2—Level #1 Worksheet (rabbit in hat)

Skill 3
Step 2—Level #1 Worksheet (robot)

Skill 3
Step 2—Level #1 Worksheet (TV screen)

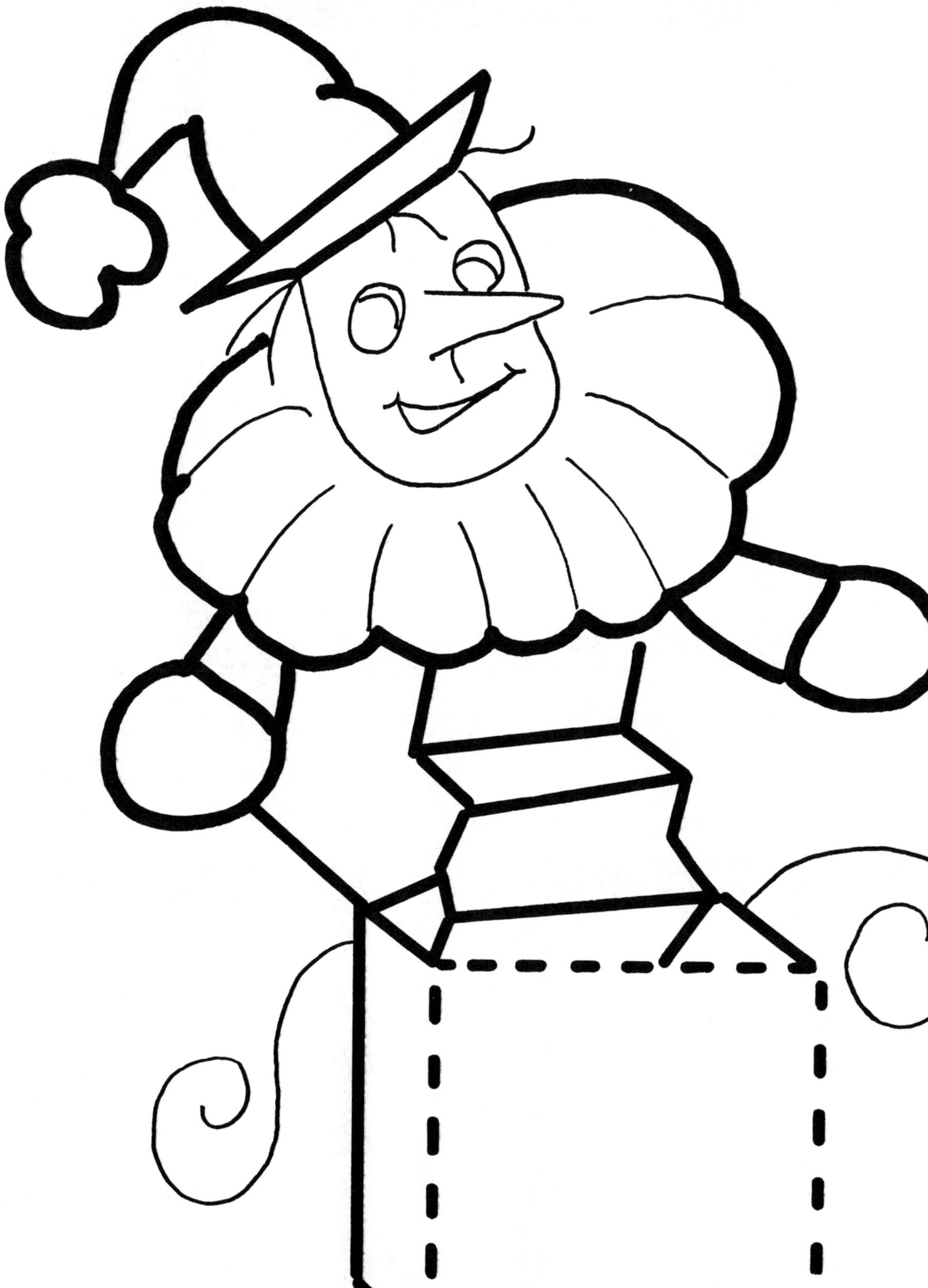

Step 2—Level #2 Worksheet

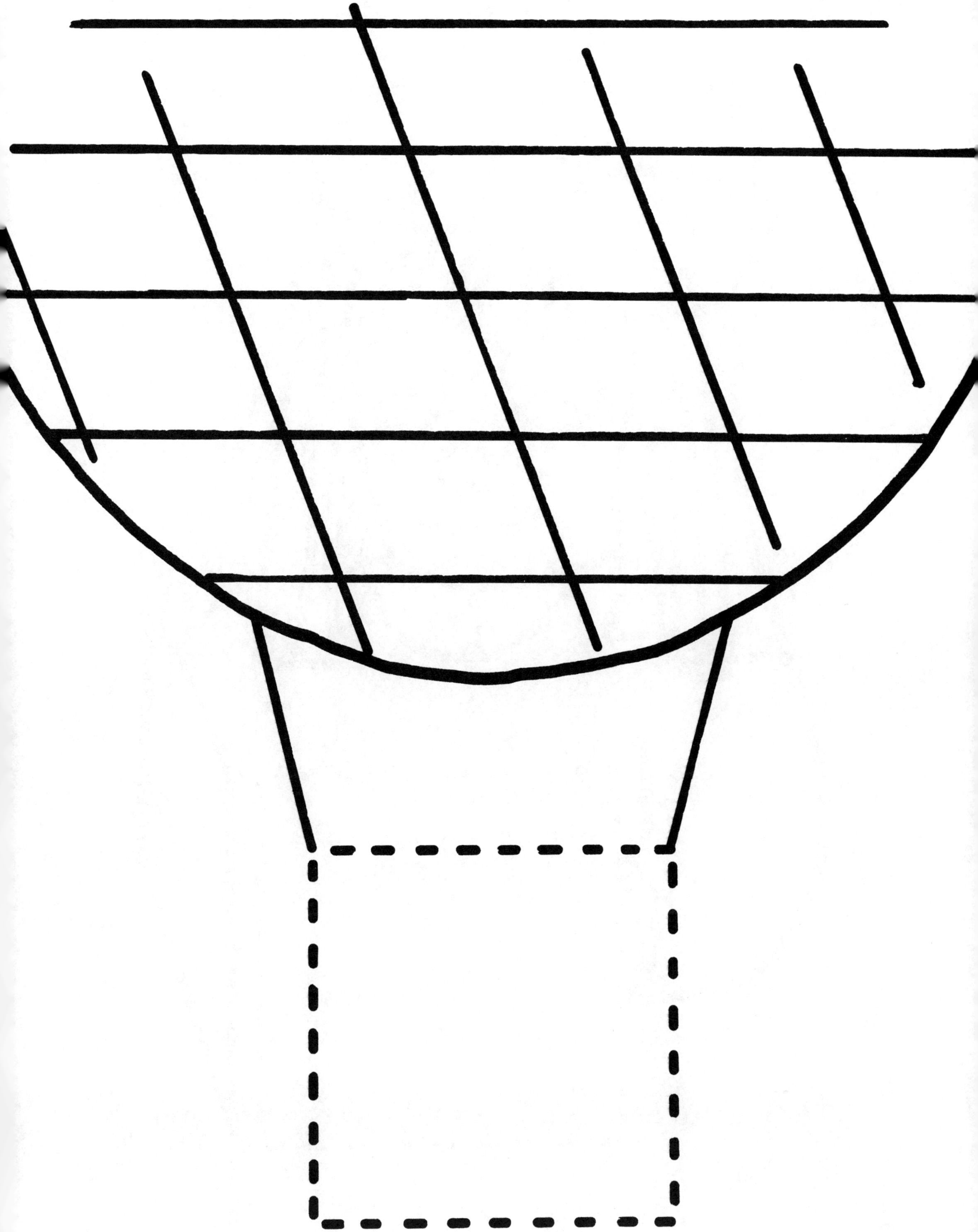

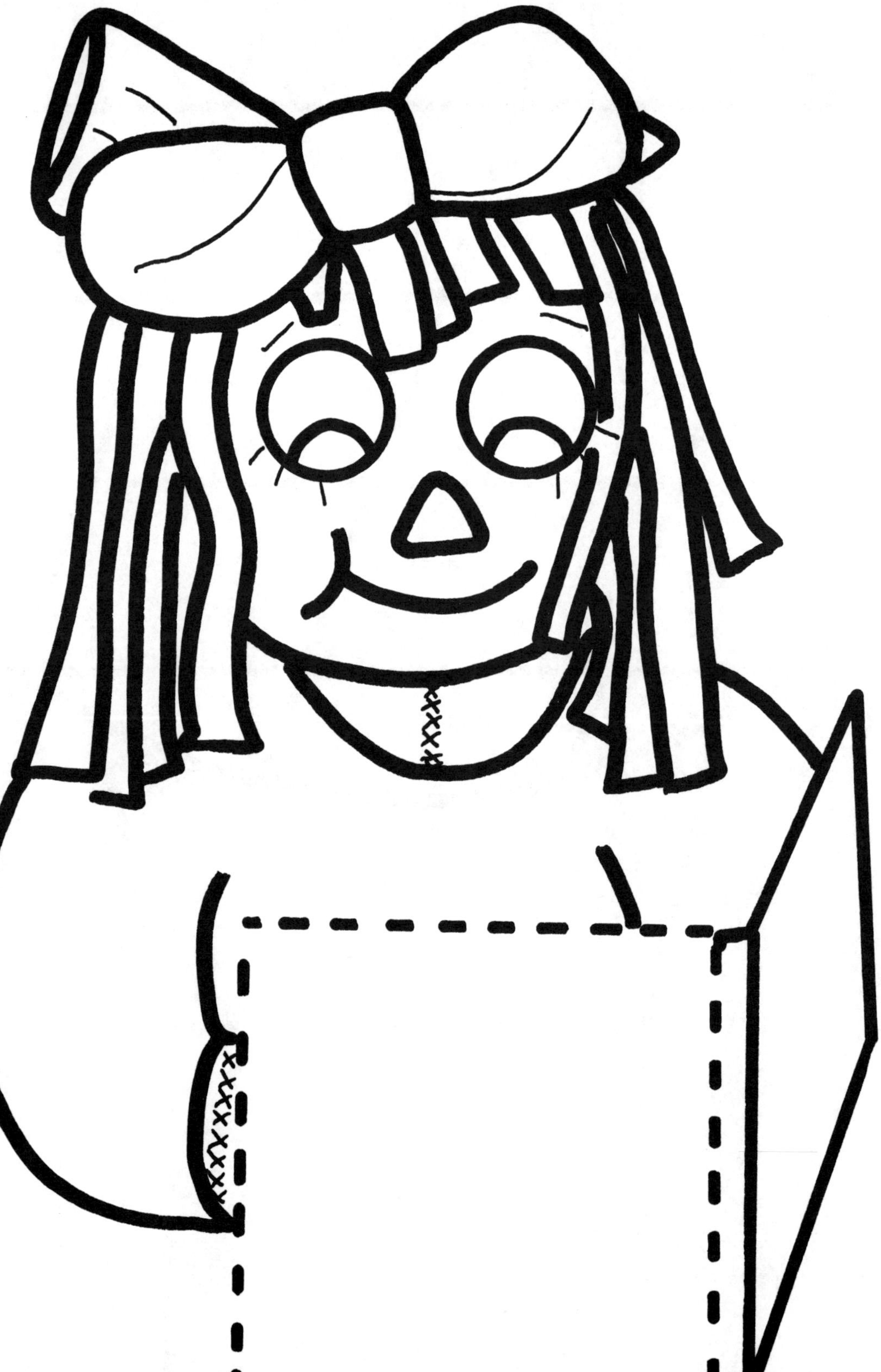

Step 2—Level #2 Worksheet

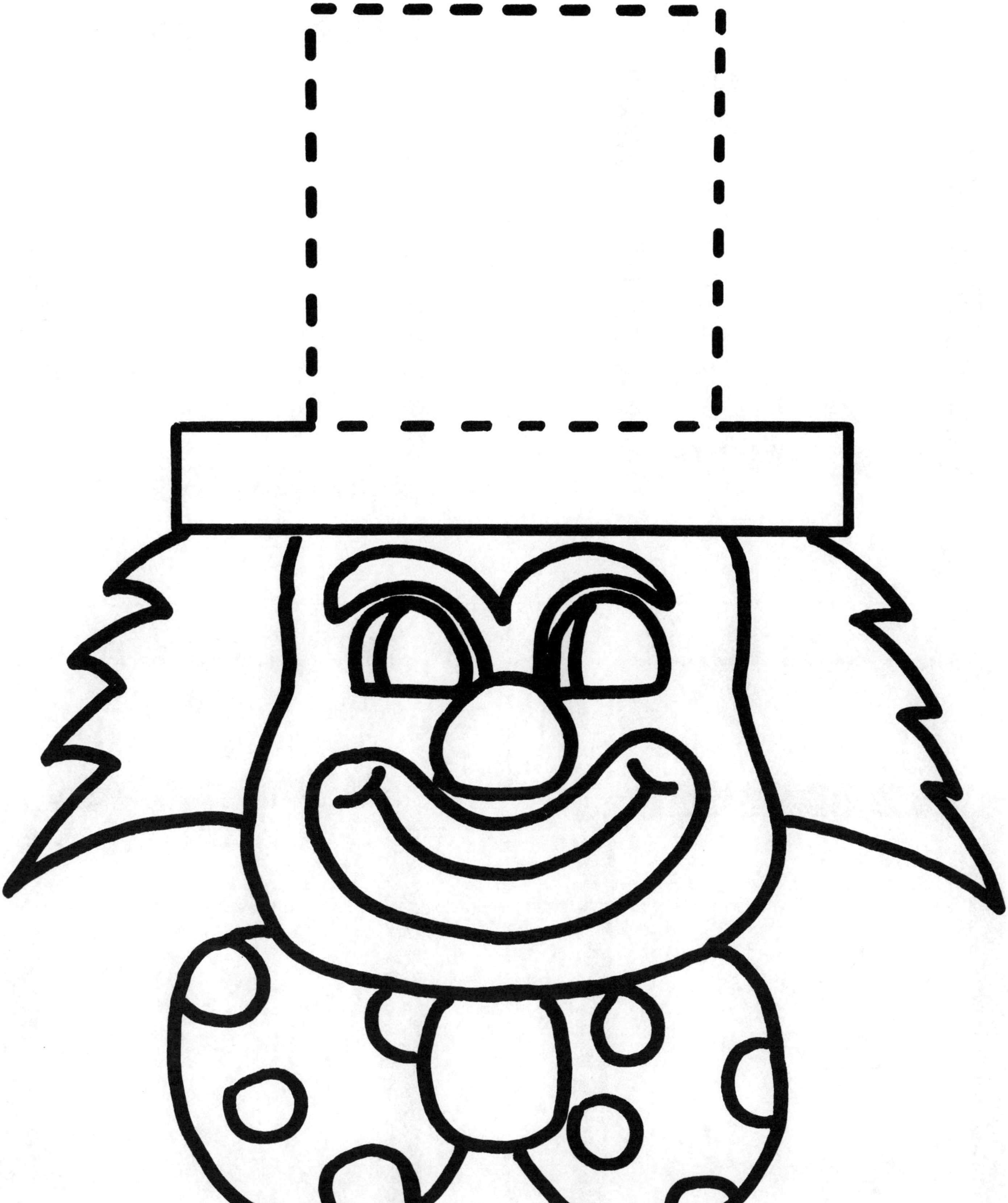

Skill 3
Step 2—Level #2 Pre/Posttest (jack-in-the-box)

Skill 3
Step 2—Level #2 Worksheet (hot air balloon)

Skill 3
Step 2—Level #2 Worksheet (book)

The End!

Skill 3
Step 2—Level #2 Worksheet (clown's hat)

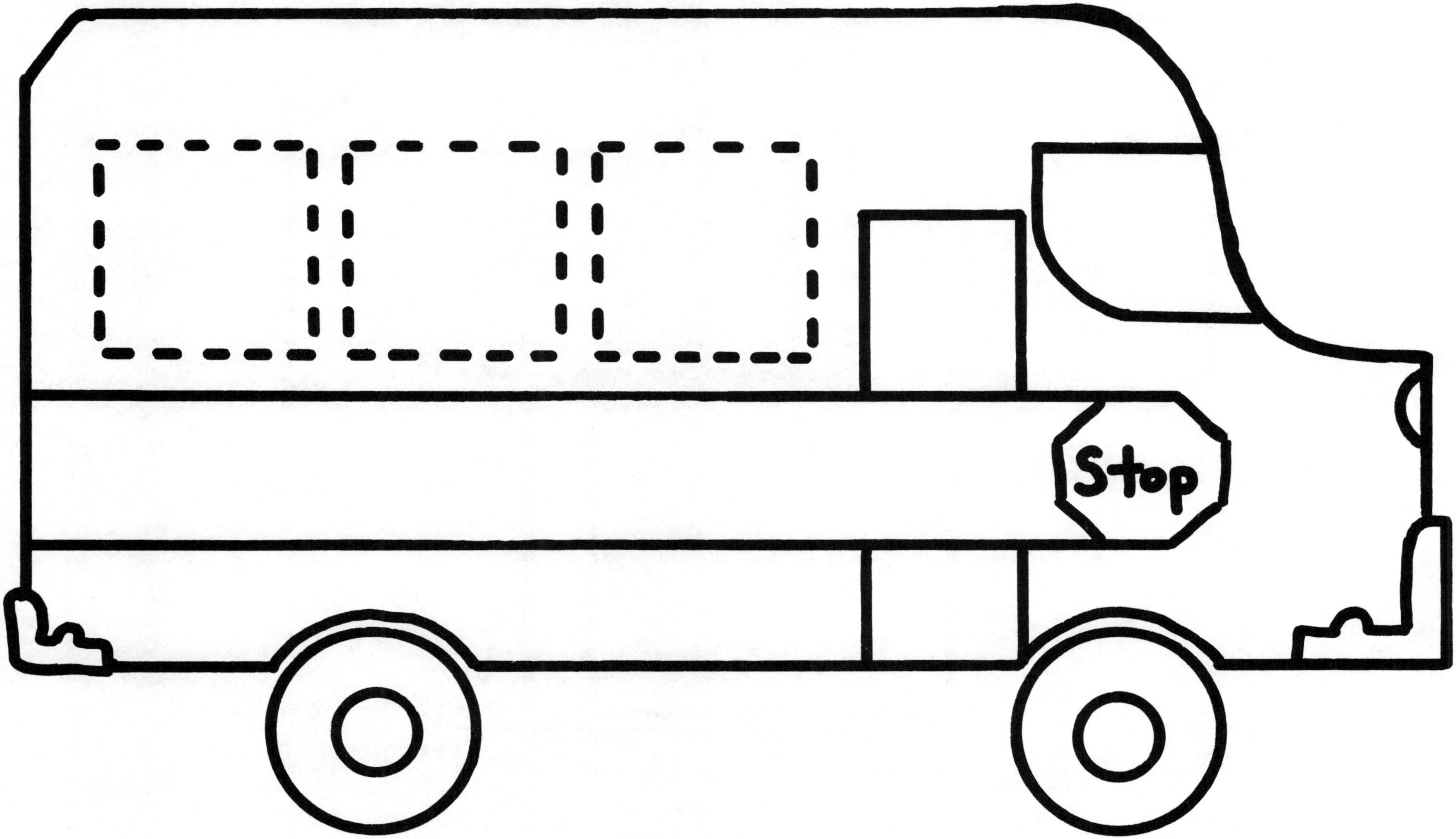
Stop

Step 2—Level #3 Worksheet

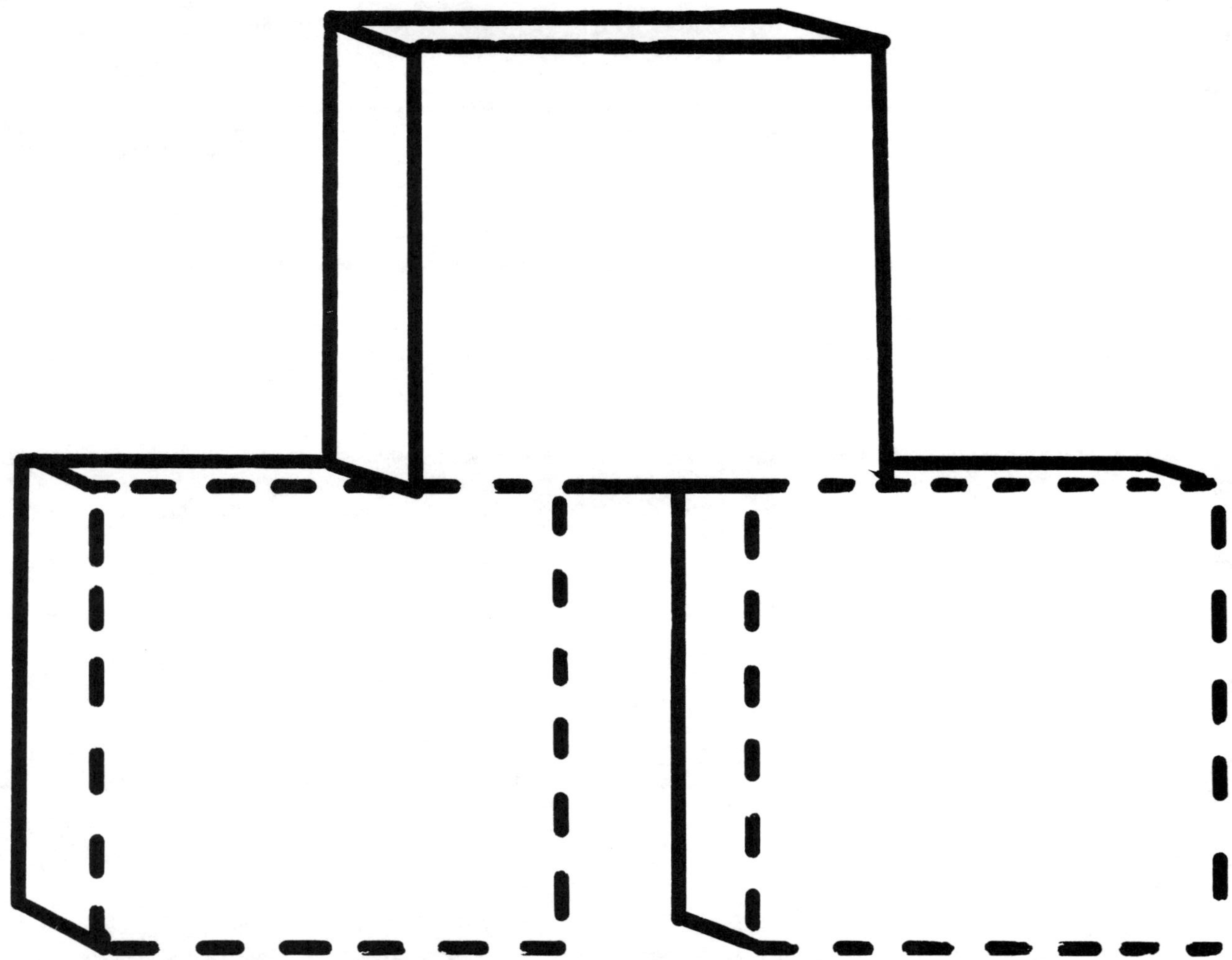

Skill 3
Step 2—Level #3 Pre/Posttest (school bus)

Skill 3
Step 2—Level #3 Worksheet (blocks)

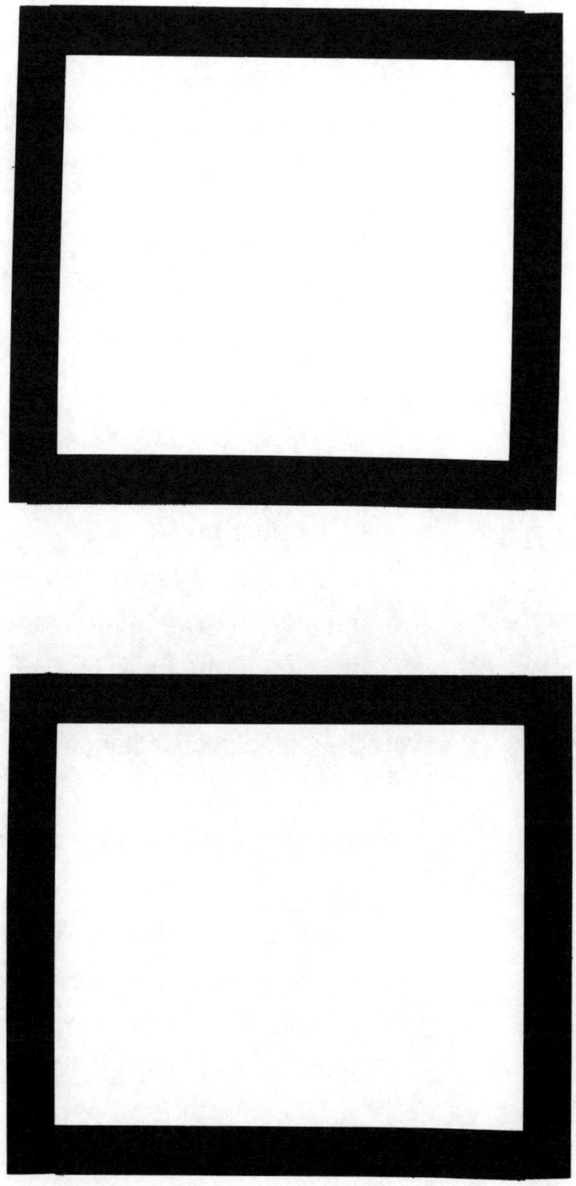

SKILL 3—STEP 3—RECTANGLES

Level #1—Rectangles, ¼" wide line
Pretest: Student takes Level #1 Pretest (train, 4½" x 3" rectangle).

If criterion met: Student advances to Level #2.

If criterion not met:
1. Student cuts Level #1 worksheets:
   helicopter—6" x 4"
   wagon—7" x 3"
   truck—5½" x 3½"
2. Student takes Level #1 Posttest (train).
   If criterion met: Student advances to Level #2.
   If criterion not met: Student repeats Level #1 worksheets and Posttest.

Level #2—Smaller Rectangles, ¼" wide line
Pretest: Student takes Level #2 Pretest (bear with gift—3" x 2" rectangle).

If criterion met: Student advances to Level #3.

If criterion not met:
1. Student cuts Level #2 worksheets:
   hobby horse—4" x 2"
   spaceship—2" x 3½"
   tree trunk—2" x 3"
2. Student takes Level #2 Posttest (bear with gift).
   If criterion met: Student advances to Level #3.
   If criterion not met: Student repeats Level #2 worksheets and Posttest.

Level #3—Combined Rectangles, ¼" wide line
Pretest: Student takes Level #3 Pretest (birthday cake—five rectangles, 1" x 2").

If criterion met: Student advances to Step 4—Triangles.

If criterion not met:
1. Student cuts Level #3 worksheet (giraffe—four rectangles, 1" x 1½").
2. Student takes Level #3 Posttest (birthday cake).
   If criterion met: Student advances to Step 4—Triangles.
   If criterion not met: Student repeats Level #3 worksheet and Posttest.

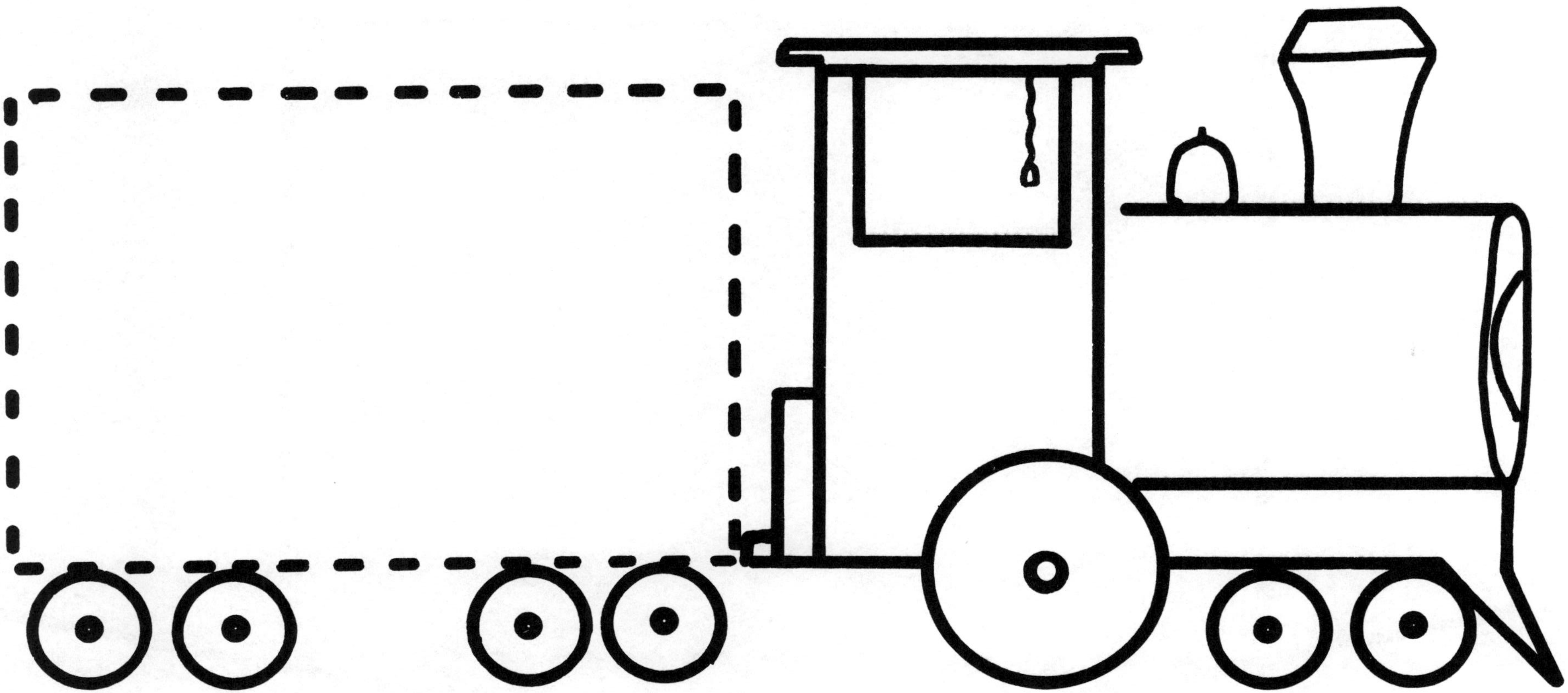

Step 3—Level #1 Worksheet

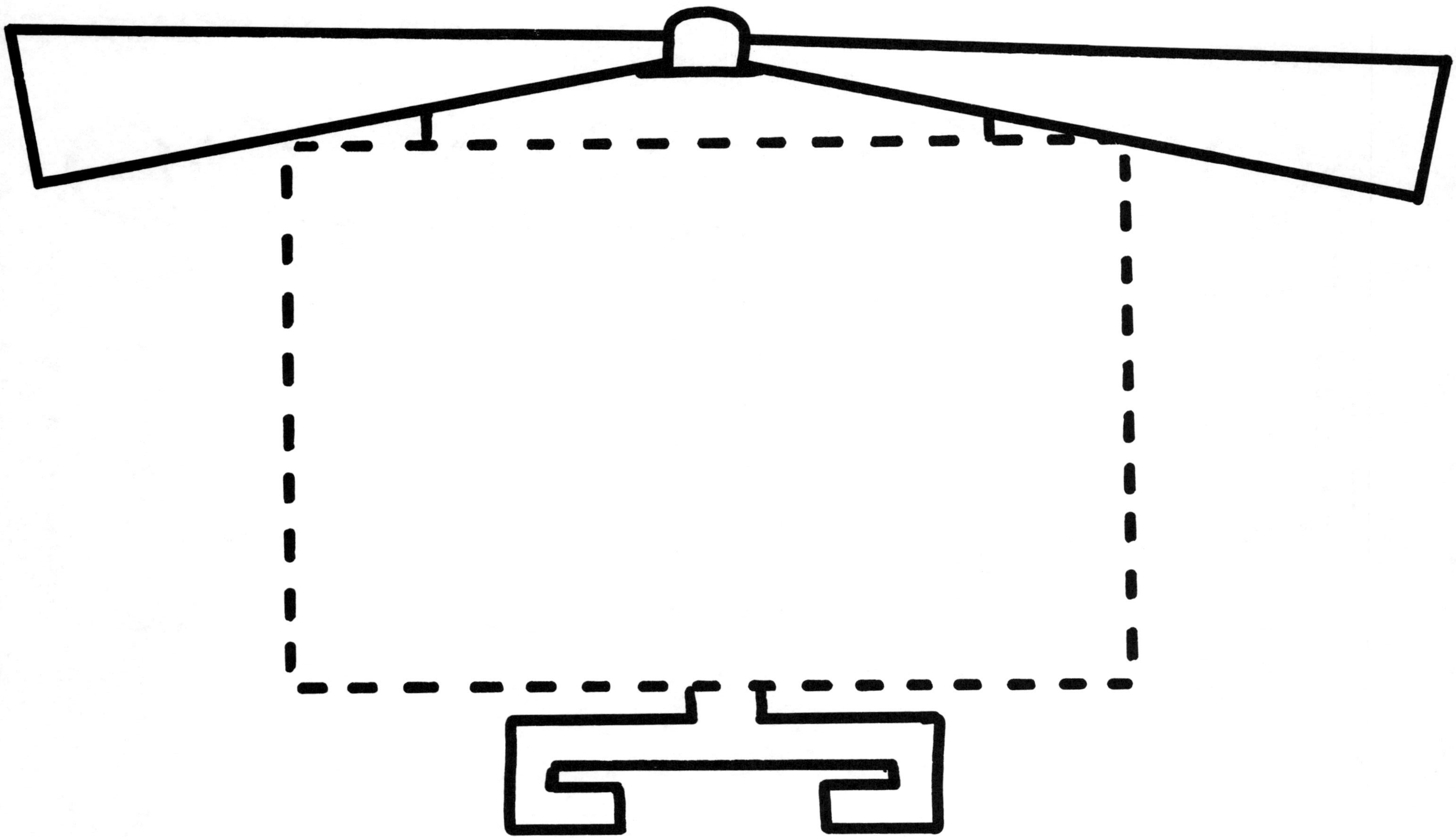

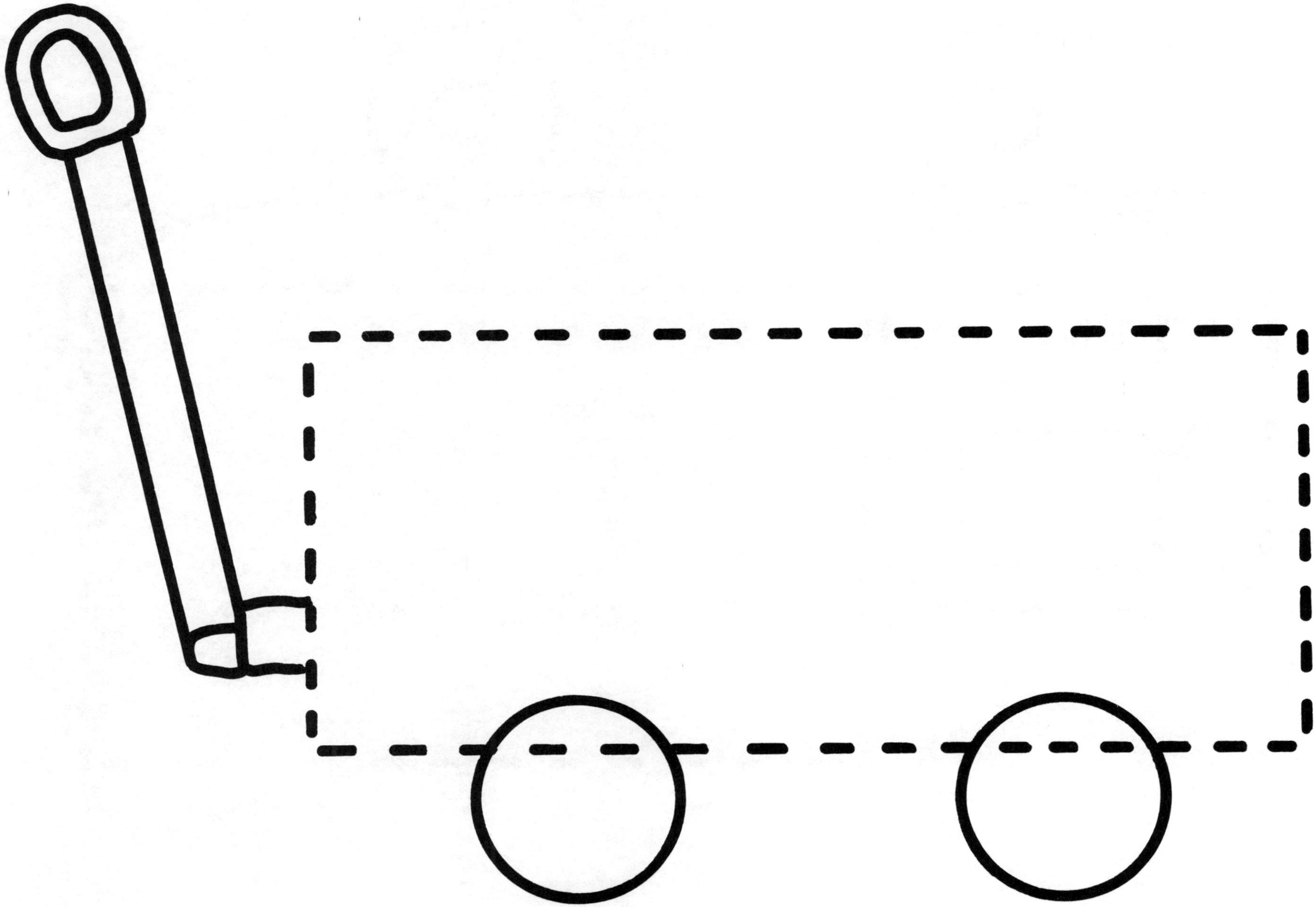

Step 3—Level #1 Worksheet

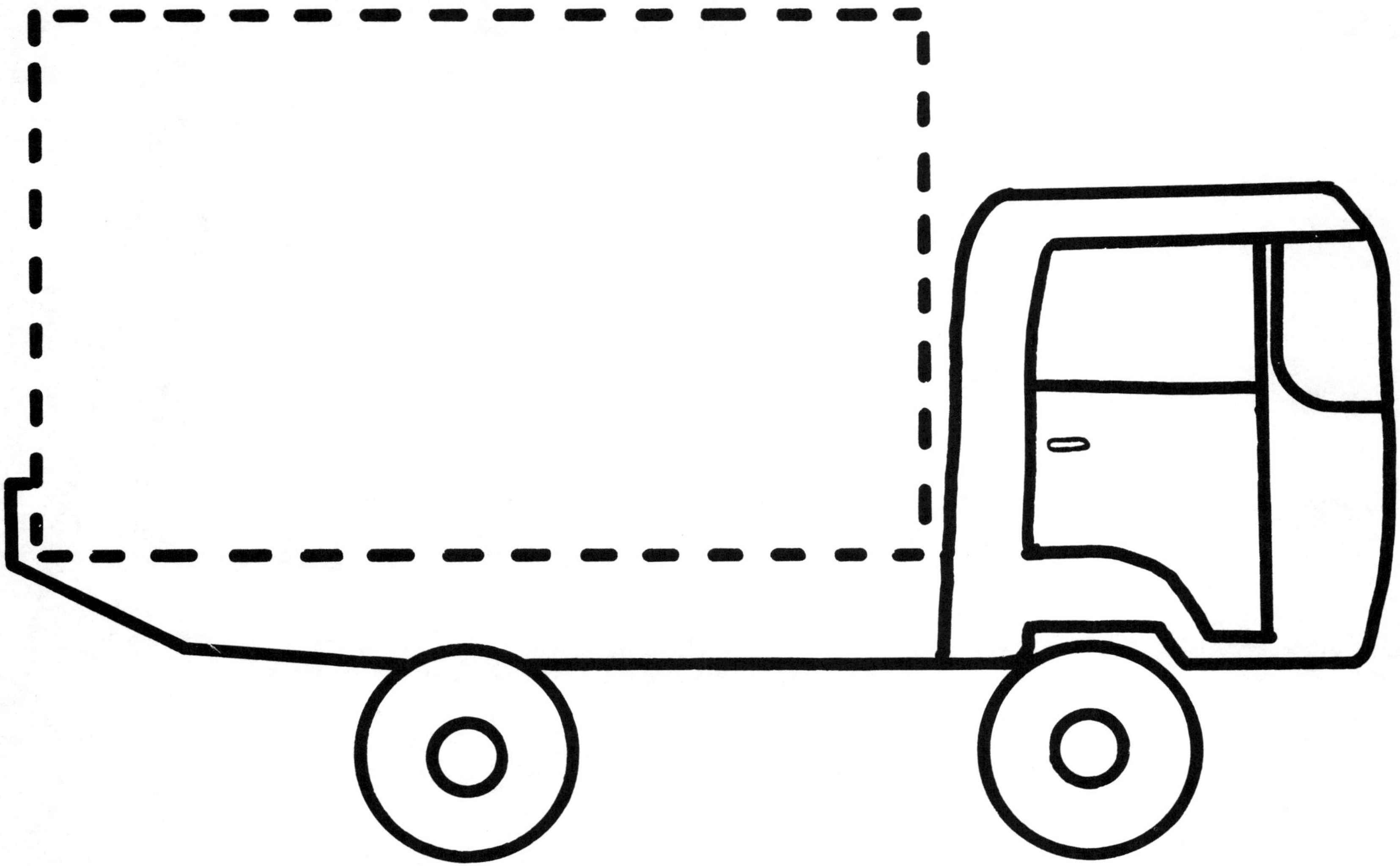

Skill 3
Step 3—Level #1 Pre/Posttest (train)

Skill 3
Step 3—Level #1 Worksheet (helicopter)

Skill 3
Step 3—Level #1 Worksheet (wagon)

Skill 3
Step 3—Level #1 Worksheet (truck)

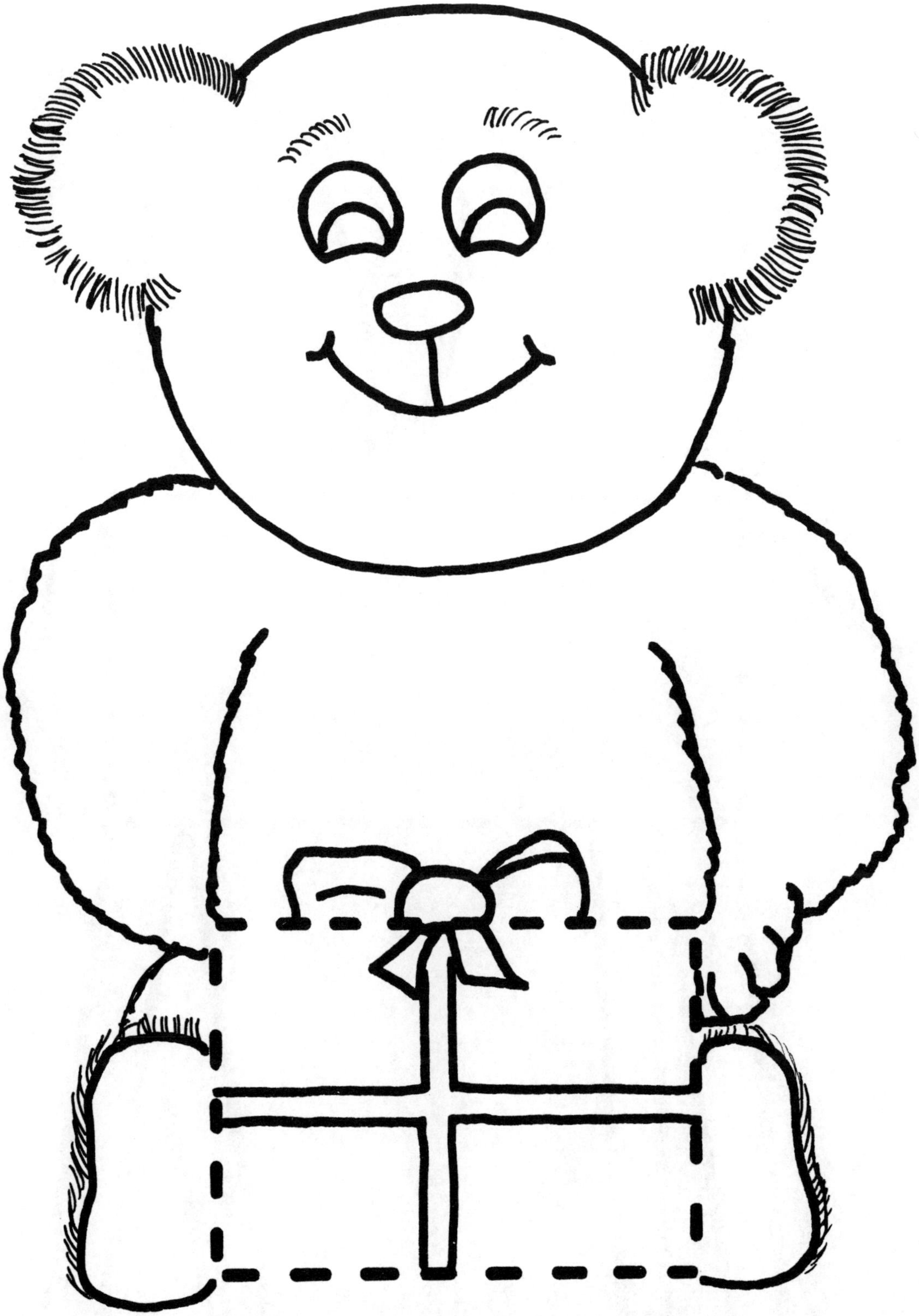

Step 3—Level #2 Worksheet

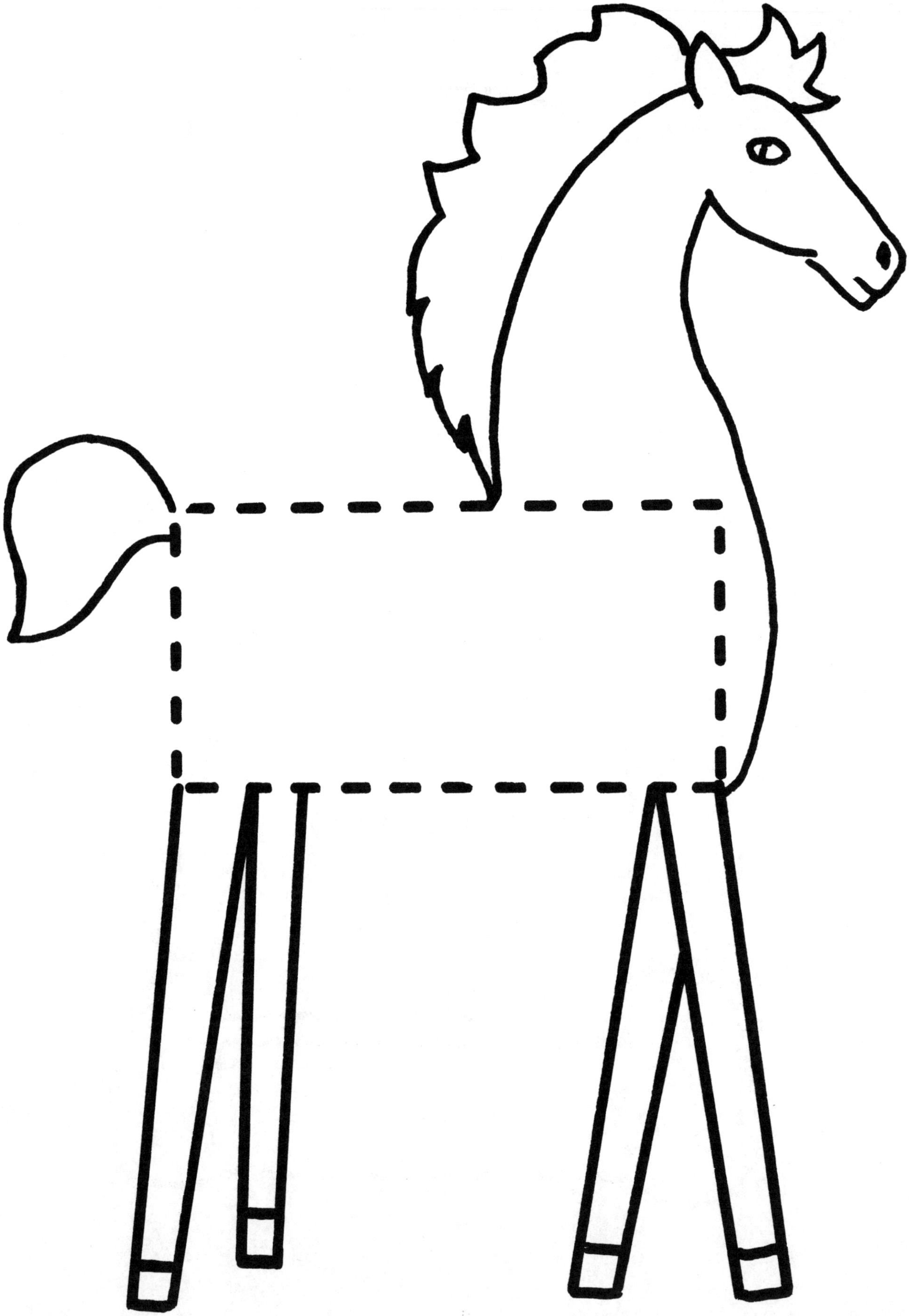

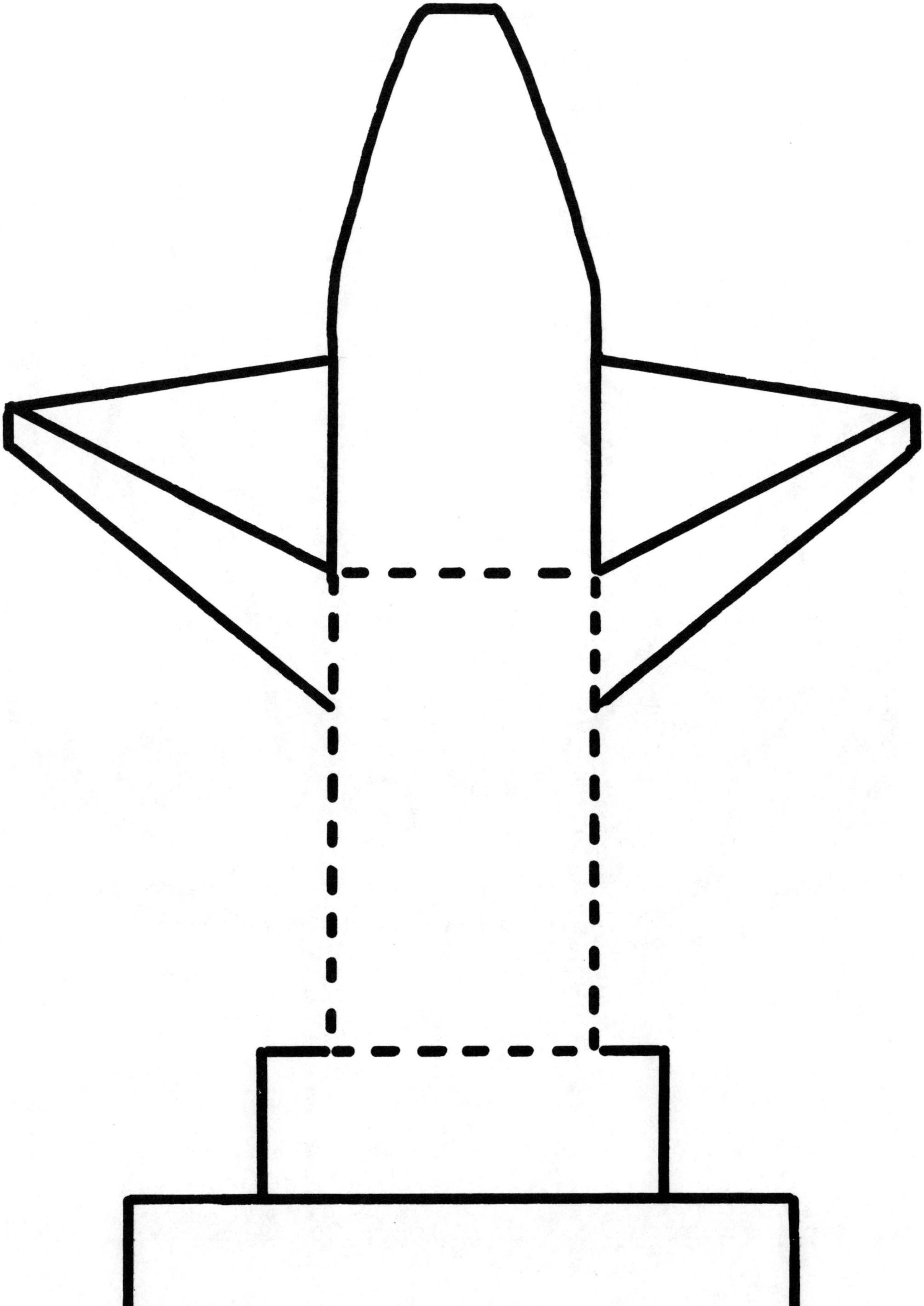

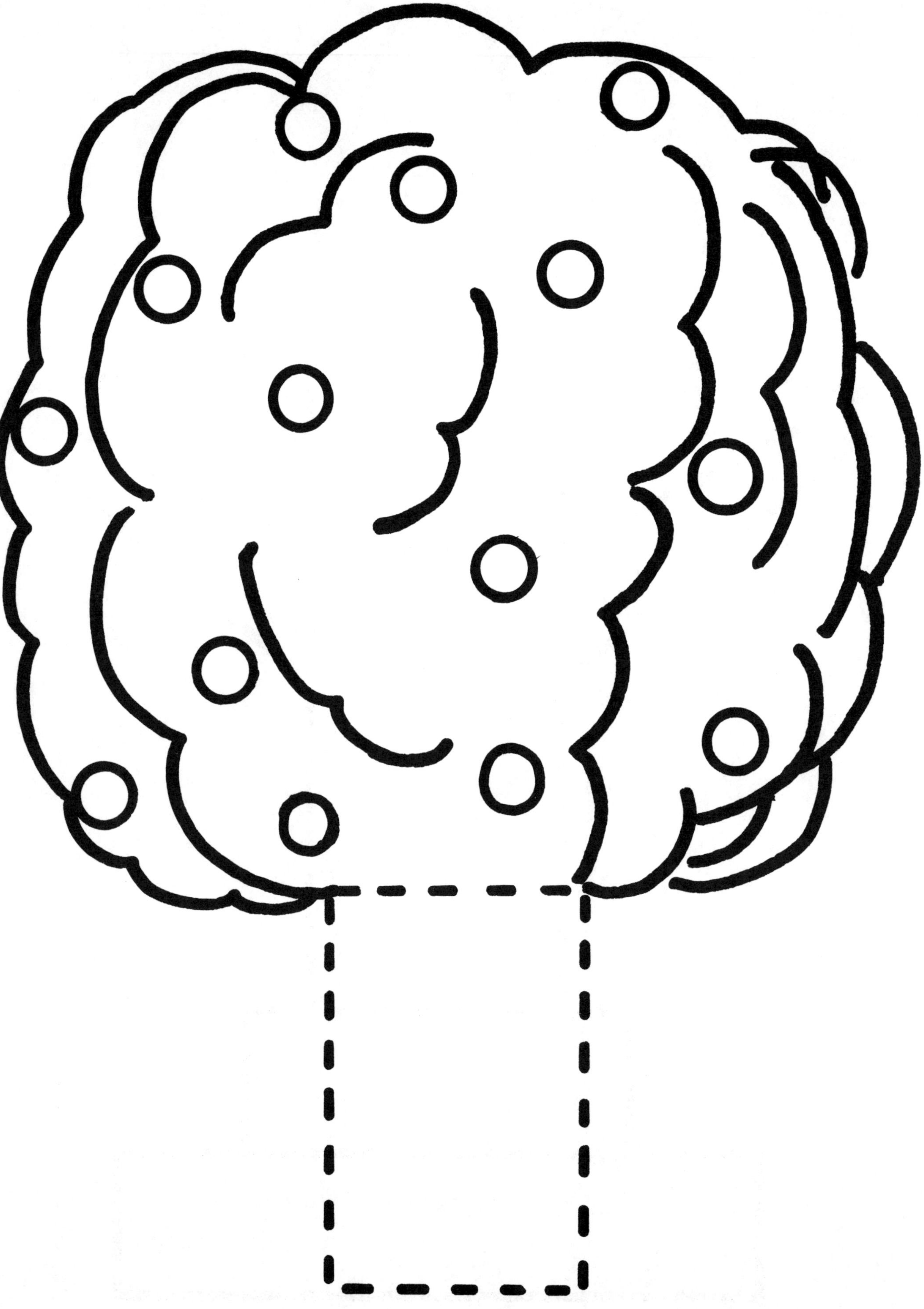

Skill 3
Step 3—Level #2 Pre/Posttest (bear with gift)

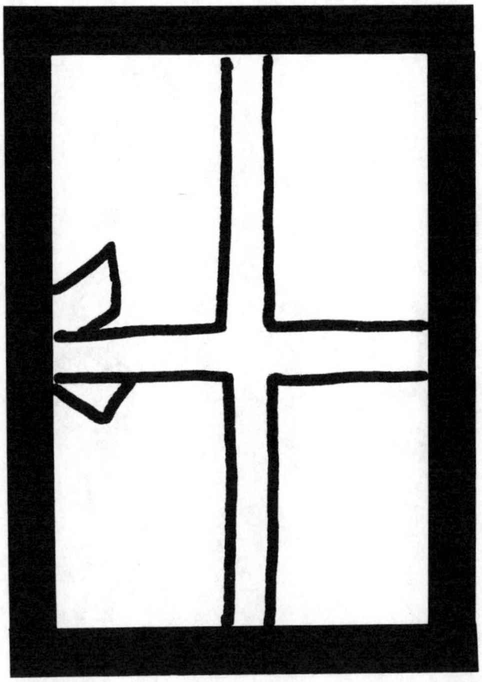

Skill 3
Step 3—Level #2 Worksheet (hobby horse)

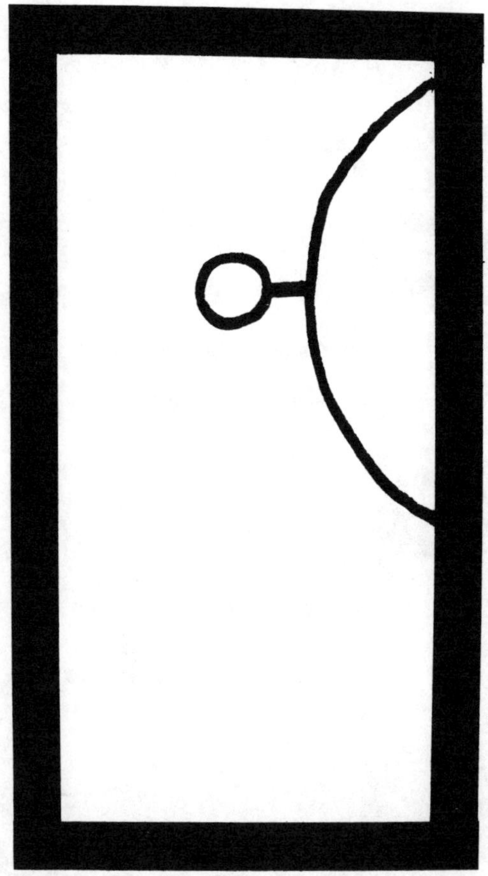

Skill 3
Step 3—Level #2 Worksheet (spaceship)

Skill 3
Step 3—Level #2 Worksheet (tree trunk)

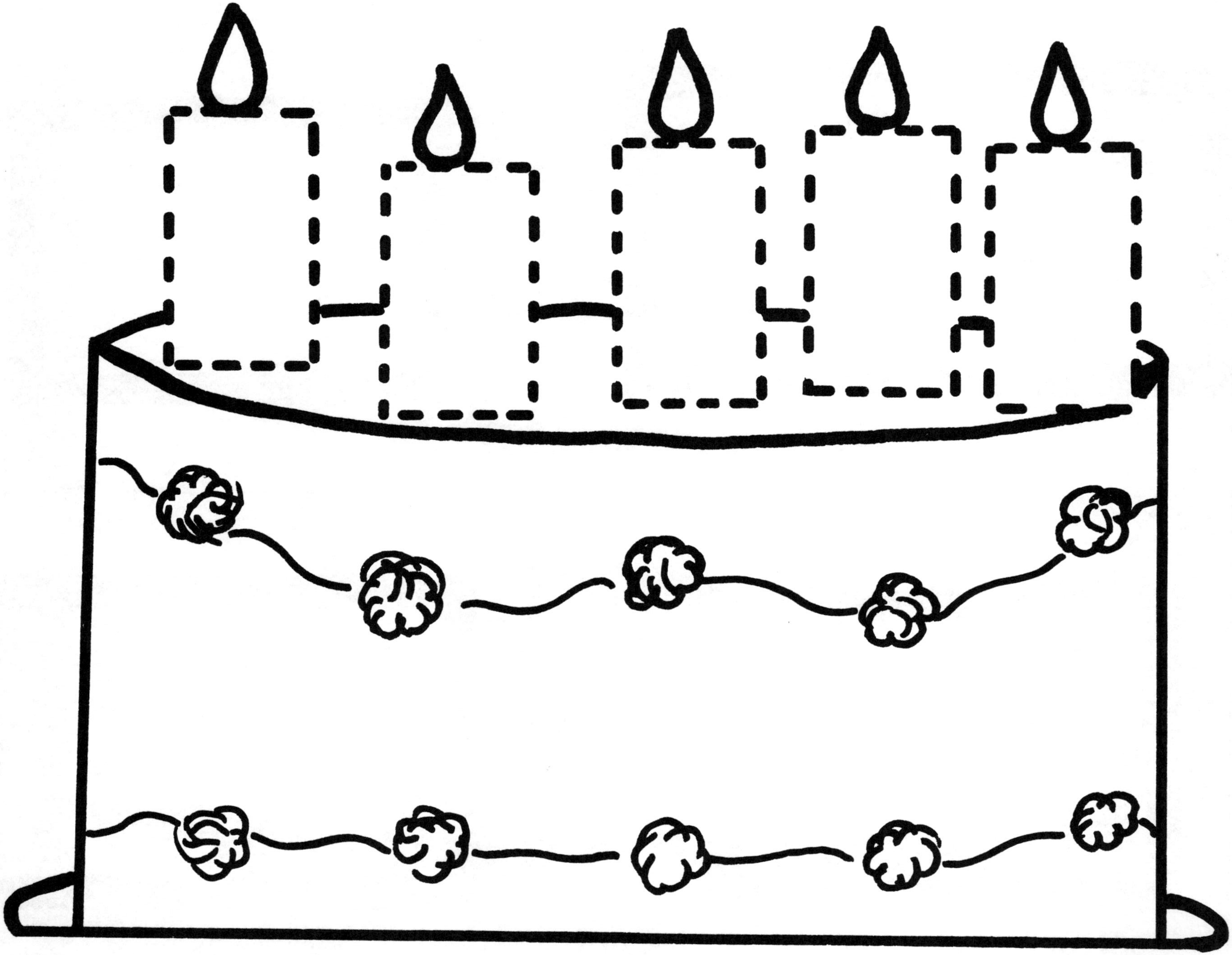

Step 3—Level #3 Pre/Posttest

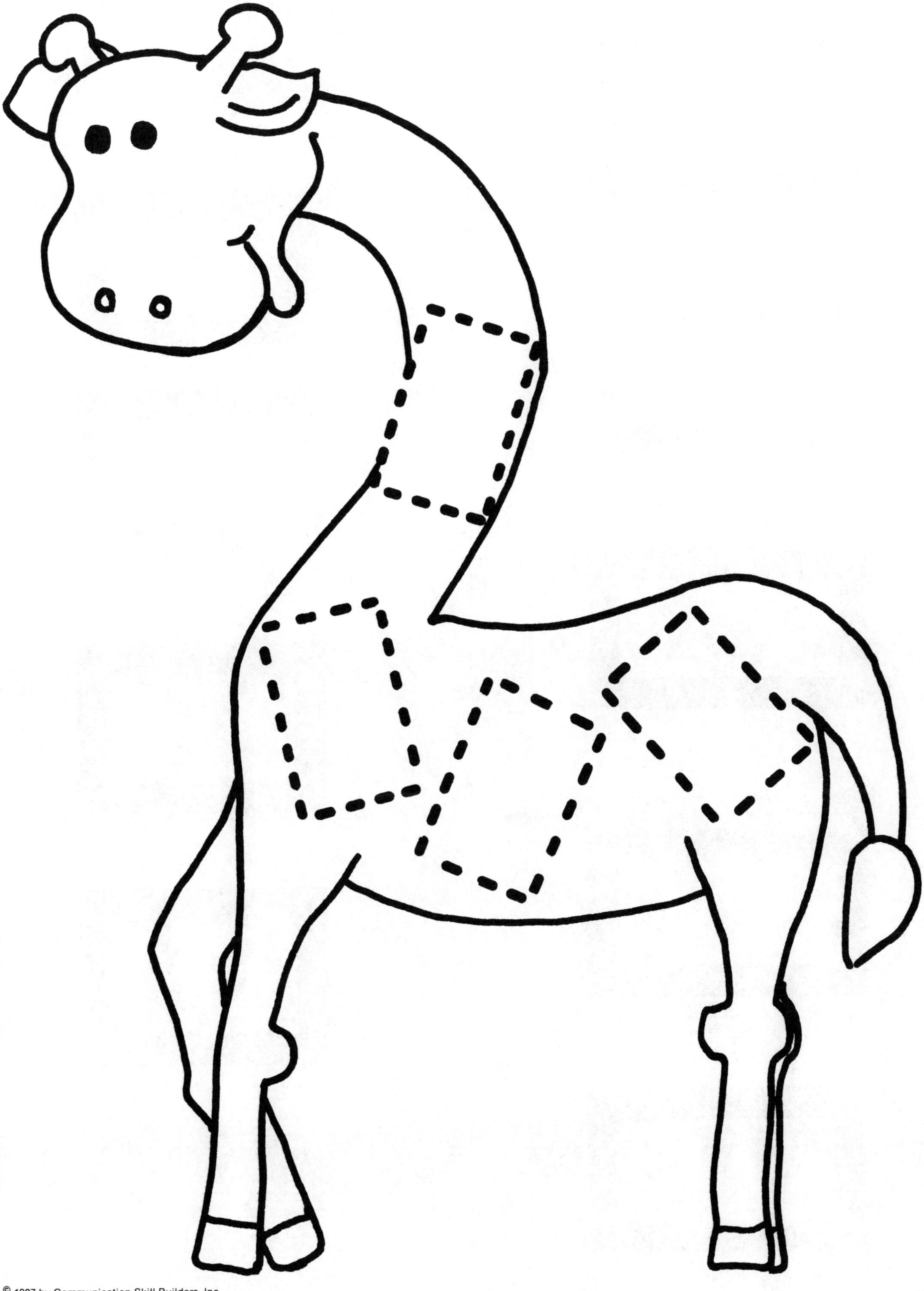

Skill 3
Step 3—Level #3 Pre/Posttest (birthday cake)

Skill 3
Step 3—Level #3 Worksheet (giraffe)

SKILL 3—STEP 4—TRIANGLES

Level #1—Triangles, 1/4" wide line
Pretest: Student takes Level #1 Pretest (barn—triangle with 4" base).

If criterion met: Student advances to Level #2.

If criterion not met:
1. Student cuts Level #1 worksheets:
   dog house—5" base
   tepee—5" base
   kite—4" base
2. Student takes Level #1 Posttest (barn).
   If criterion met: Student advances to Level #2.
   If criterion not met: Student repeats Level #1 worksheets and Posttest.

Level #2—Smaller Triangles, 1/4" wide line
Pretest: Student takes Level #2 Pretest (drum, triangle with 2½" base).

If criterion met: Student advances to Level #3.

If criterion not met:
1. Student cuts Level #2 worksheets:
   party hat—4" base
   carrot—3½" base
   clown's hat—2½" base
2. Student takes Level #2 Posttest (drum).
   If criterion met: Student advances to Level #3.
   If criterion not met: Student repeats Level #2 worksheets and Posttest.

Level #3—Combined Triangles, 1/4" wide line
Pretest: Student takes Level #3 Pretest (walrus—two triangles, 1" base).

If criterion met: Student advances to Step 5—Diamonds.

If criterion not met:
1. Student cuts Level #3 worksheet (sailboat—two triangles, 3" base and 1½" base).
2. Student takes Level #2 Posttest (walrus).
   If criterion met: Student advances to Step 5—Diamonds.
   If criterion not met: Student repeats worksheet and Posttest.

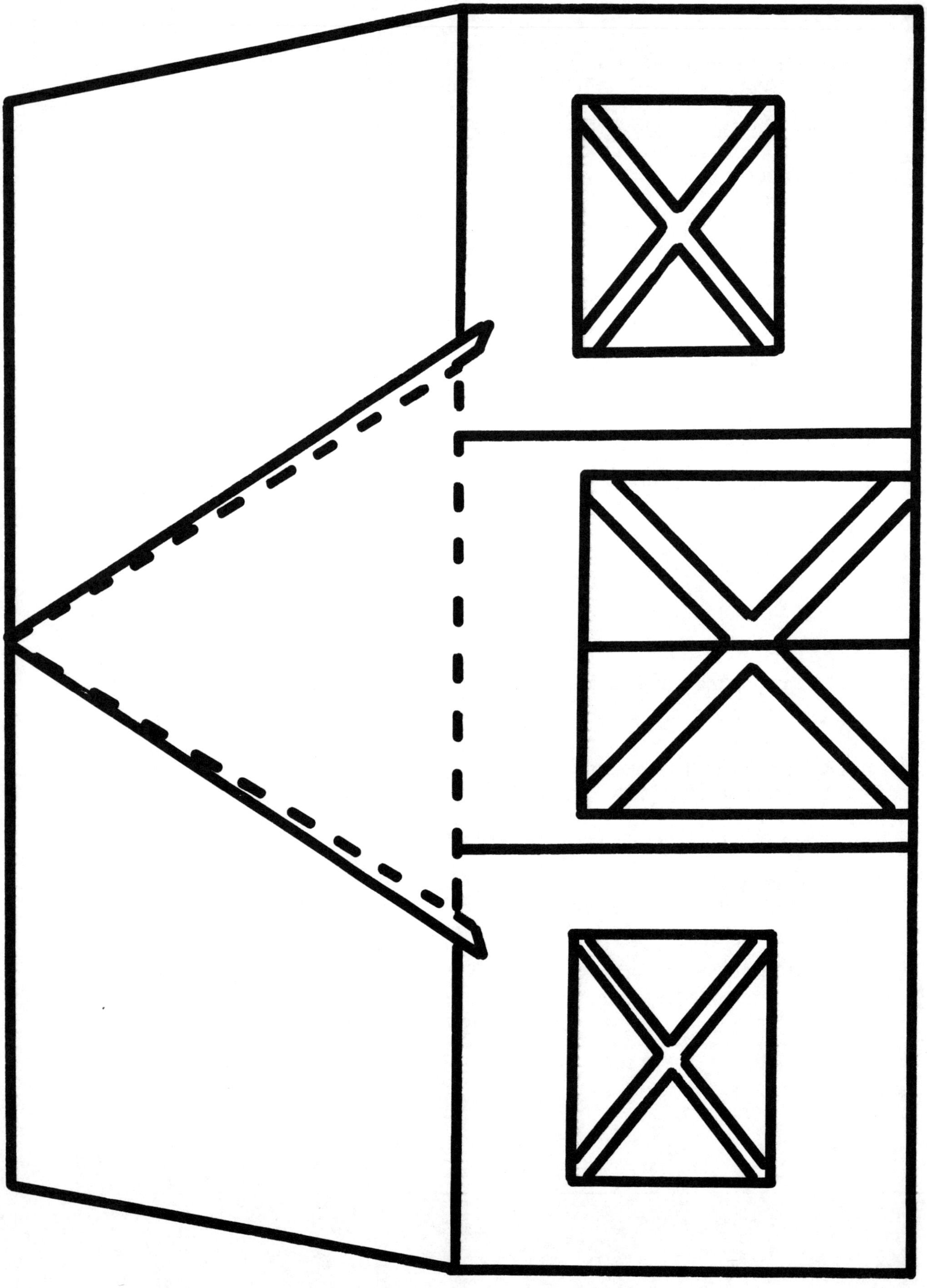

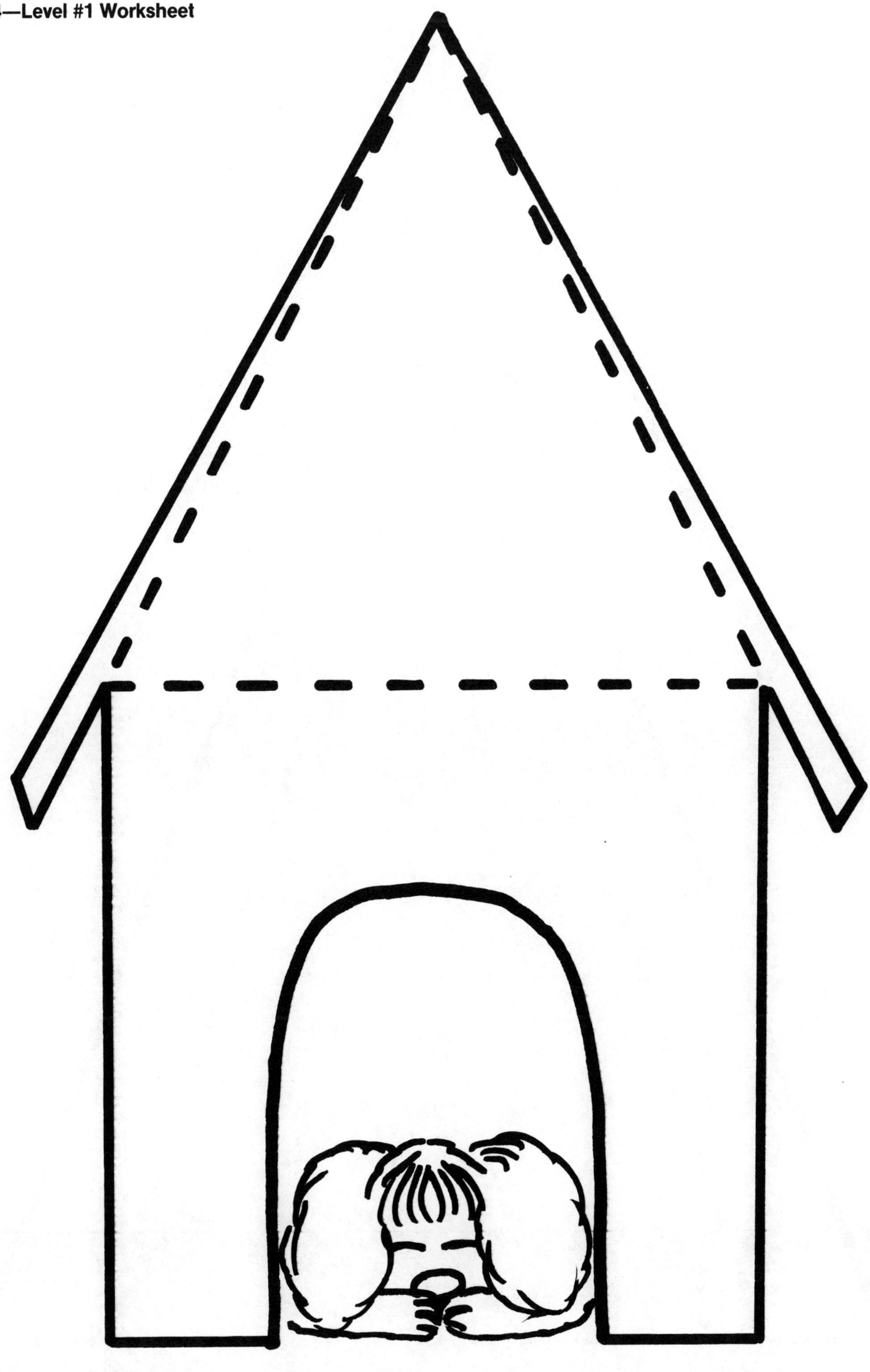

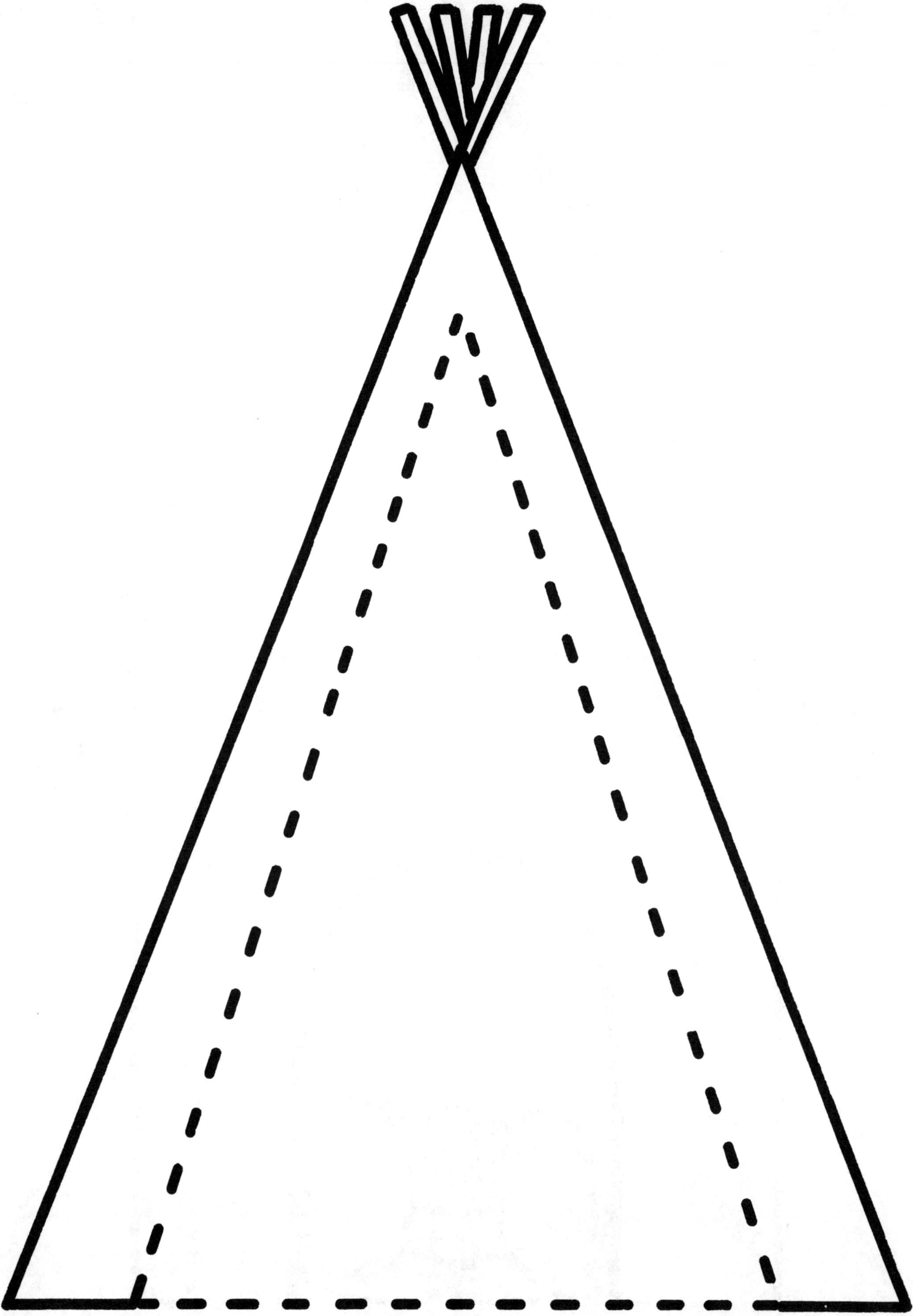

Step 4—Level #1 Worksheet

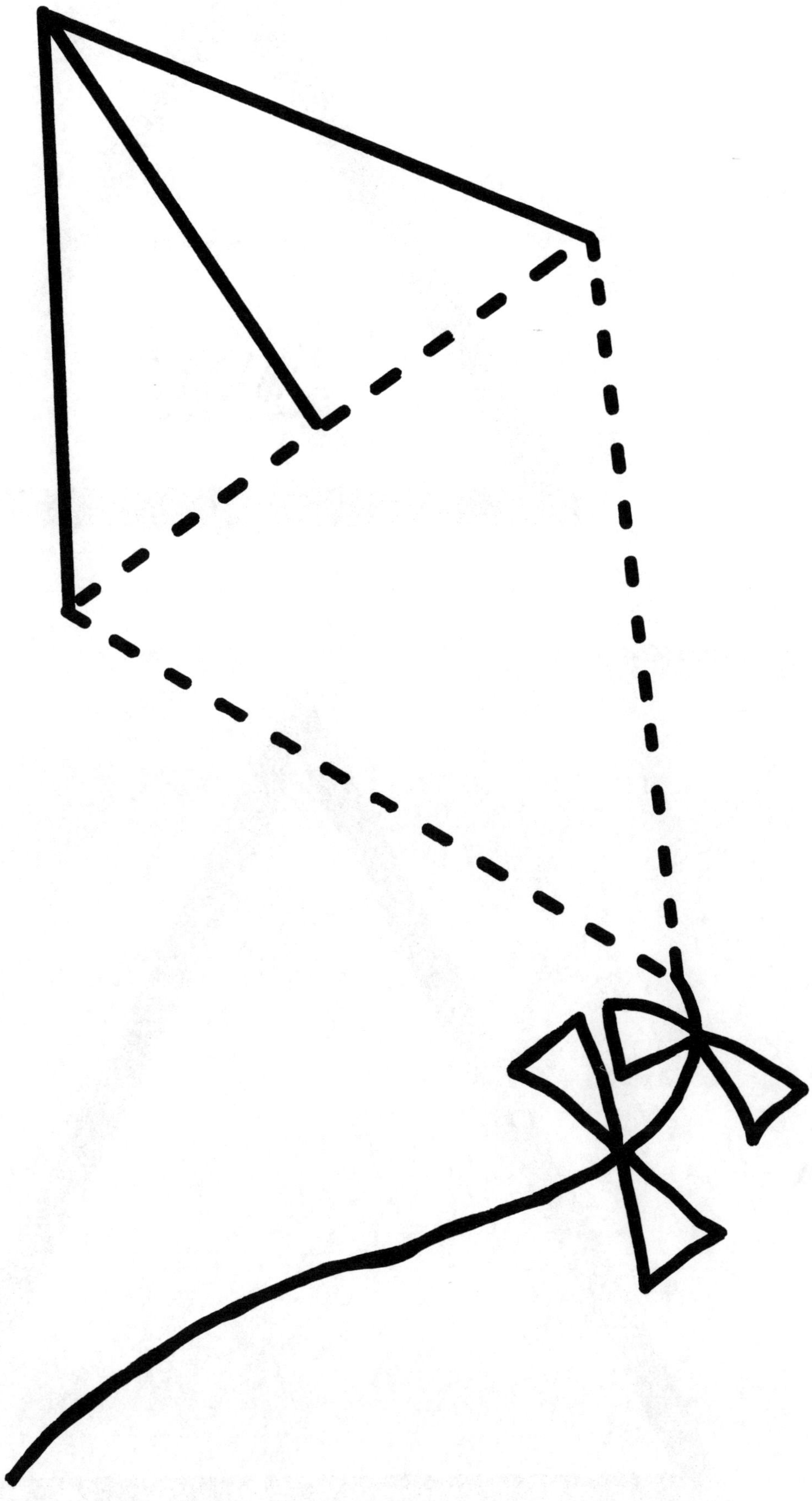

Skill 3
Step 4—Level #1 Pre/Posttest (barn)

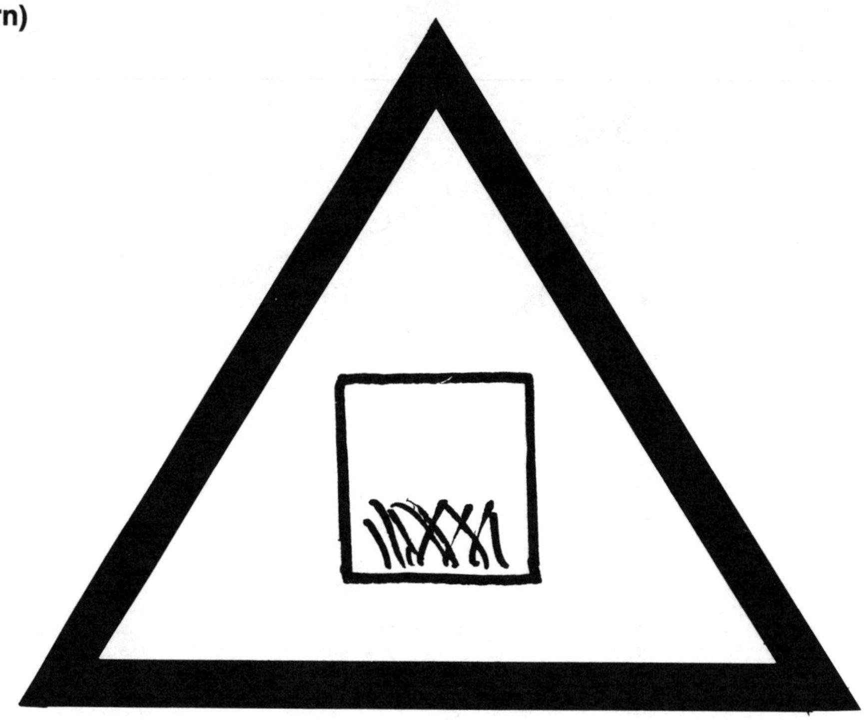

Skill 3
Step 4—Level #1 Worksheet (dog house)

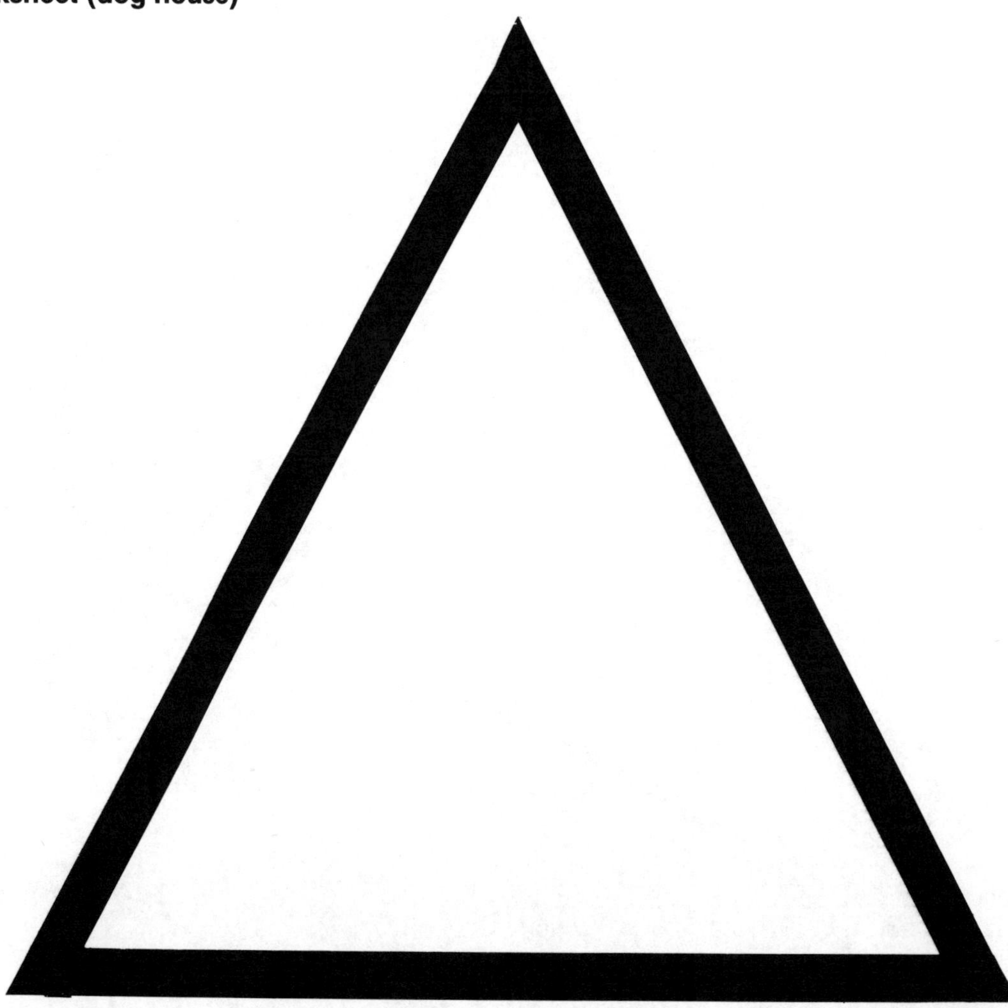

Skill 3
Step 4—Level #1 Worksheet (tepee)

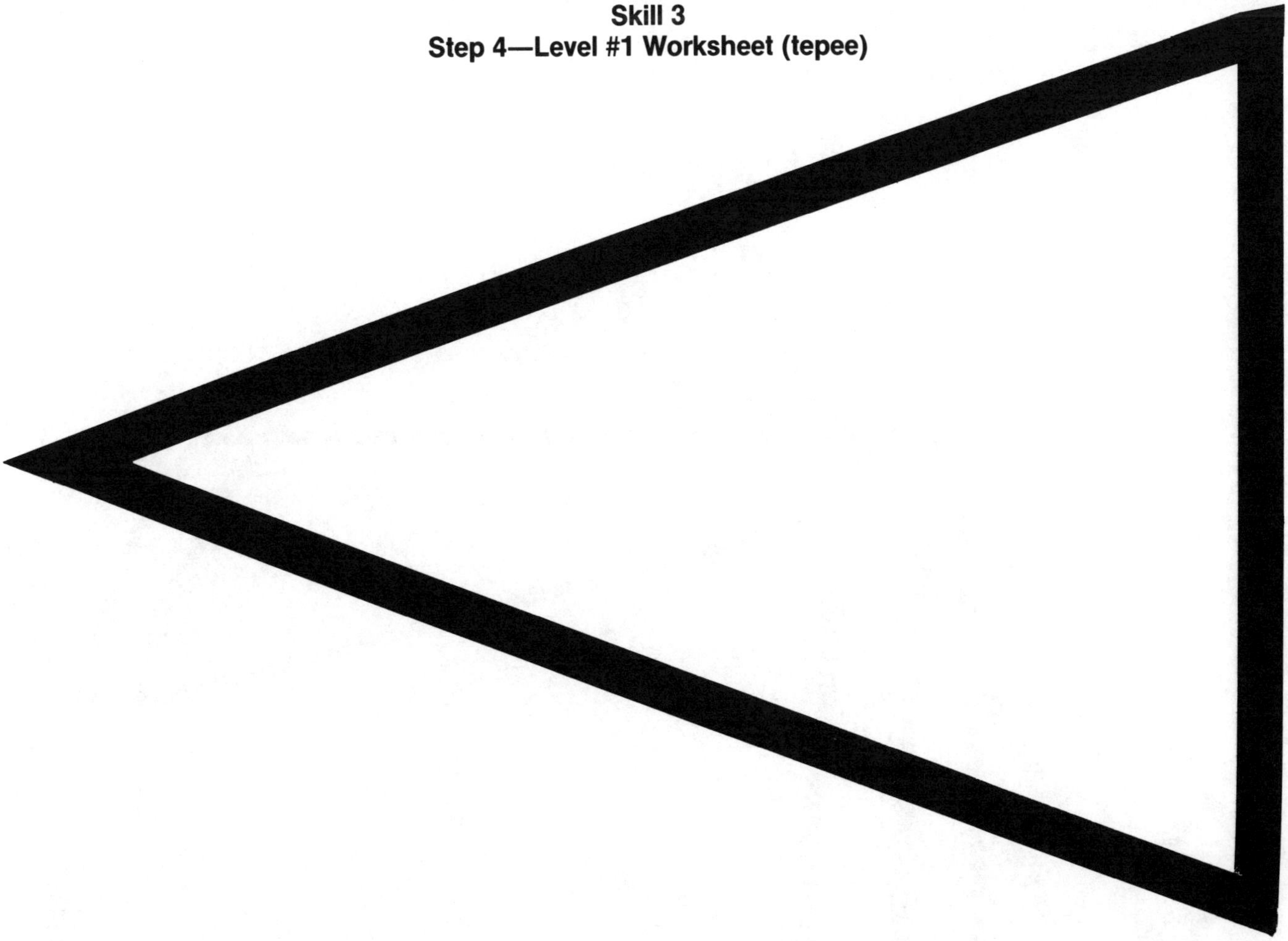

Skill 3
Step 4—Level #1 Worksheet (kite)

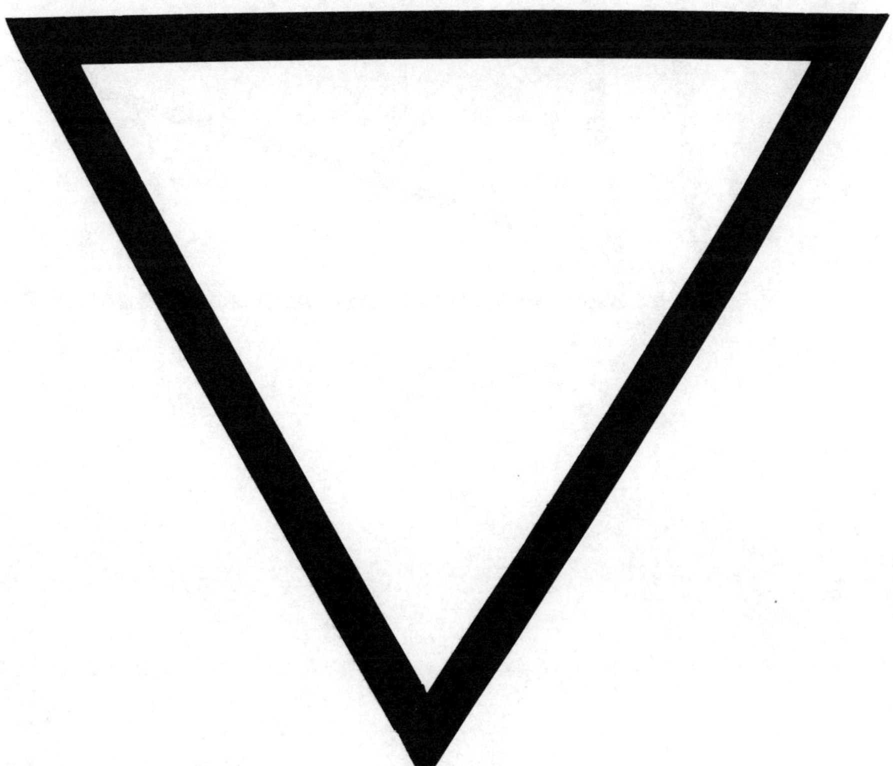

Step 4—Level #2 Pre/Posttest

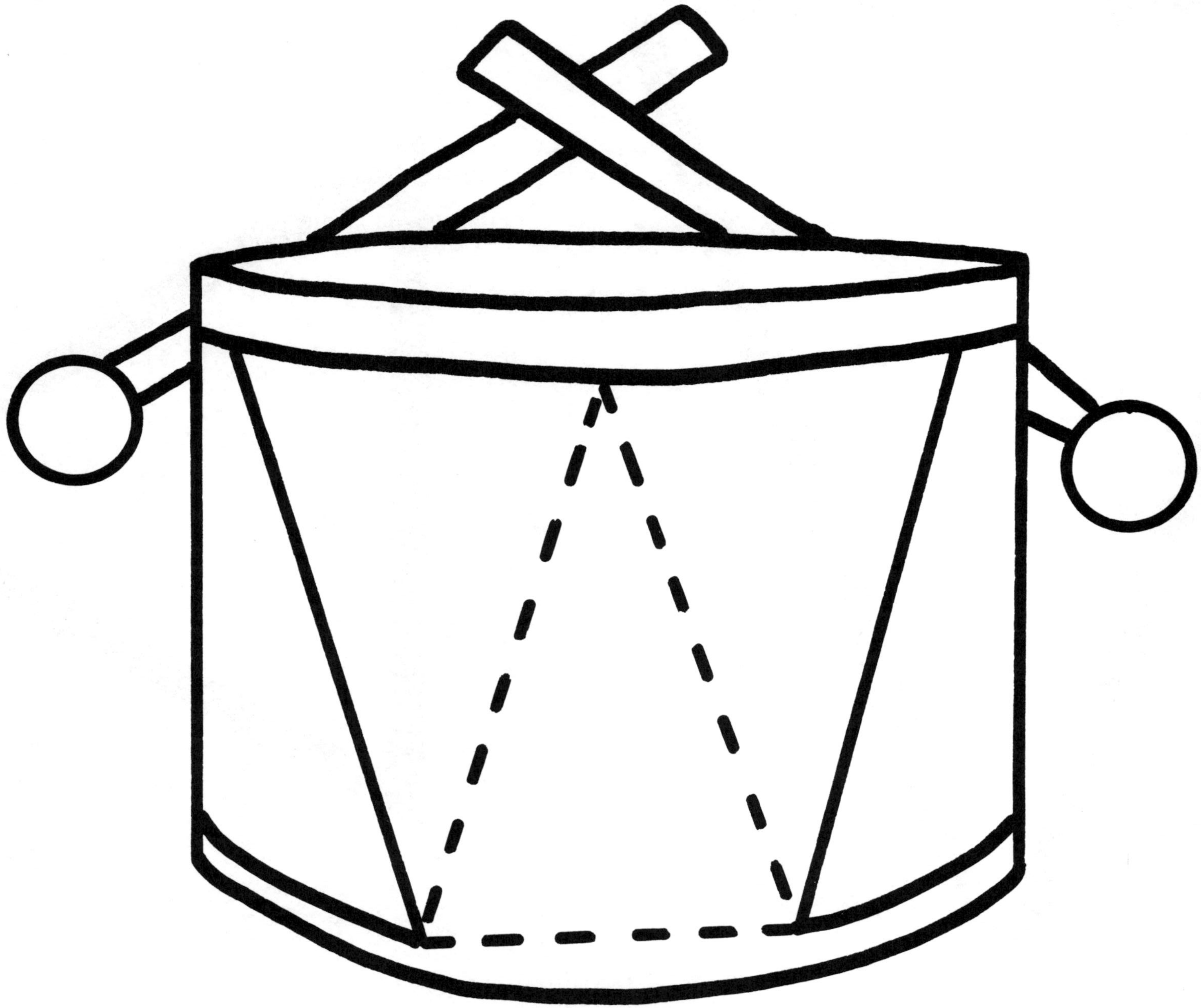

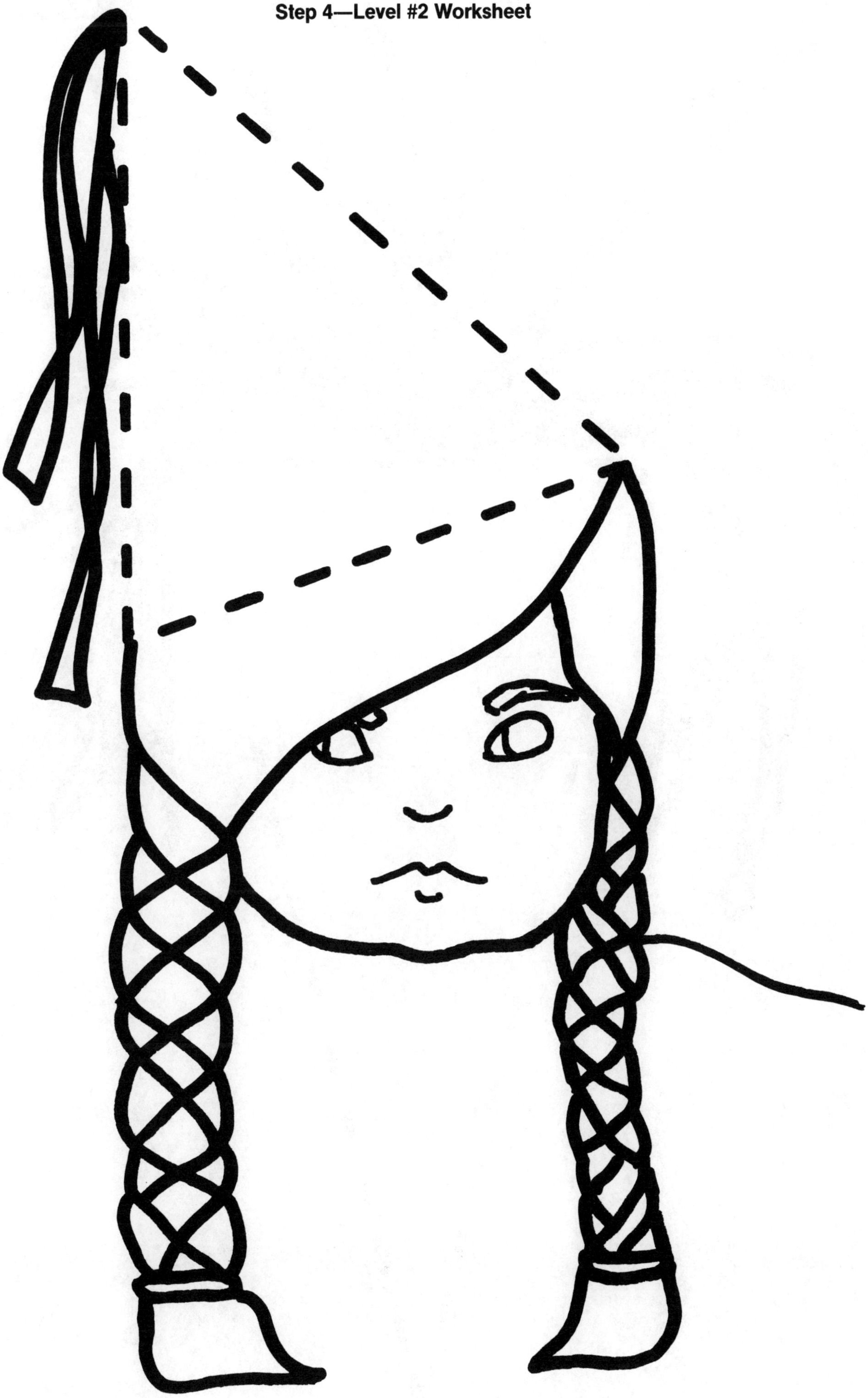

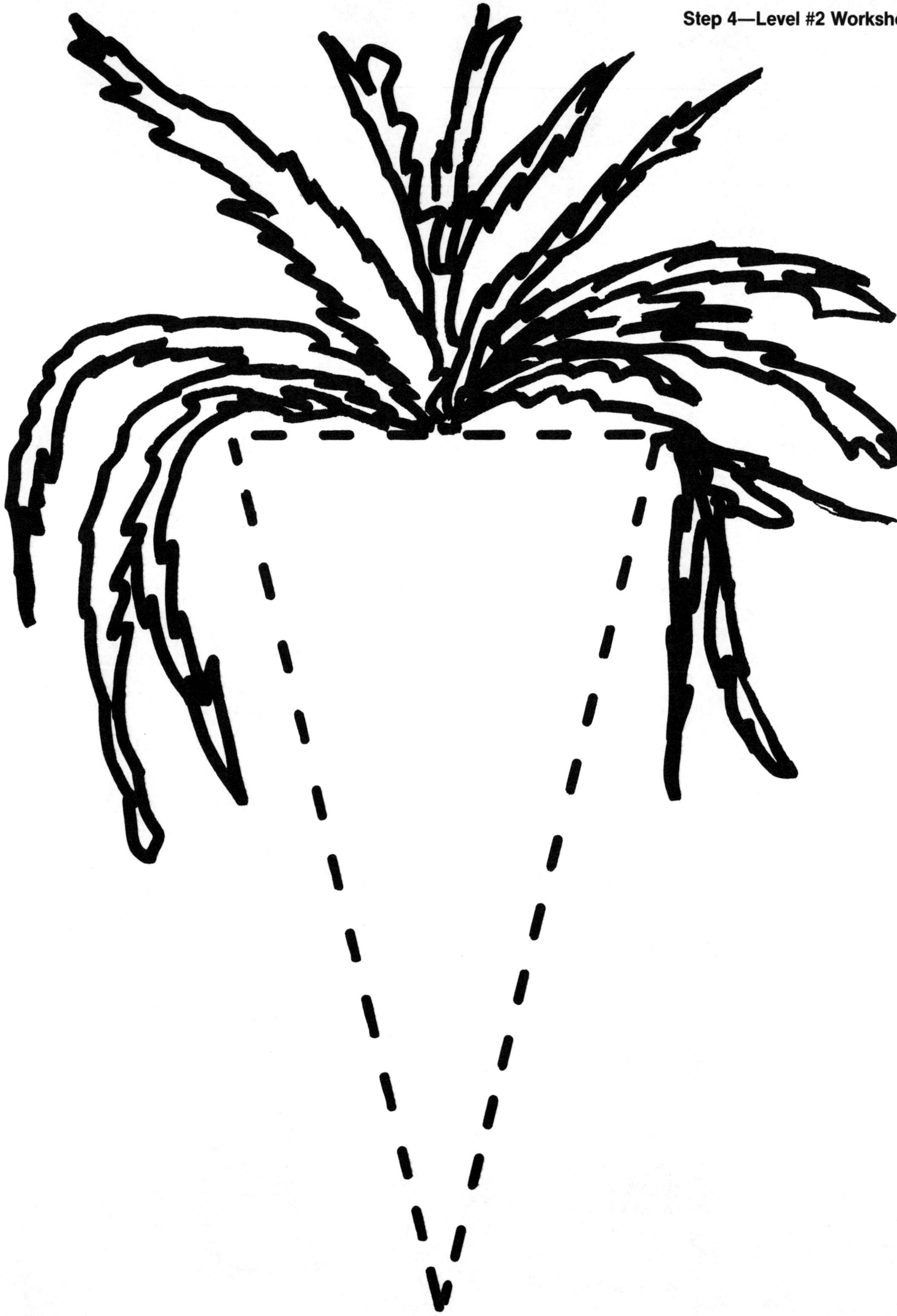

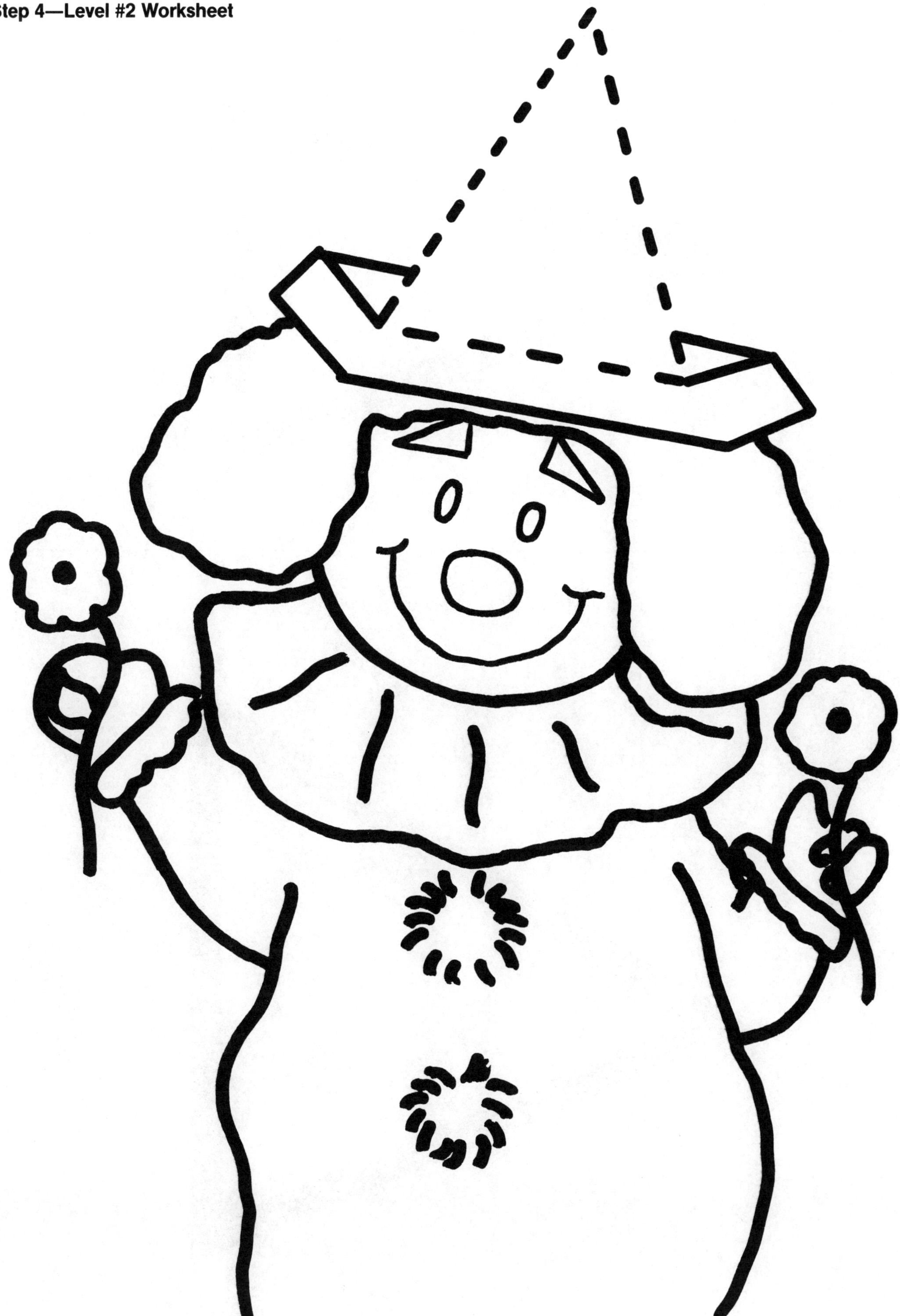

Skill 3
Step 4—Level #2 Pre/Posttest (drum)

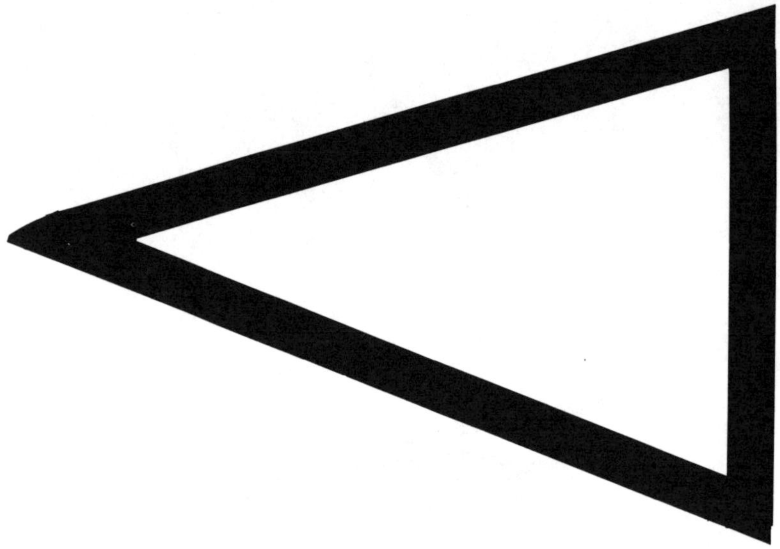

Skill 3
Step 4—Level #2 Worksheet (party hat)

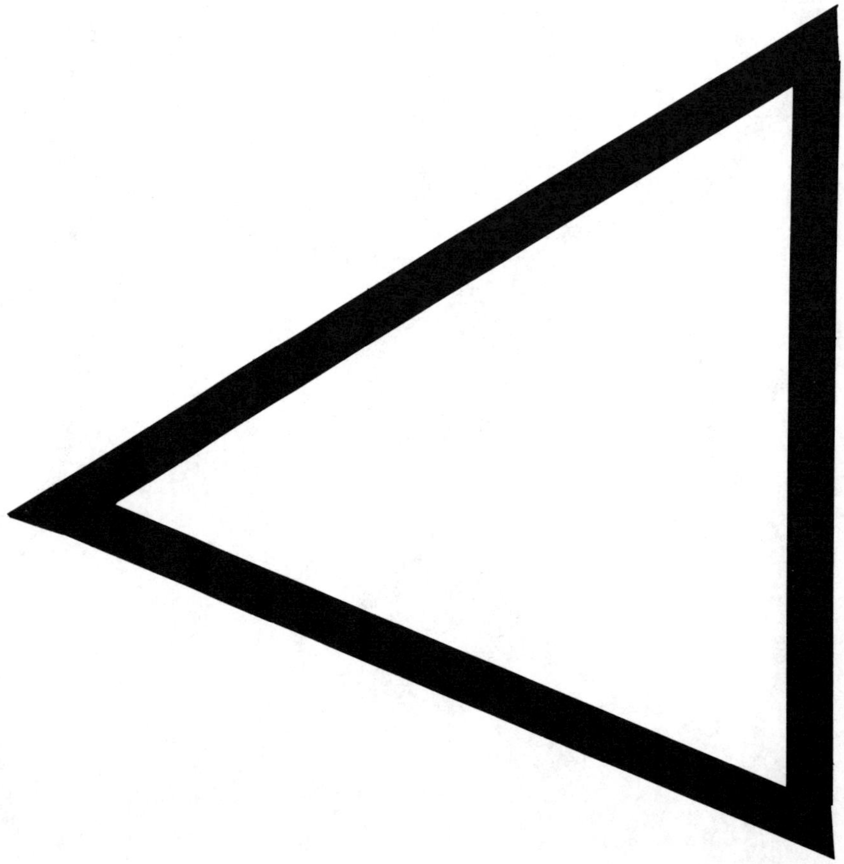

Skill 3
Step 4—Level #2 Worksheet (carrot)

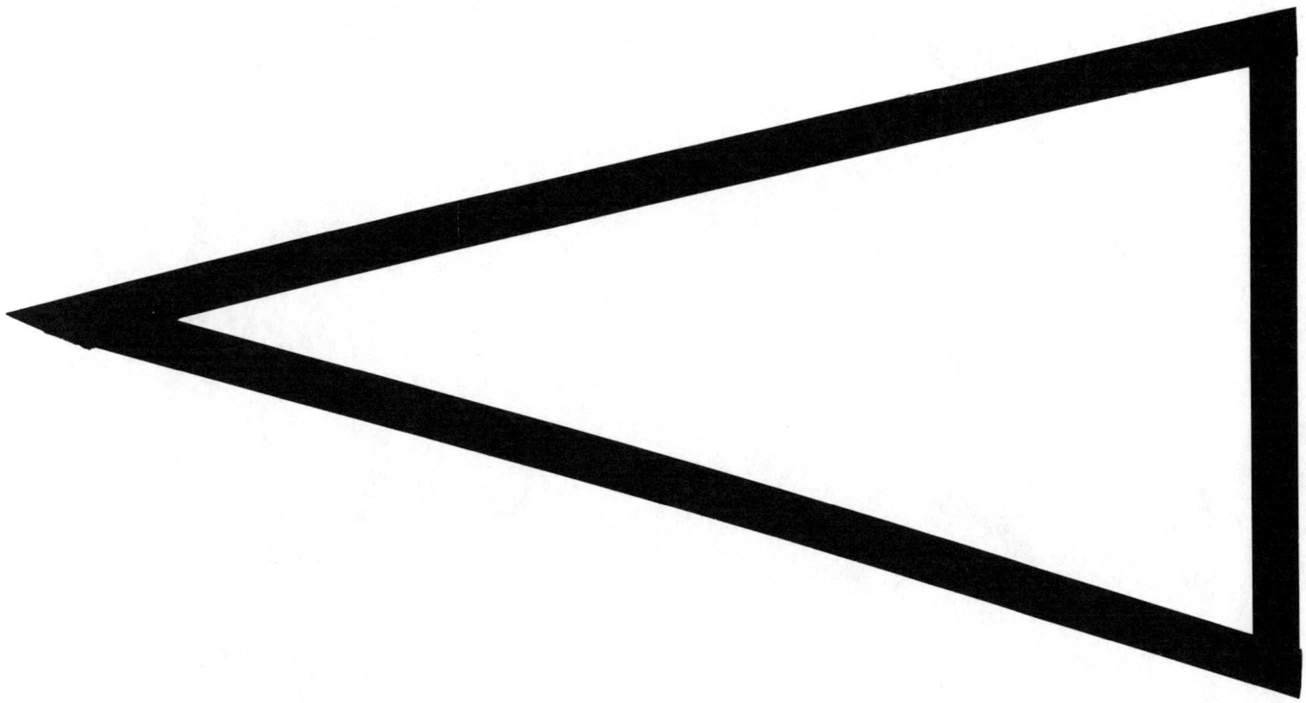

Skill 3
Step 4—Level #2 Worksheet (clown's hat)

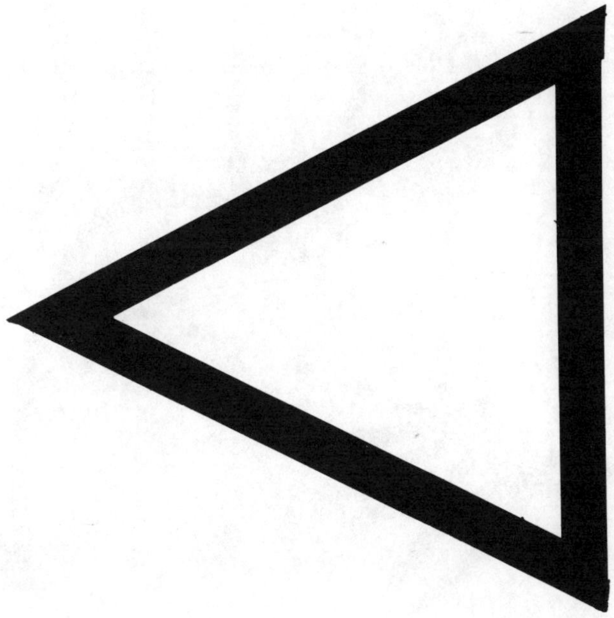

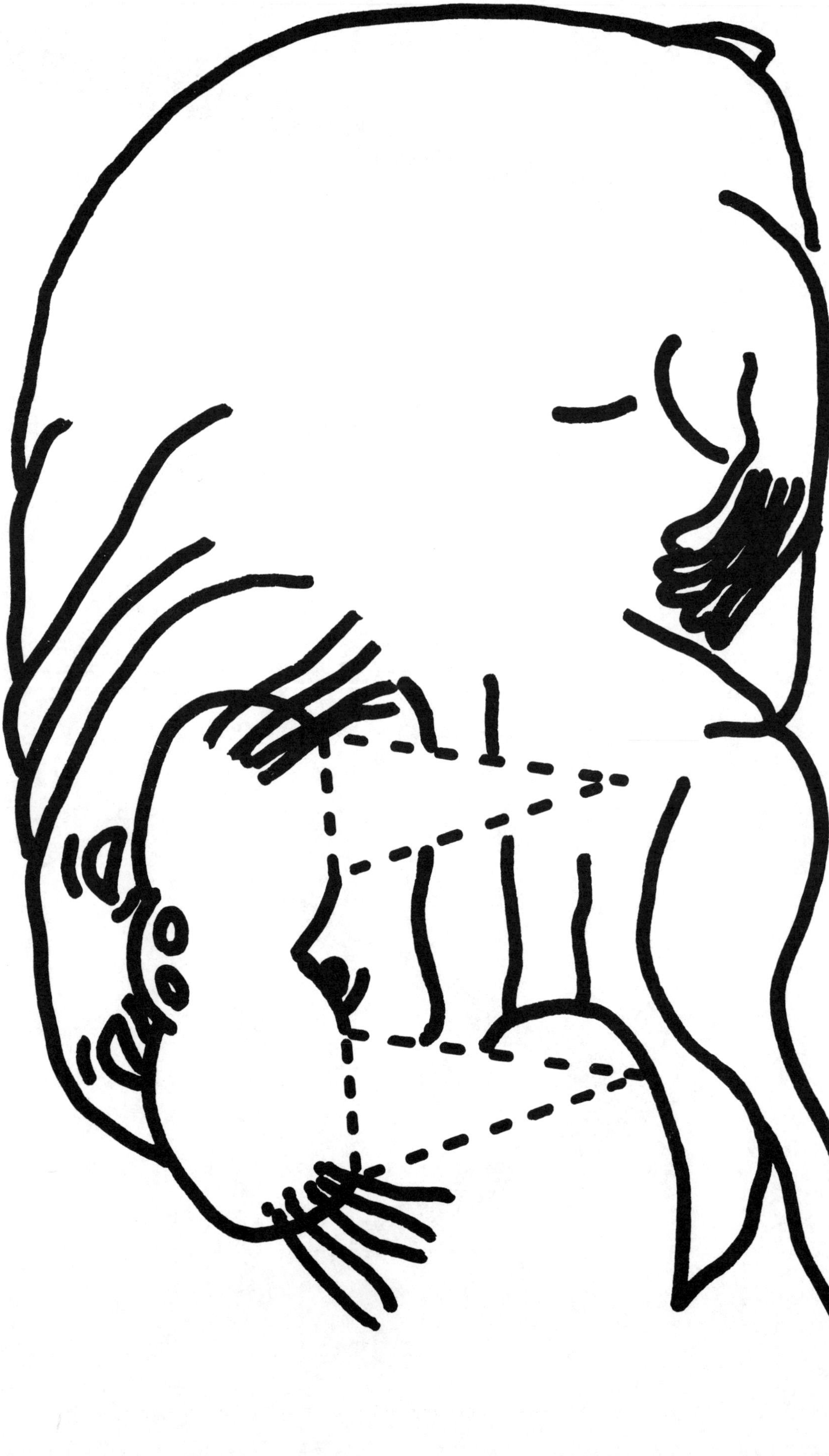

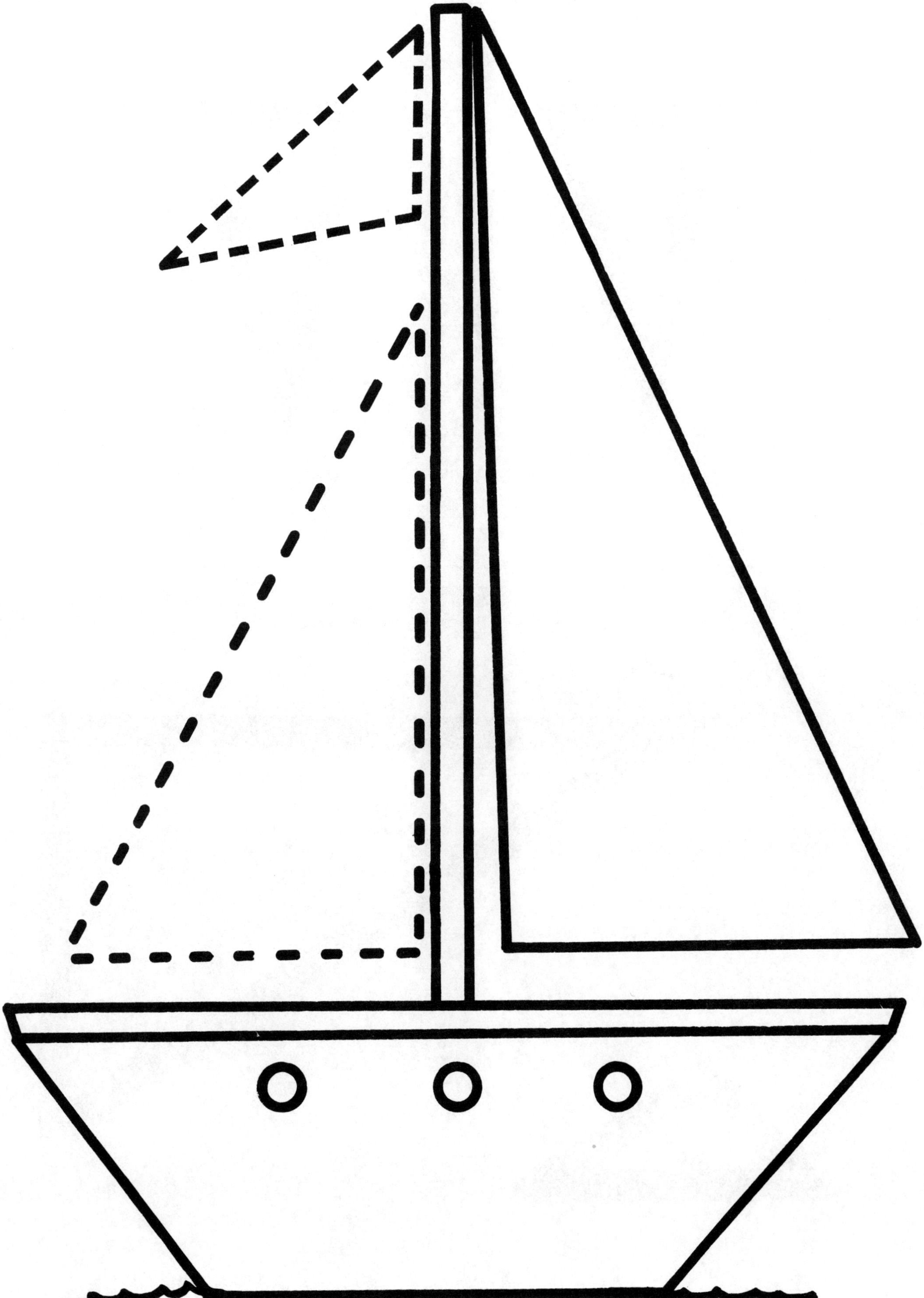

Skill 3
Step 4—Level #3 Pre/Posttest (walrus)

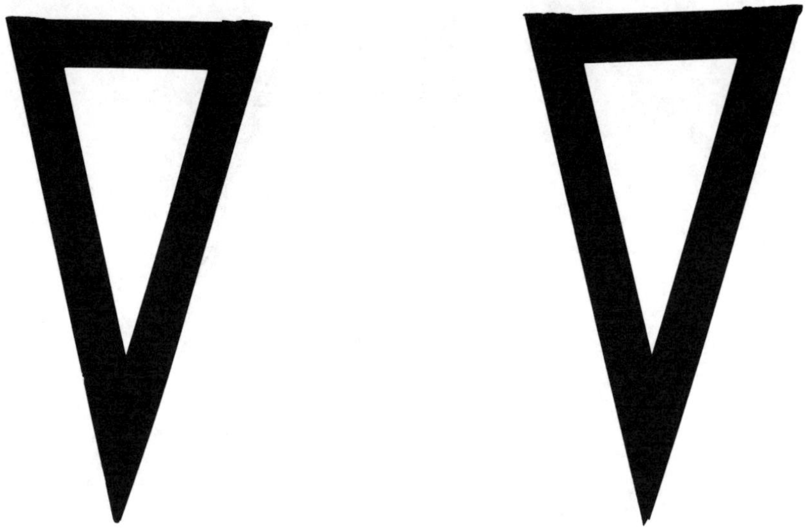

Skill 3
Step 4—Level #3 Worksheet (sailboat)

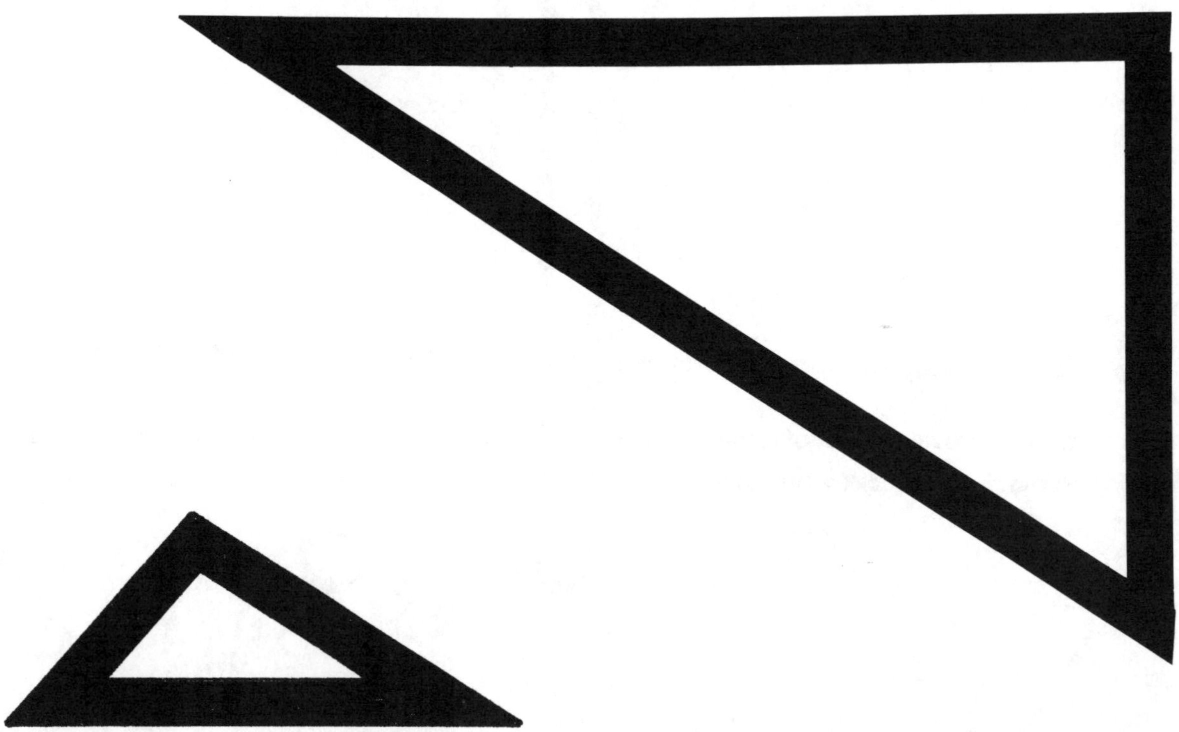

SKILL 3—STEP 5—DIAMONDS

Level #1—Diamonds, 1/4" wide line
Pretest: Student takes Level #1 Pretest (door—diamond with 2¾" base).

If criterion met: Student advances to Level #2.

If criterion not met:

1. Student cuts Level #1 worksheets:
   kite—4" base
   wishing well—3¼" base
   cookie in sundae—3" base
   shape man—3" base
2. Student takes Level #1 Posttest (door).
   If criterion met: Student advances to Level #2.
   If criterion not met: Student repeats Level #1 worksheets and Posttest.

Level #2—Diamonds, 1/4" wide line
Pretest: Student takes Level #2 Pretest (candle—diamond with 1¾" base).

If criterion met: Student advances to Level #3.

If criterion not met:

1. Student cuts Level #2 worksheets:
   bird—2½" base
   donkey—2" base
2. Student takes Level #2 Posttest (candle).
   If criterion met: Student advances to Level #3.
   If criterion not met: Student repeats Level #3 worksheets and Posttest.

Level #3—Combined Diamonds, 1/4" wide line
Pretest: Student takes Level #3 Pretest (overalls—two diamonds, 2¼" base and 1" base).

If criterion met: Student advances to Skill 4.

If criterion not met:

1. Student cuts Level #3 worksheet (flower—two diamonds, 2" base).
2. Student takes Level #3 Posttest (overalls).
   If criterion met: Student advances to Skill 4.
   If criterion not met: Student repeats Level #3 worksheet and Posttest.

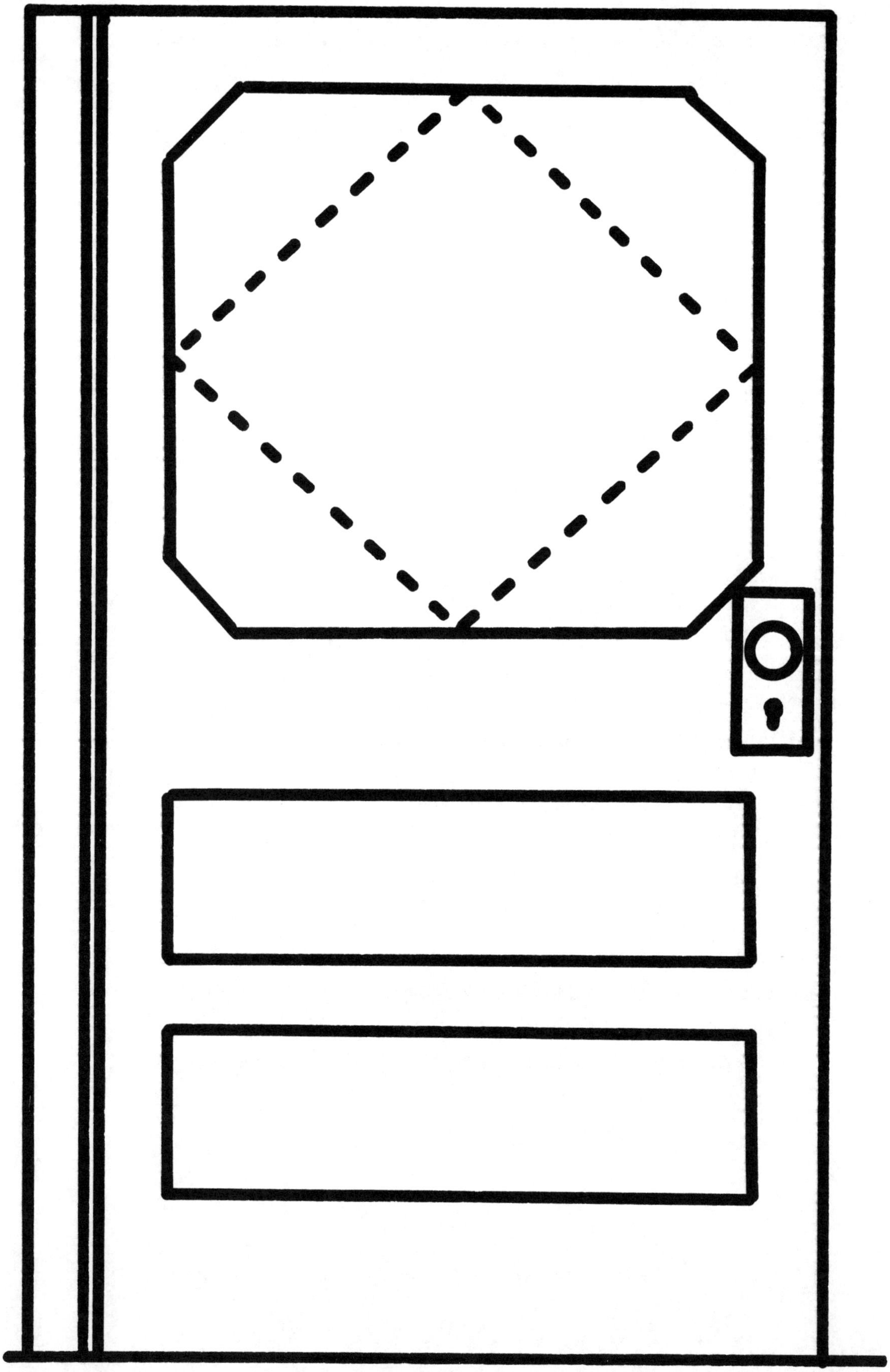

Step 5—Level #1 Worksheet

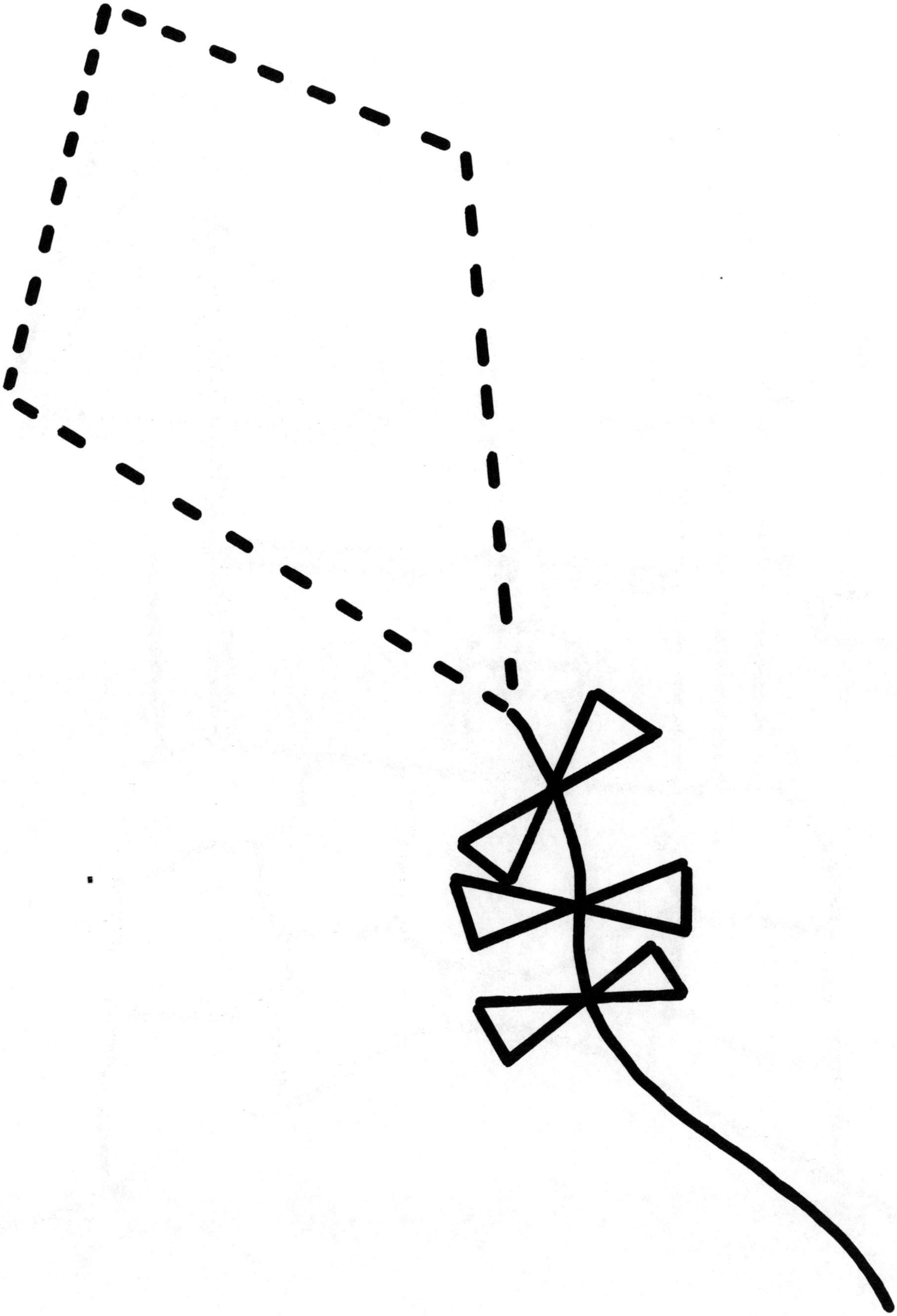

Step 5—Level #1 Worksheet

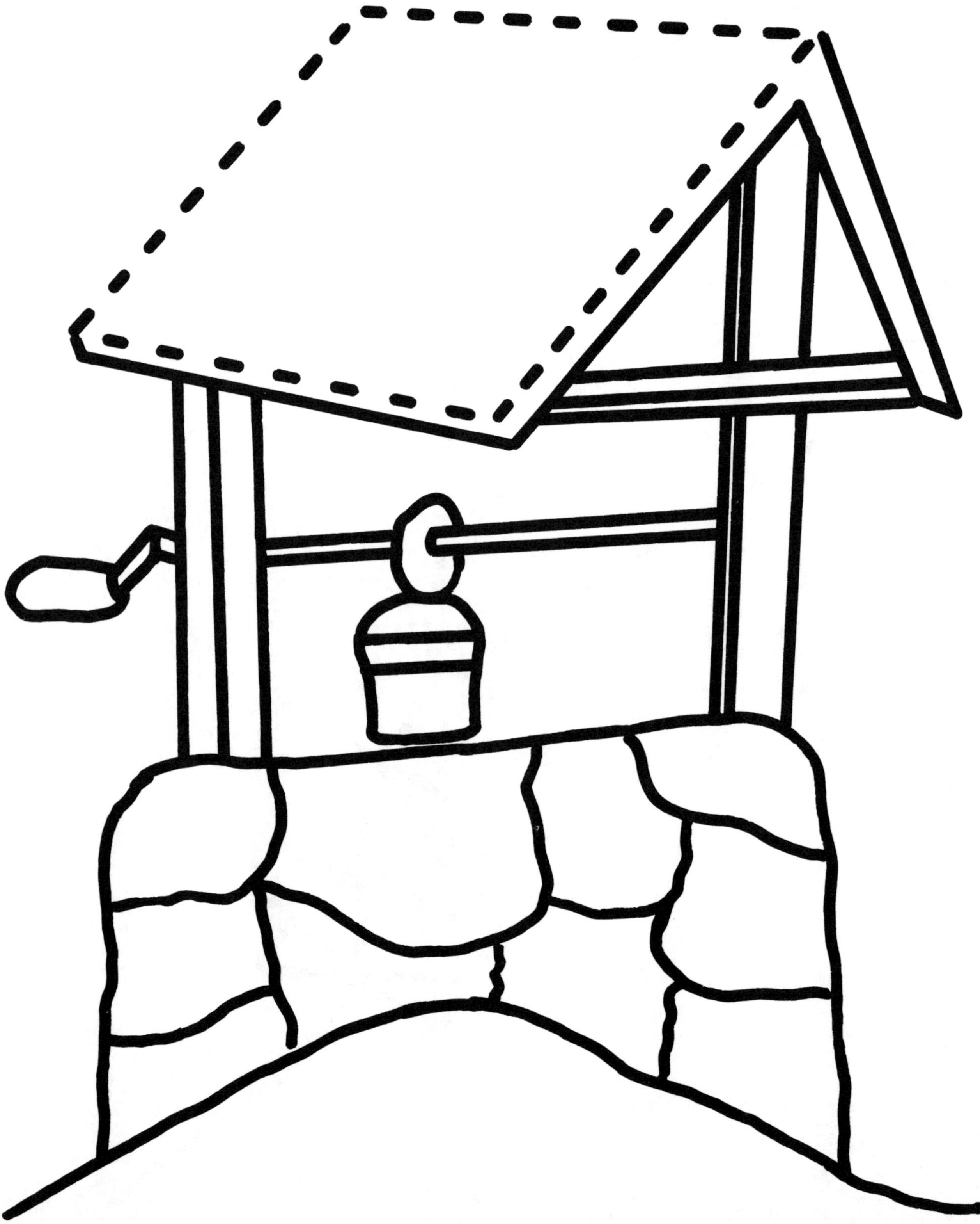

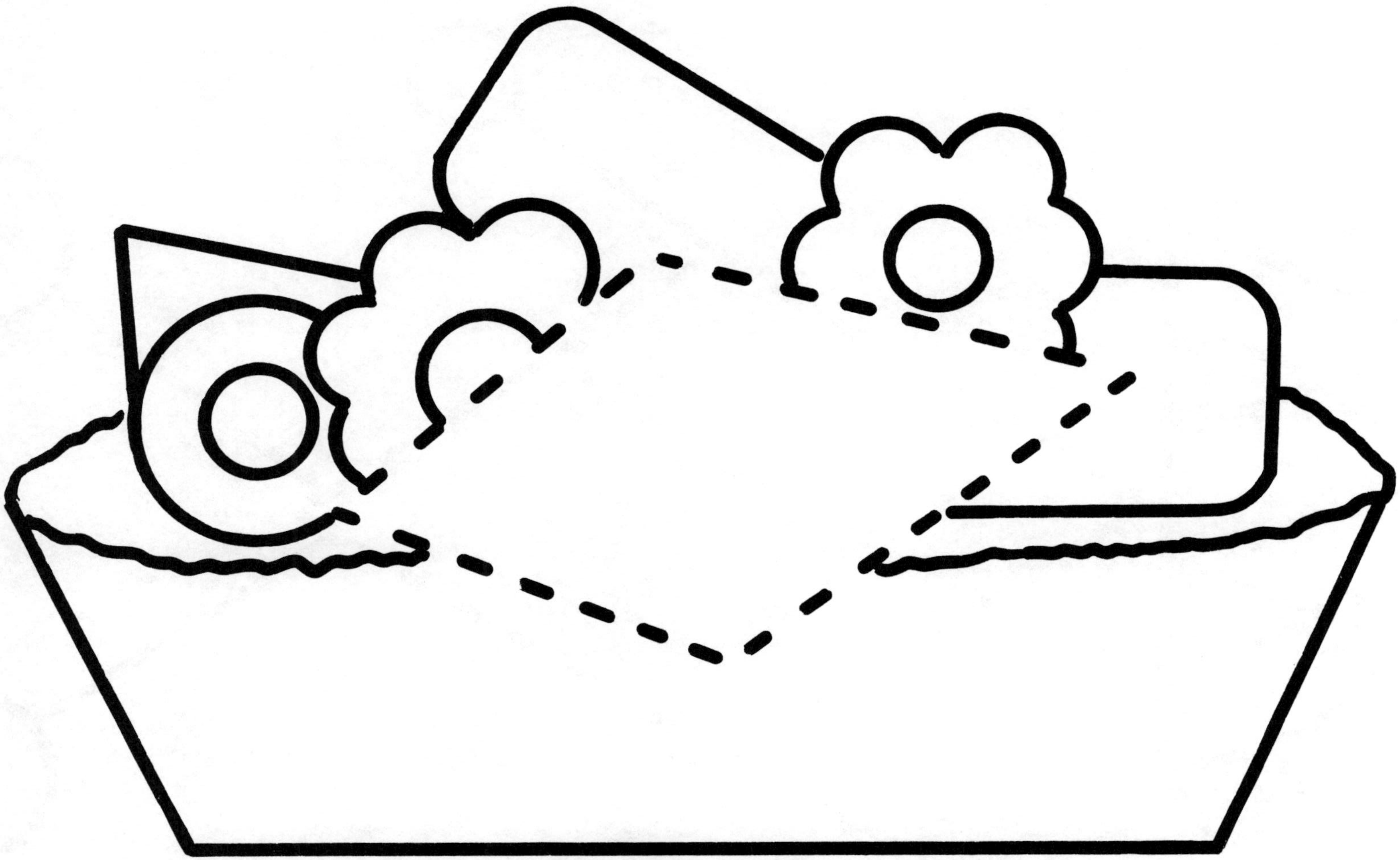

Step 5—Level #1 Worksheet

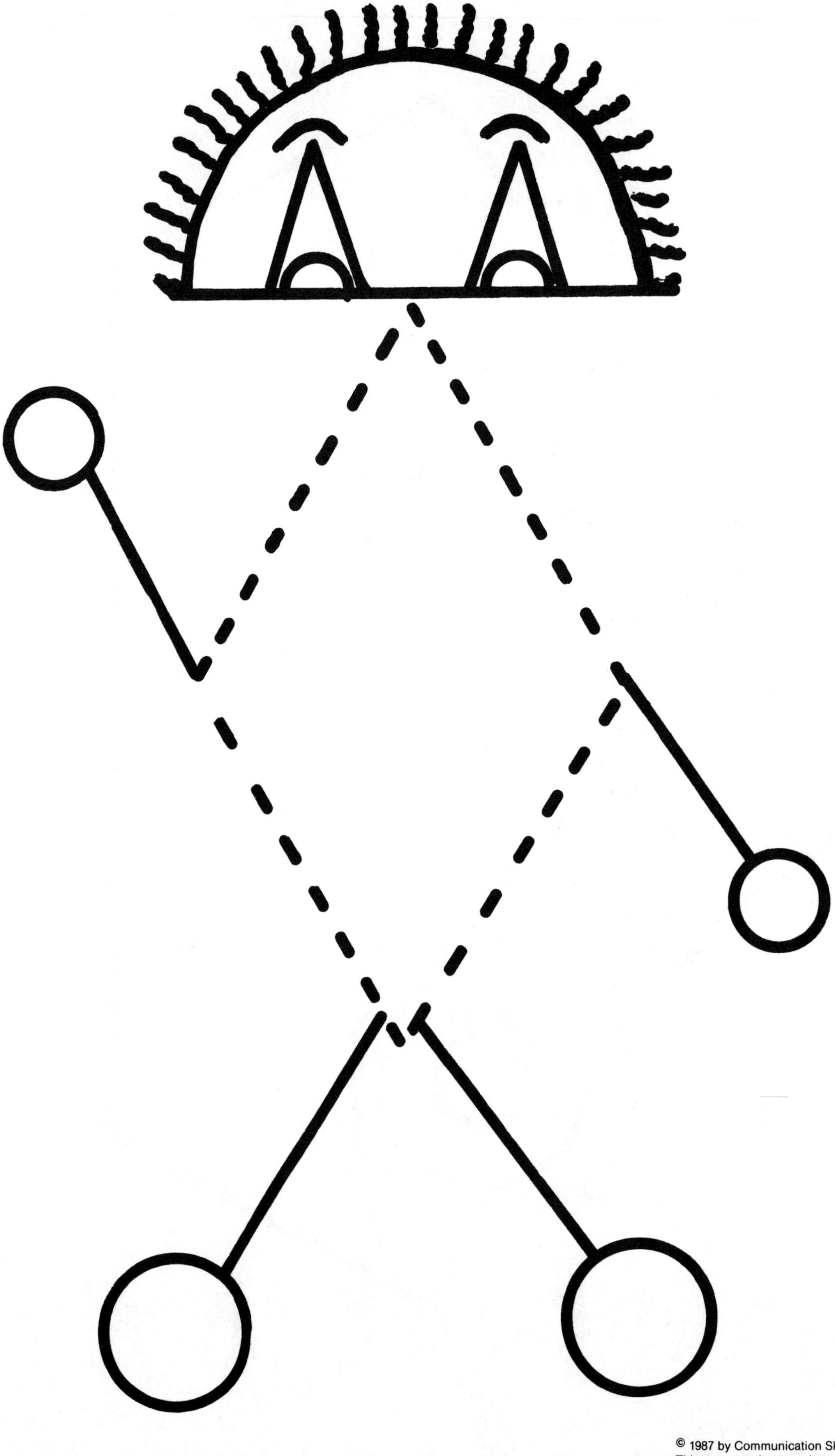

Skill 3
Step 5—Level #1 Pre/Posttest (door)

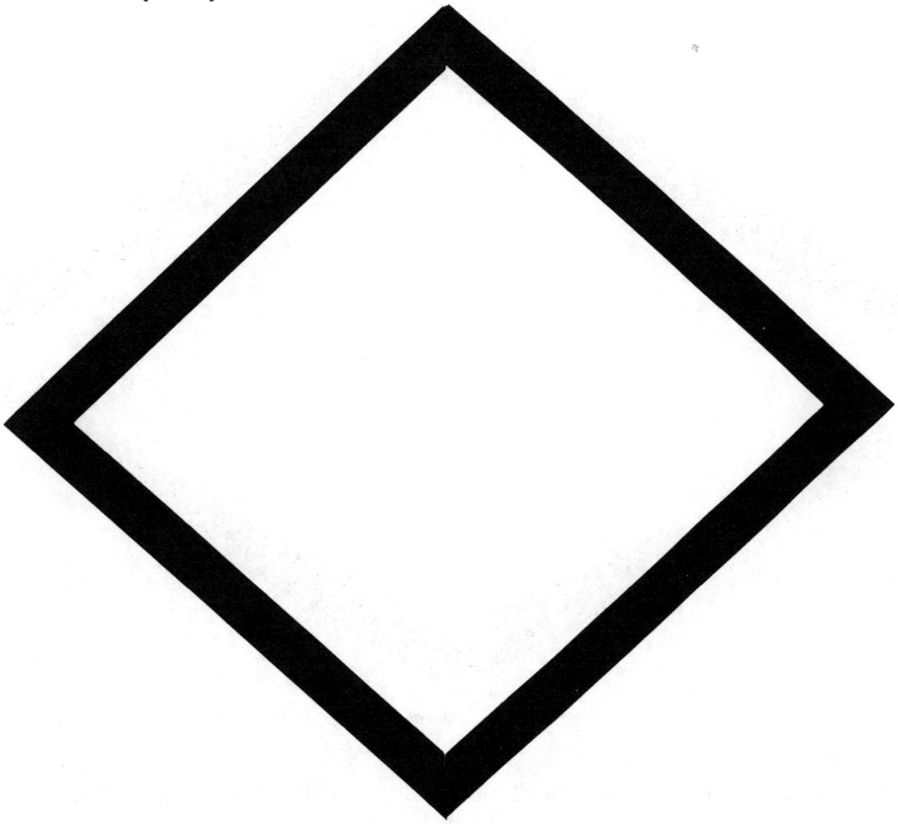

Skill 3
Step 5—Level #1 Worksheet (kite)

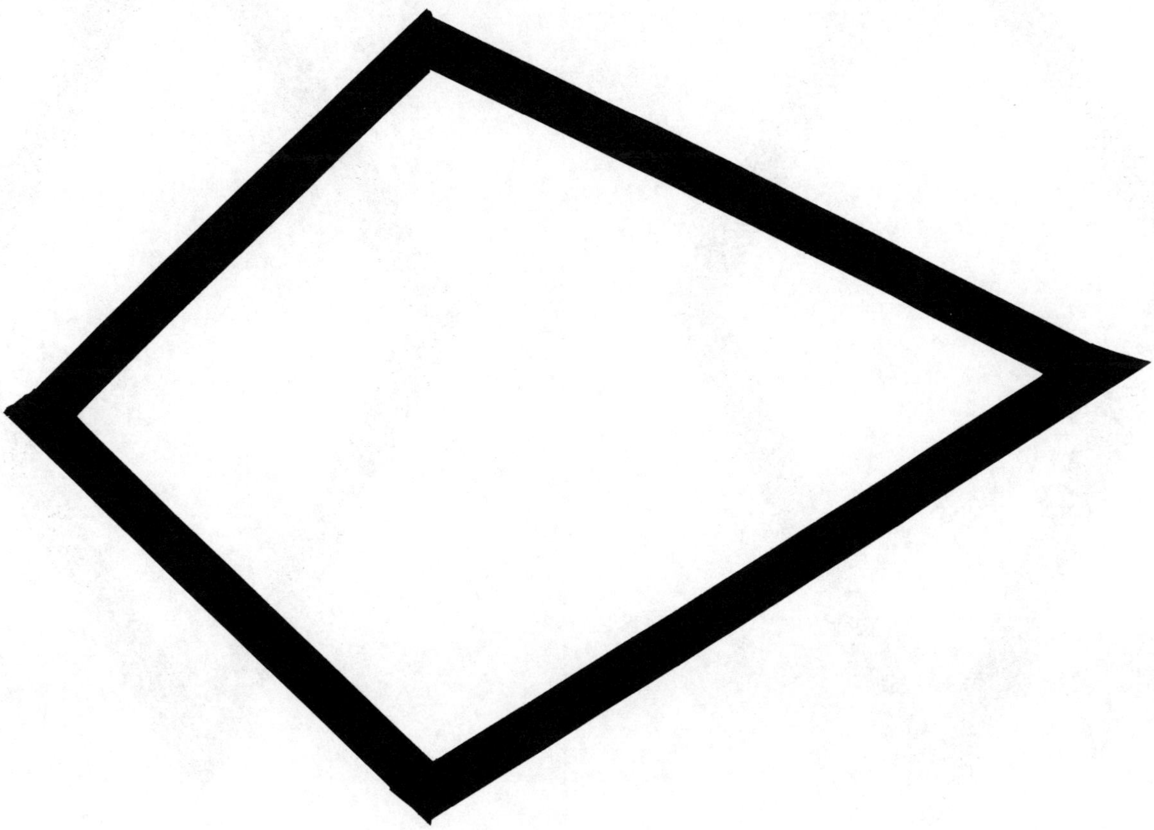

Skill 3
Step 5—Level #1 Worksheet (wishing well)

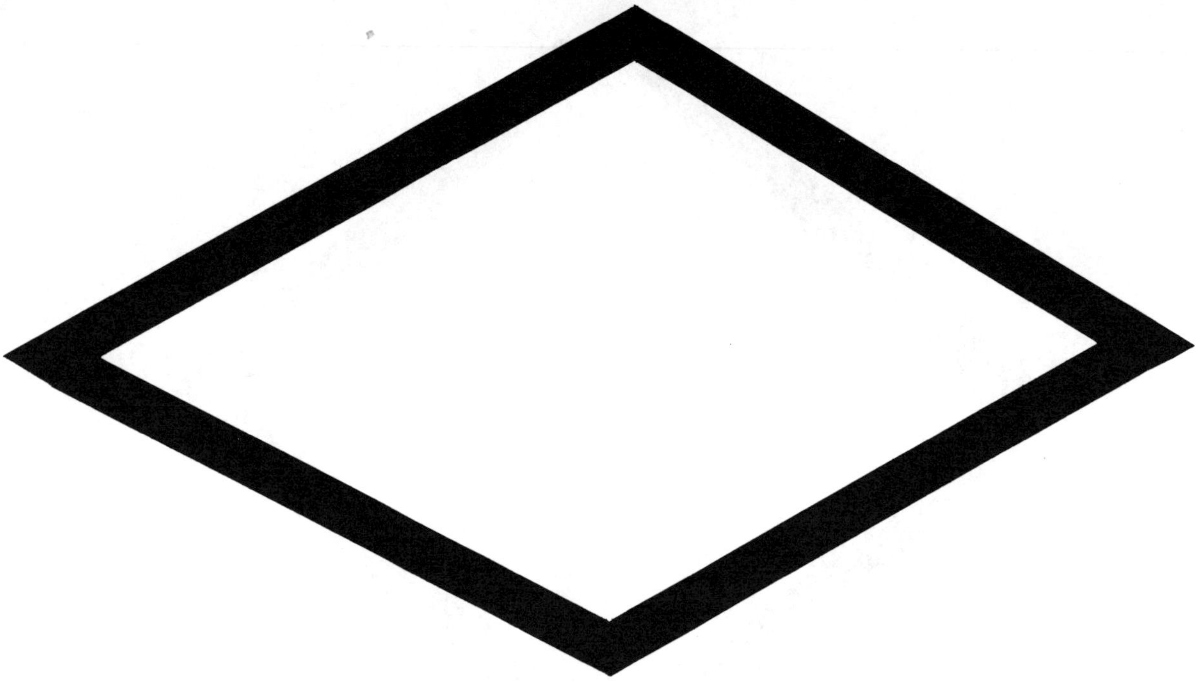

Skill 3
Step 5—Level #1 Worksheet (cookie in sundae)

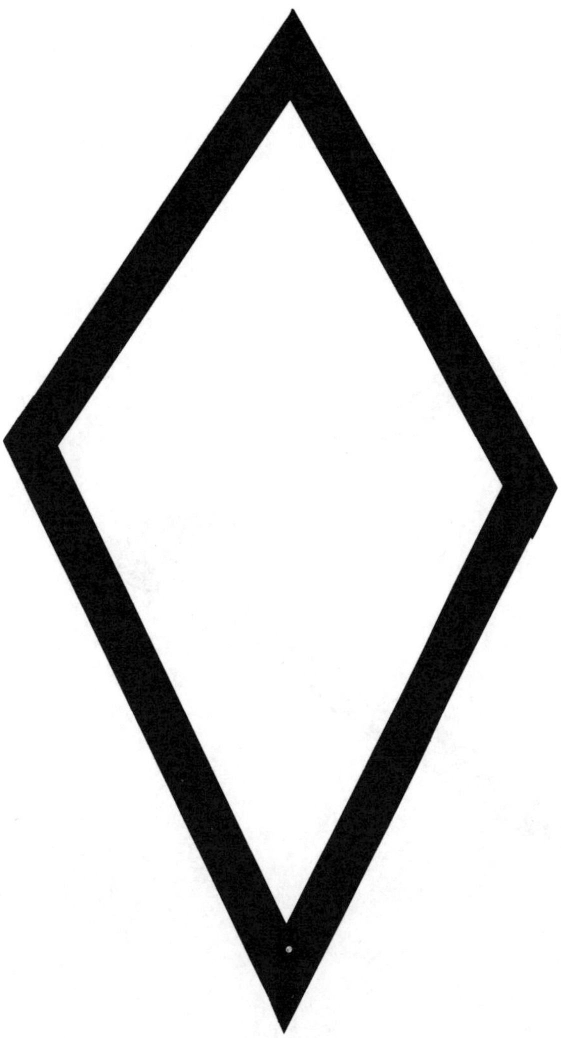

Skill 3
Step 5—Level #1 Worksheet (shape man)

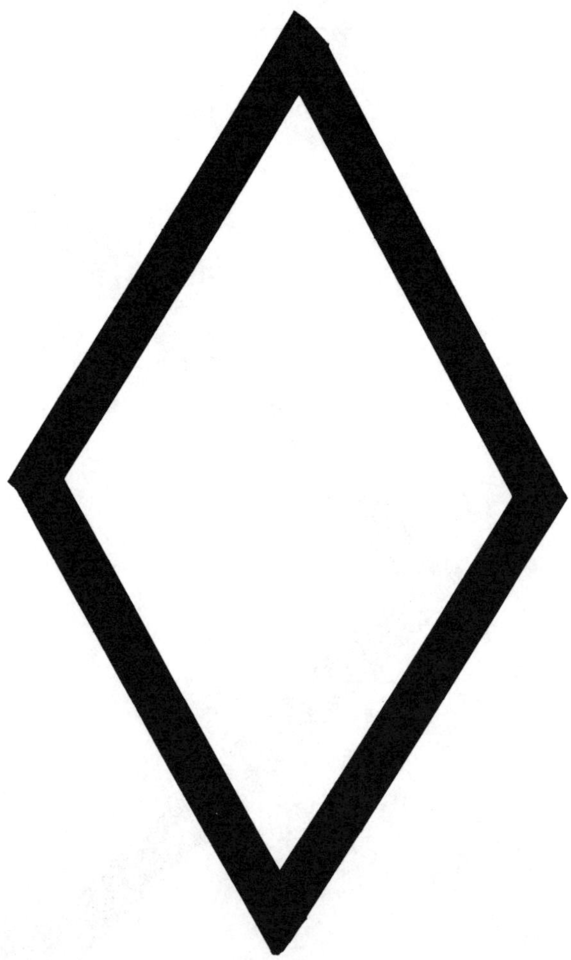

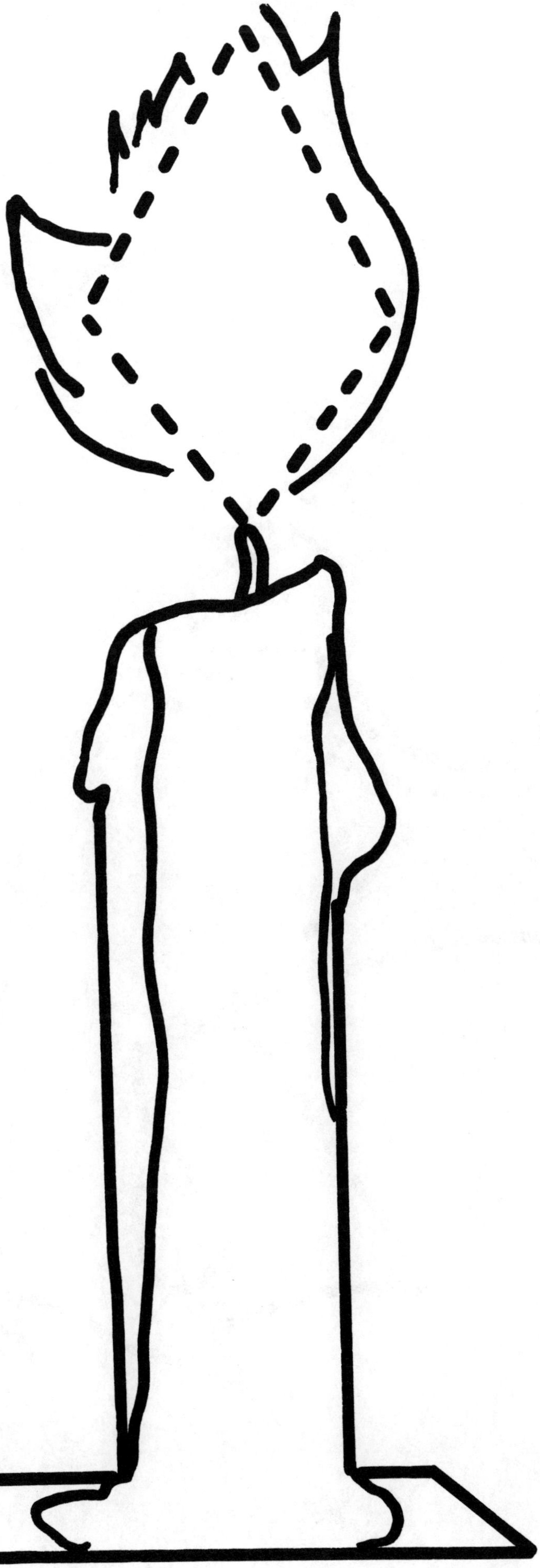

Step 5—Level #2 Worksheet

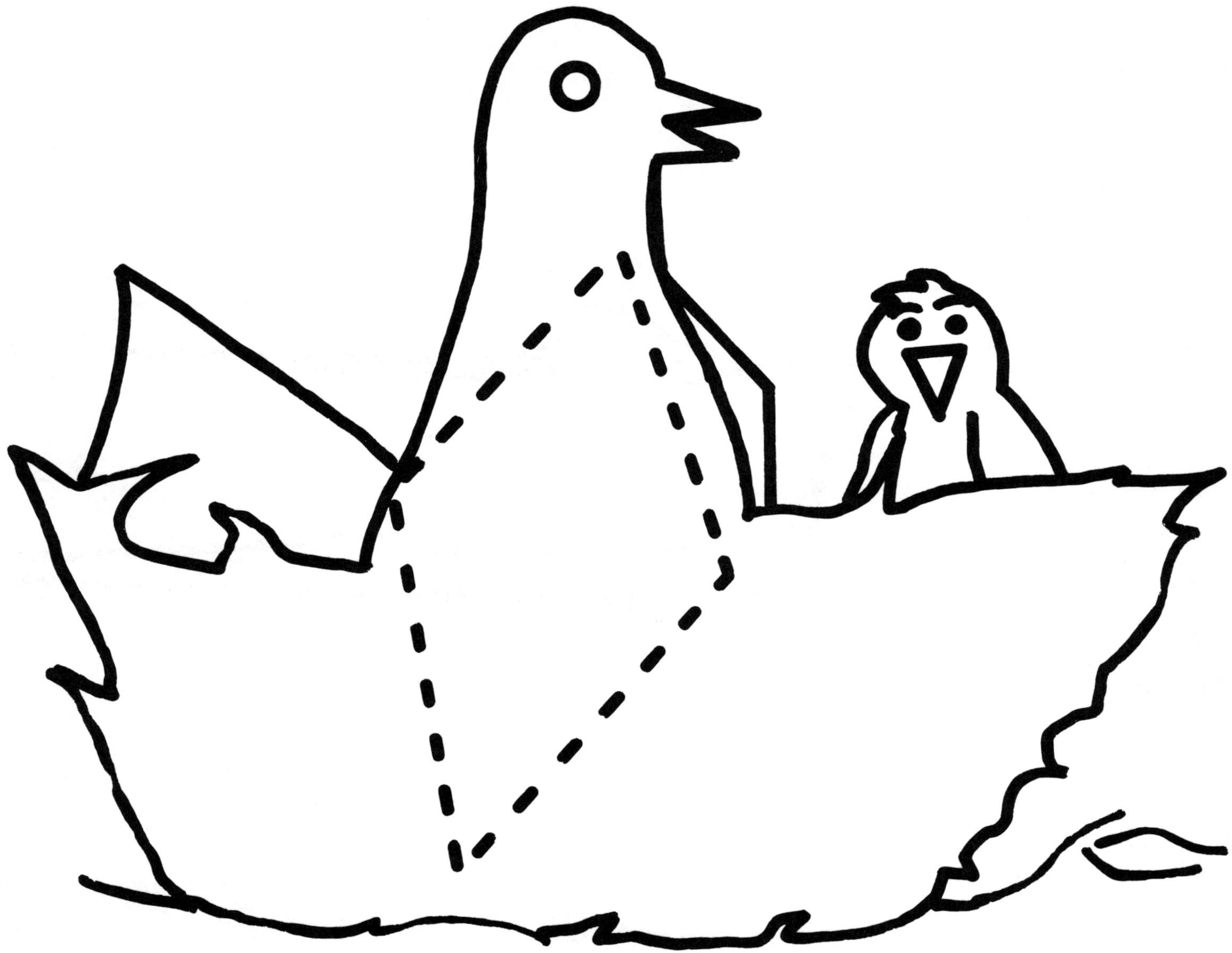

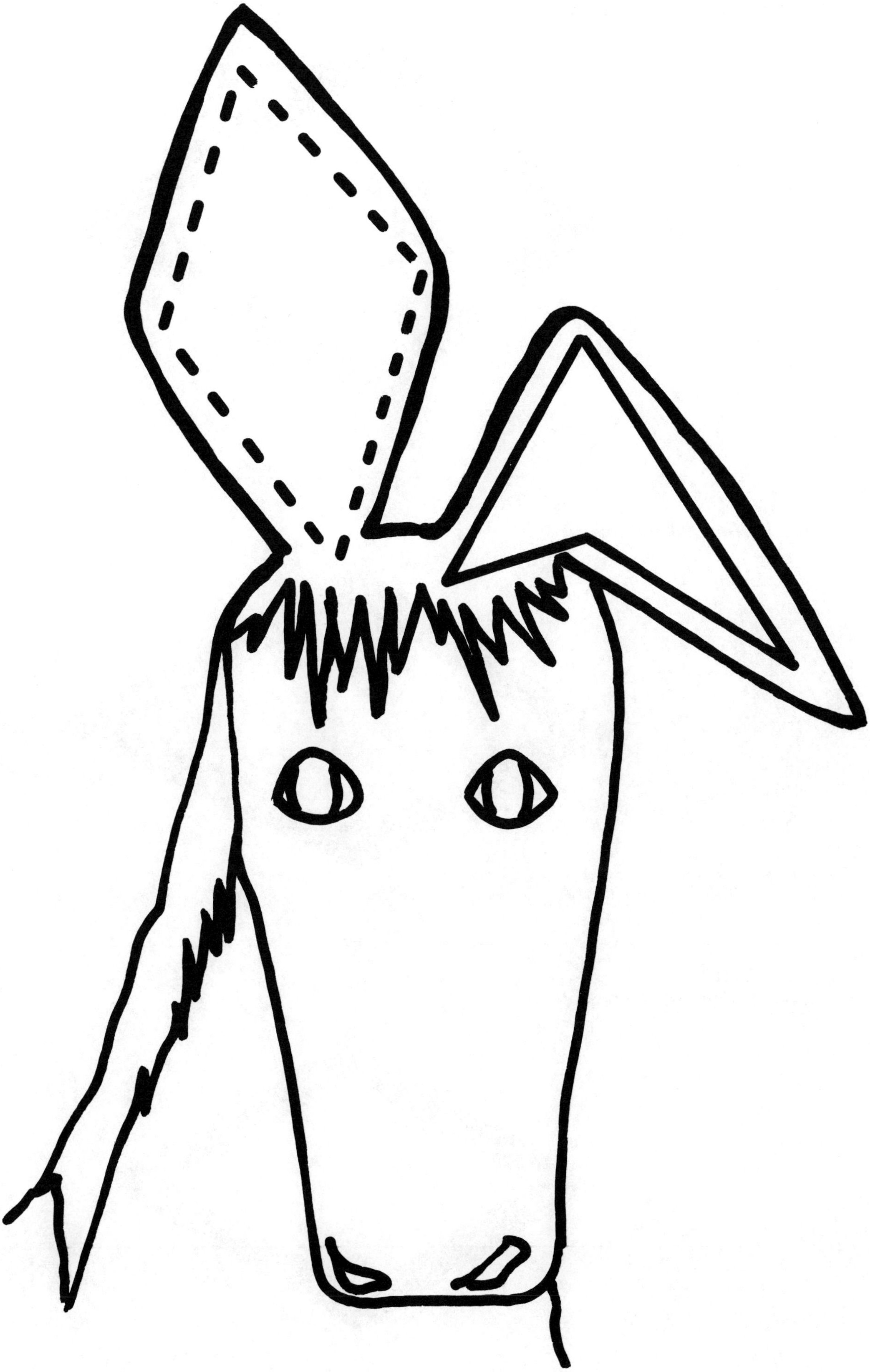

Skill 3
Step 5—Level #2 Pre/Posttest (candle)

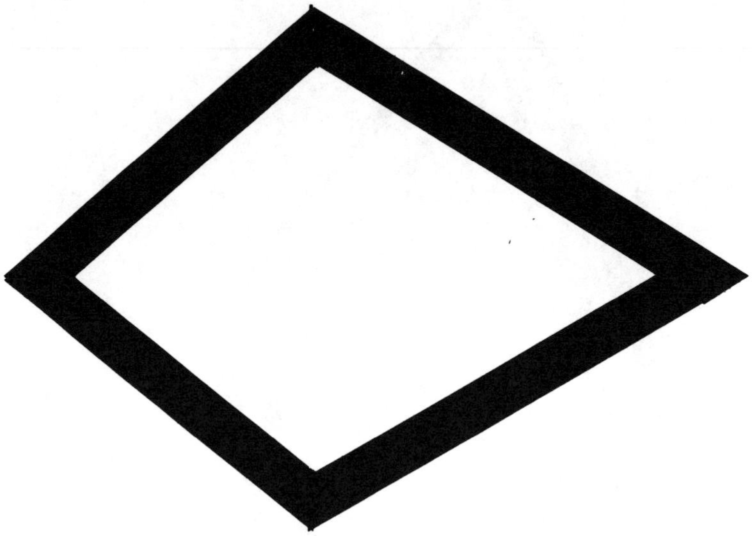

Skill 3
Step 5—Level #2 Worksheet (bird)

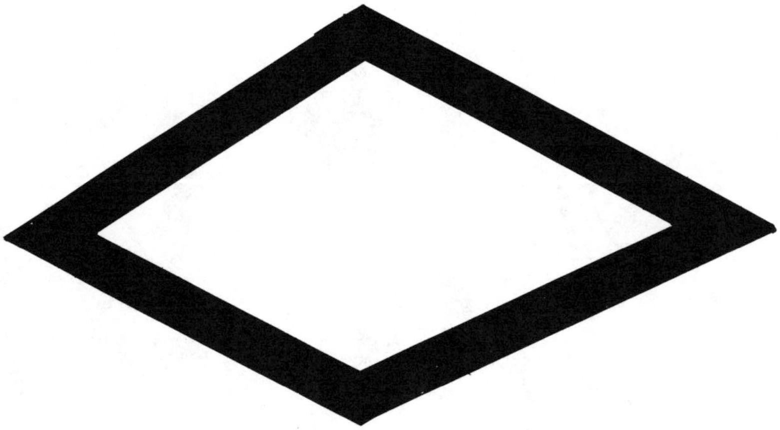

Skill 3
Step 5—Level #2 Worksheet (donkey)

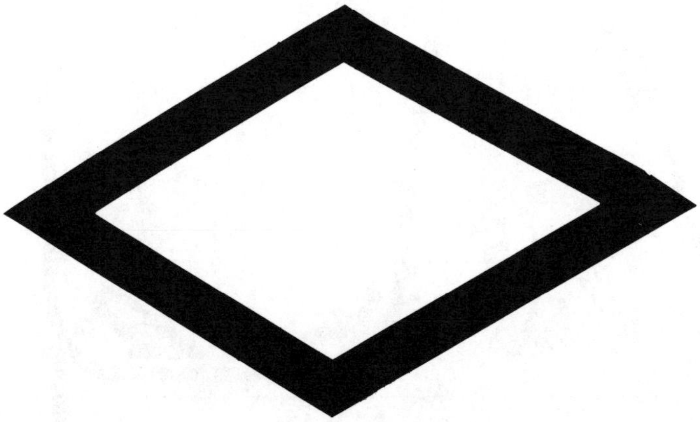

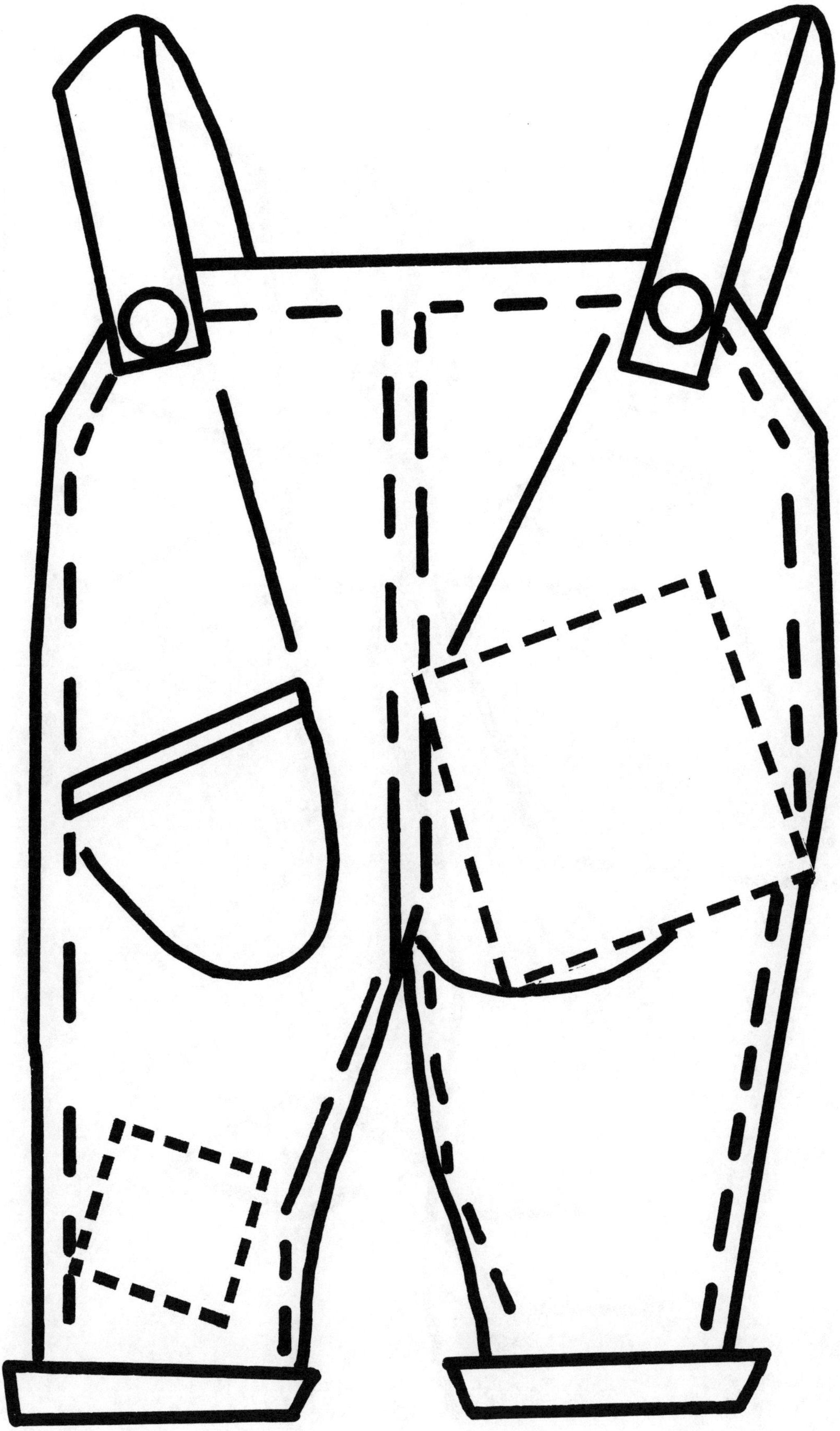

Step 5—Level #3 Worksheet

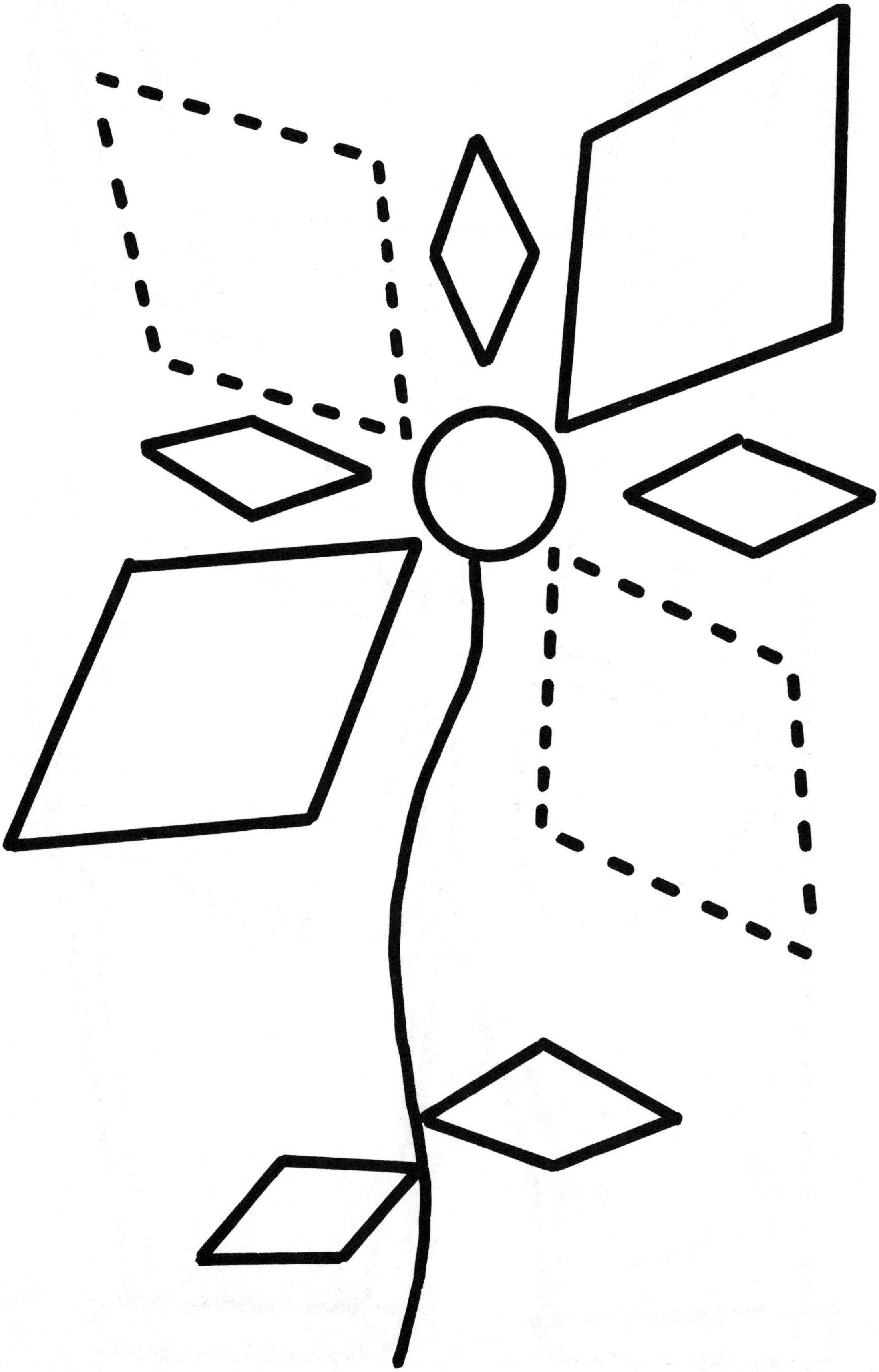

Skill 3
Step 5—Level #3 Pre/Posttest (overalls)

Skill 3
Step 5—Level #3 Worksheet (flower)

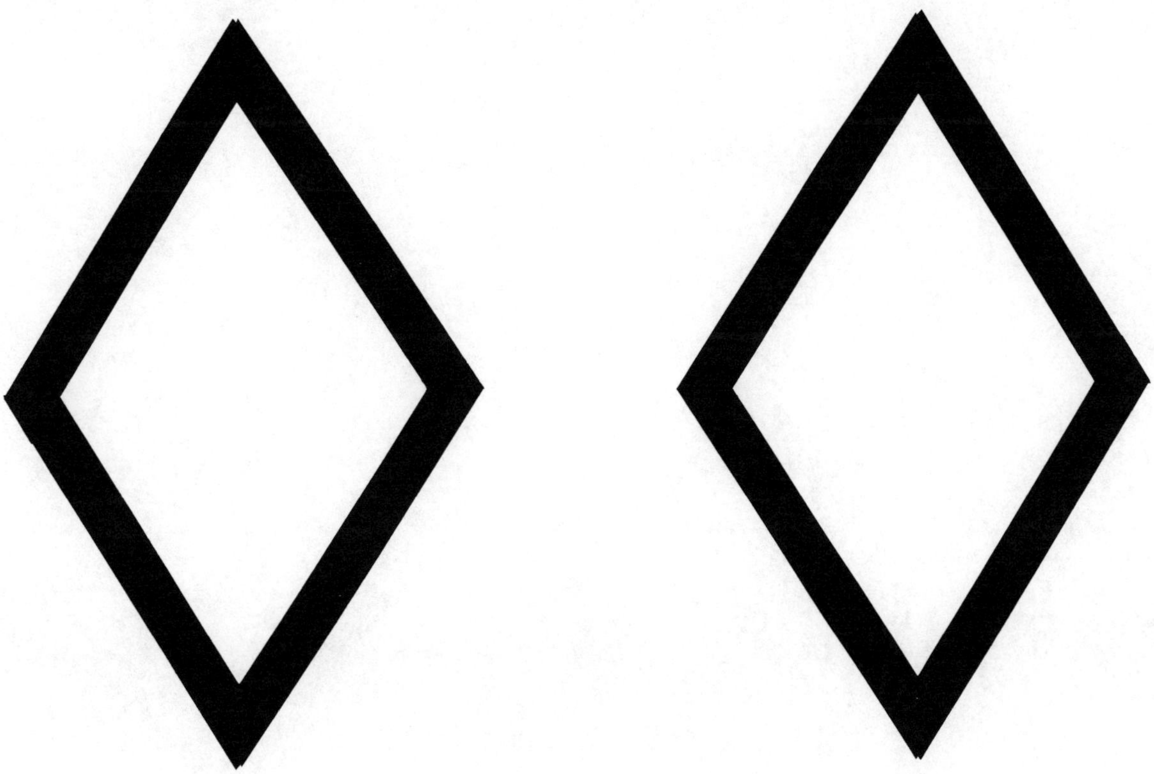

Skill 4—Cutting a Simple Shape—⅛″ Line

Objective: Student cuts out a simple shape with a line ⅛″ wide, and pastes it on a fixed outline, with 80% accuracy.

Procedure

All Skill 3 Steps and Levels are repeated, but the line is reduced to ⅛″ wide.

To prepare Pre/Posttests and worksheets for Skill 4:

1. Reproduce the worksheets (pictures only) from Skill 3 at each Step and Level:

   Step 1: pages 18-21, 24-28, 31-34, 37-38

   Step 2: pages 41-45, 48-51, 53-54

   Step 3: pages 57-60, 63-66, 68-69

   Step 4: pages 72-75, 78-81, 84-85

   Step 5: pages 88-92, 95-97, 99-100

2. DO NOT reproduce the cutouts (with ¼″ wide lines) from Skill 3.

3. Reproduce the cutouts that follow (pages 103-126). These shapes have ⅛″ wide lines needed for Skill 4.

   Use these Skill 4 shapes with the worksheets (pictures) from Skill 3.

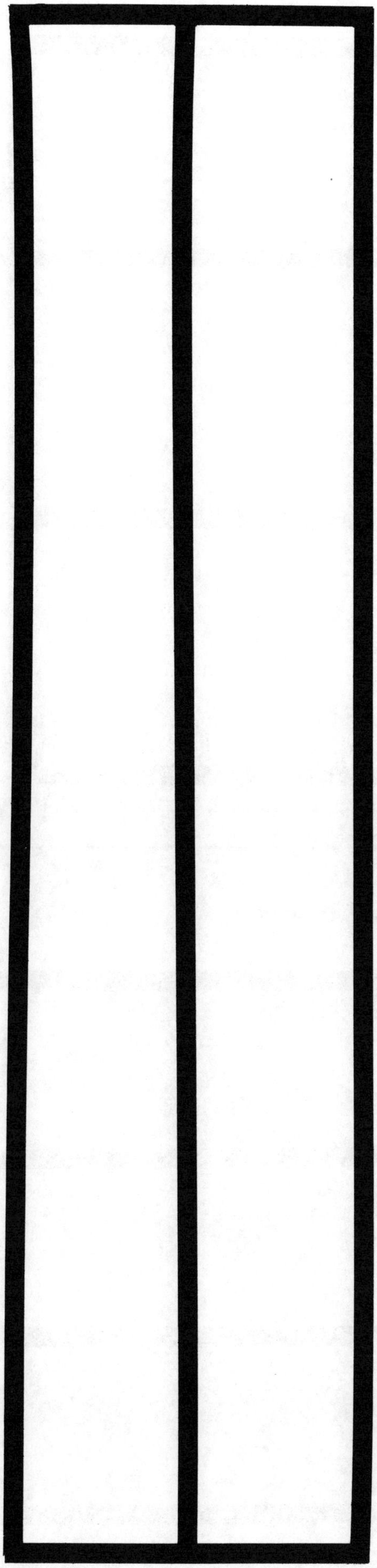

Skill 4
Step 1—Level #1 Pre/Posttest (picture frame)

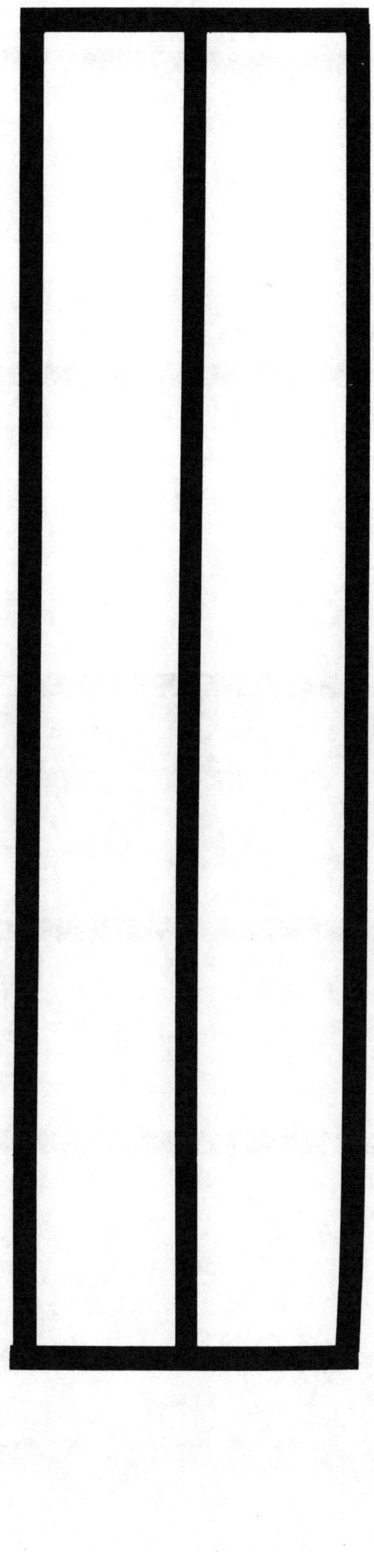

Skill 4
Step 1—Level #1 Worksheet (window)

Skill 4
Step 1—Level #1 Worksheet (crayons)

Skill 4
Step 1—Level #1 Worksheet (knife, fork, spoon)

Skill 4
Step 1—Level #2 Pre/Posttest (bird in cage)

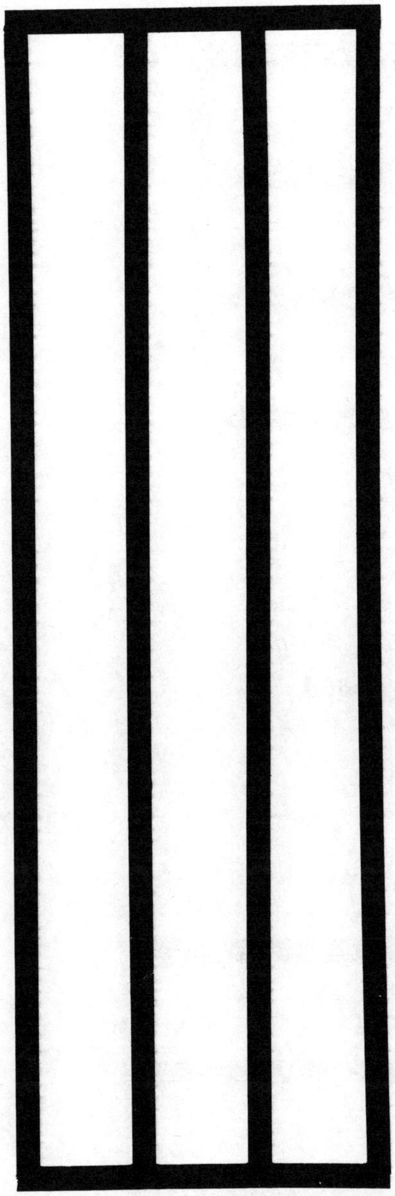

Skill 4
Step 1—Level #2 Worksheet (broom)

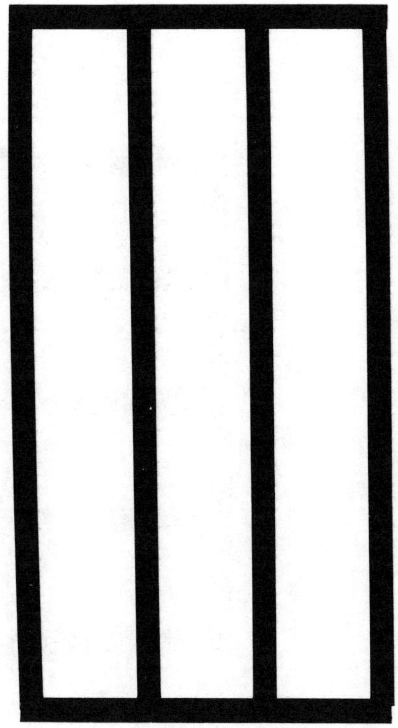

Skill 4
Step 1—Level #2 Worksheet (helicopter)

Skill 4
Step 1—Level #2 Worksheet (sunburst)

Skill 4
Step 1—Level #2 Worksheet (tiger in cage)

Skill 4
Step 1—Level #3 Pre/Posttest (guitar)

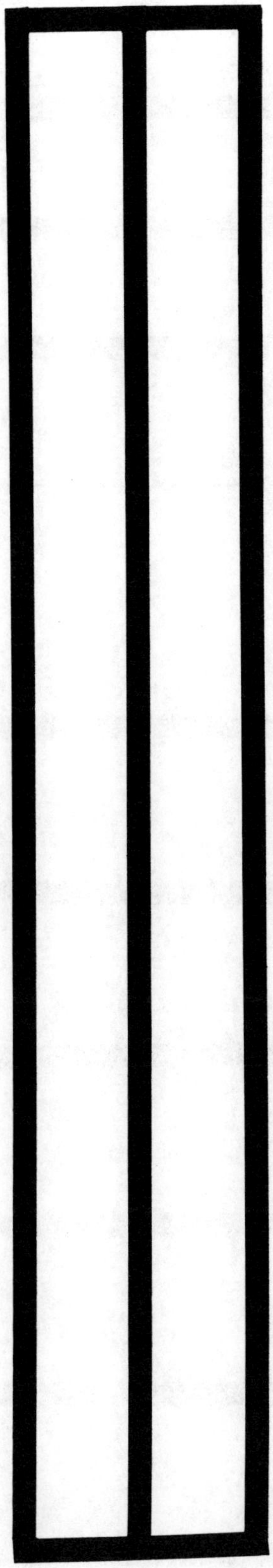

Skill 4
Step 1—Level #3 Worksheet (house)

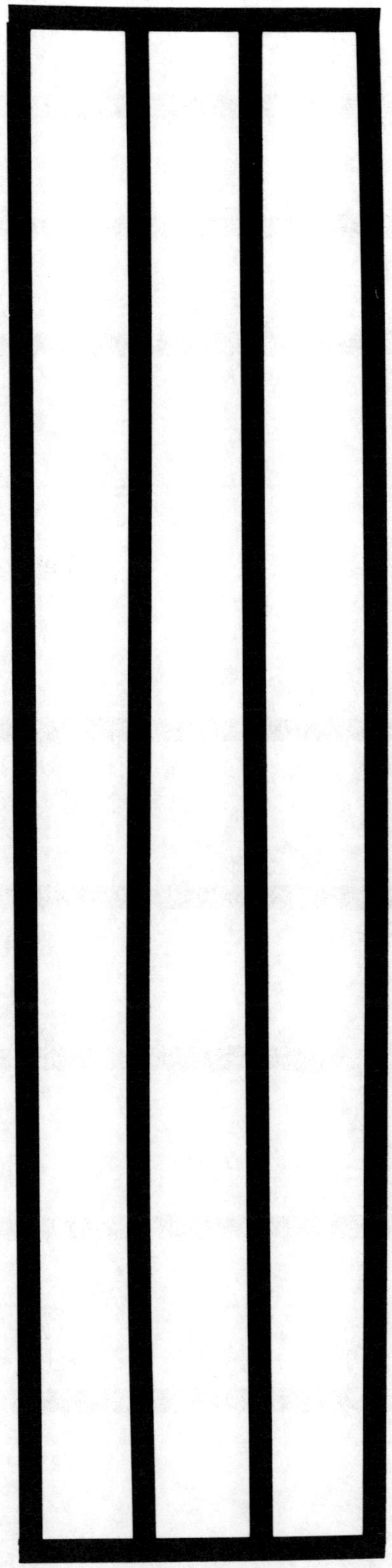

Skill 4
Step 1—Level #3 Worksheet (swing)

Skill 4
Step 1—Level #3 Worksheet (fence)

Skill 4
Step 1—Level #4 Pre/Posttest (spider)

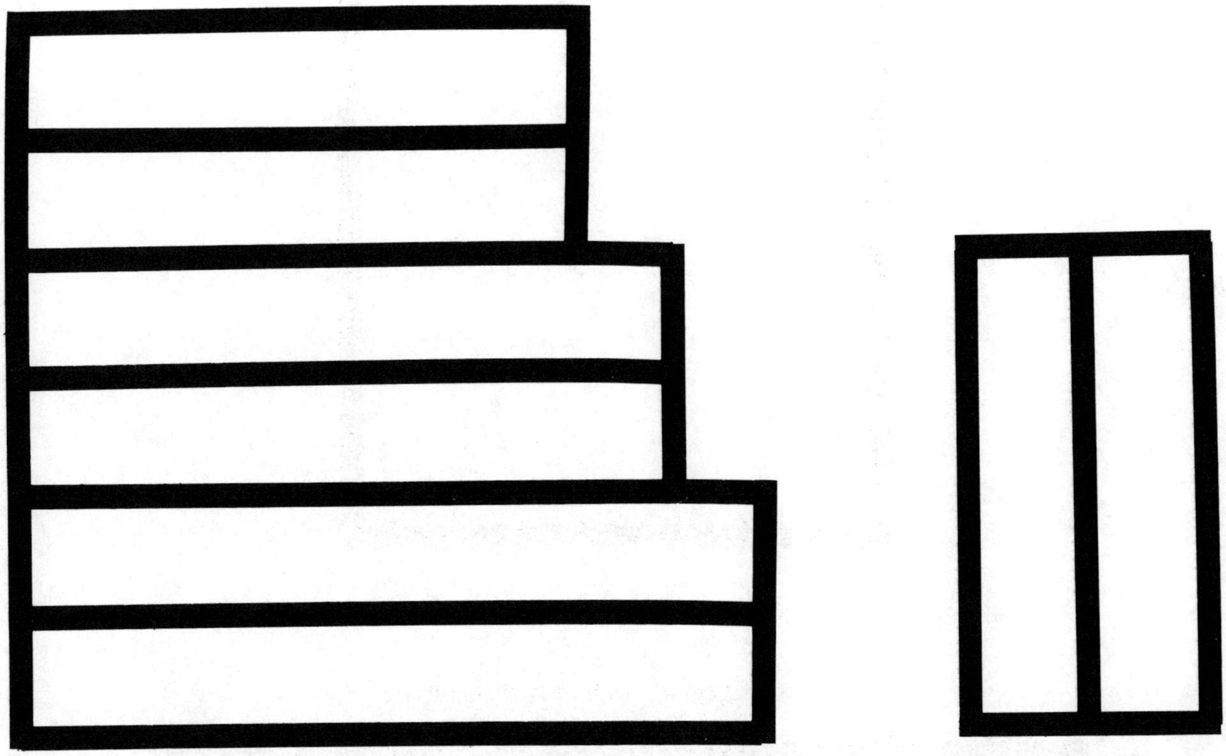

Skill 4
Step 1—Level #4 Worksheet (flowers)

Skill 4
Step 2—Level #1 Pre/Posttest (shape man)

Skill 4
Step 2—Level #1 Worksheet (house)

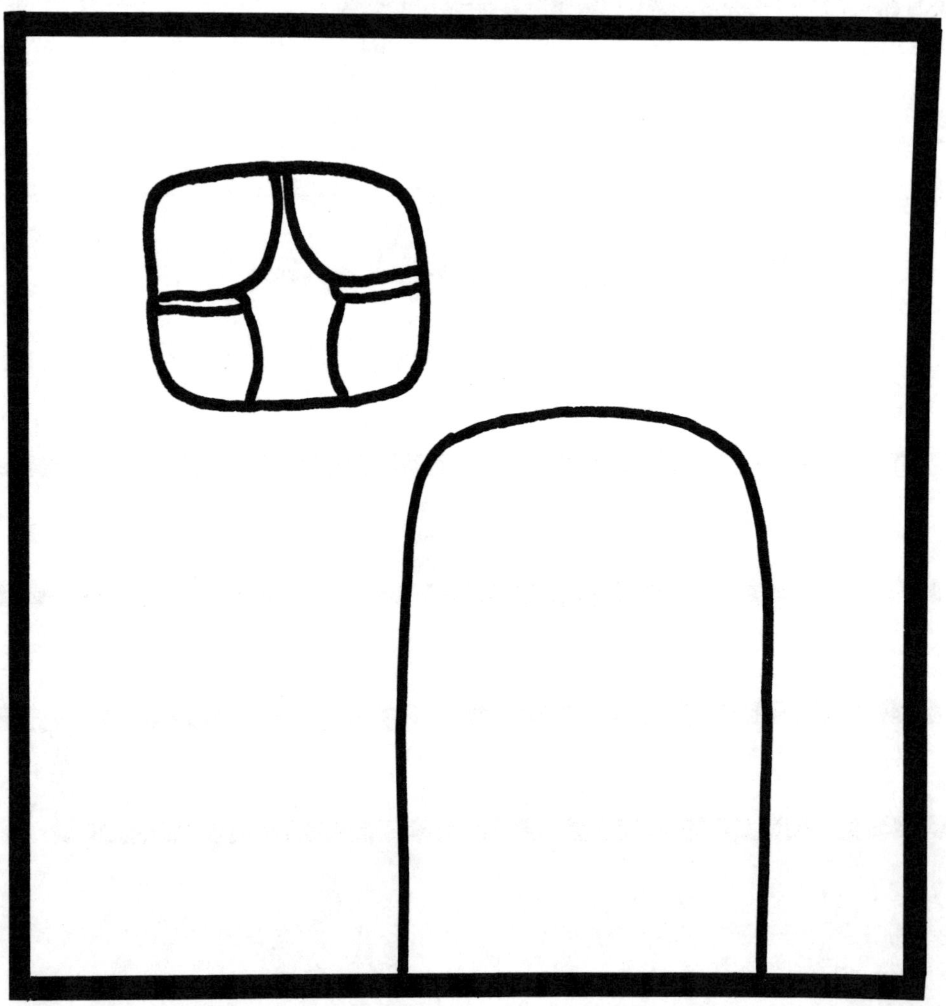

Skill 4
Step 2—Level #1 Worksheet (rabbit in hat)

Skill 4
Step 2—Level #1 Worksheet (robot)

Skill 4
Step 2—Level #1 Worksheet (TV screen)

Skill 4
Step 2—Level #2 Pre/Posttest (jack-in-the-box)

Skill 4
Step 2—Level #2 Worksheet (hot air balloon)

Skill 4
Step 2—Level #2 Worksheet (book)

The End!

Skill 4
Step 2—Level #2 Worksheet (clown's hat)

Skill 4
Step 2—Level #3 Pre/Posttest (school bus)

Skill 4
Step 2—Level #3 Worksheet (blocks)

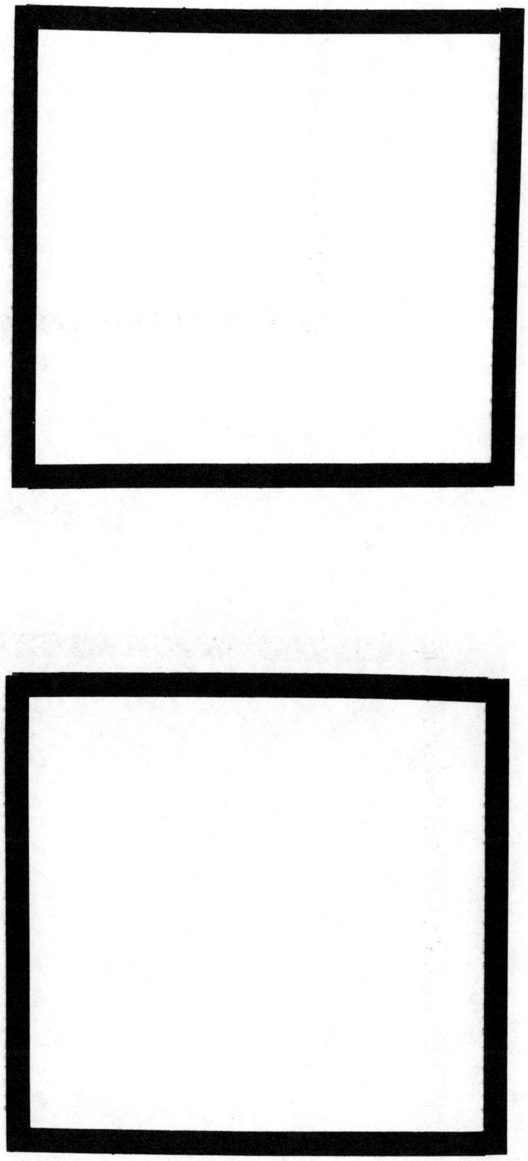

Skill 4
Step 3—Level #1 Pre/Posttest (train)

Skill 4
Step 3—Level #1 Worksheet (helicopter)

Skill 4
Step 3—Level #1 Worksheet (wagon)

Skill 4
Step 3—Level #1 Worksheet (truck)

Skill 4
Step 3—Level #2 Pre/Posttest (bear with gift)

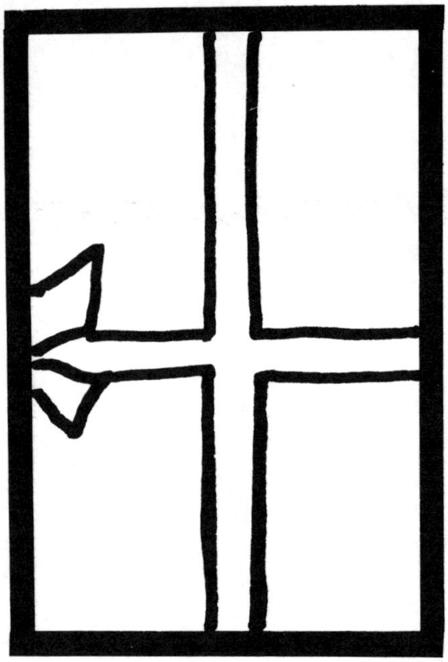

Skill 4
Step 3—Level #2 Worksheet (hobby horse)

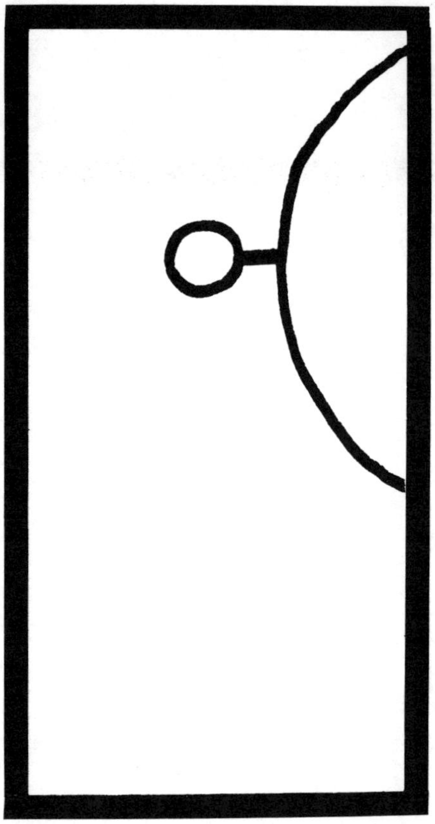

Skill 4
Step 3—Level #2 Worksheet (spaceship)

Skill 4
Step 3—Level #2 Worksheet (tree trunk)

Skill 4
Step 3—Level #3 Pre/Posttest (birthday cake)

Skill 4
Step 3—Level #3 Worksheet (giraffe)

Skill 4
Step 4—Level #1 Pre/Posttest (barn)

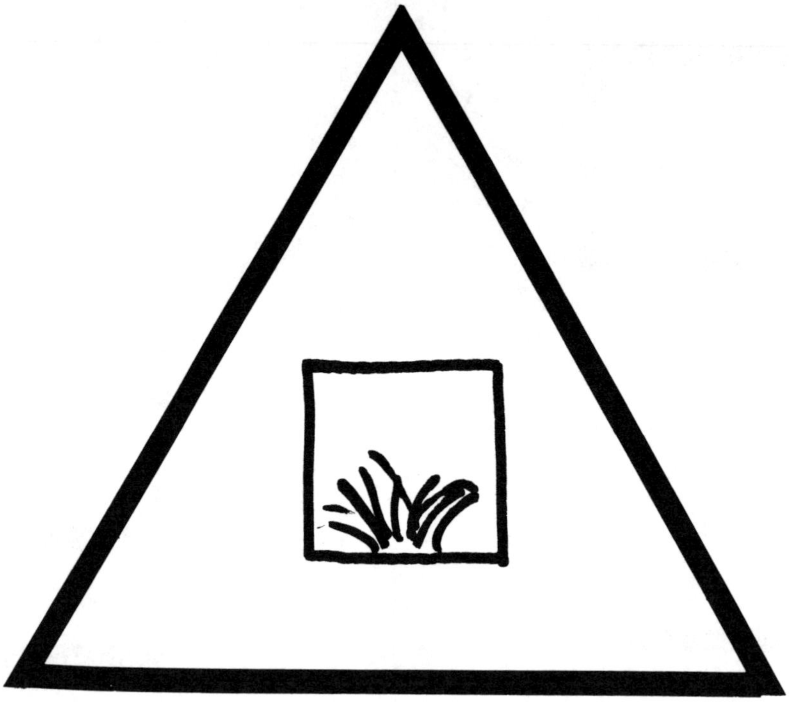

Skill 4
Step 4—Level #1 Worksheet (dog house)

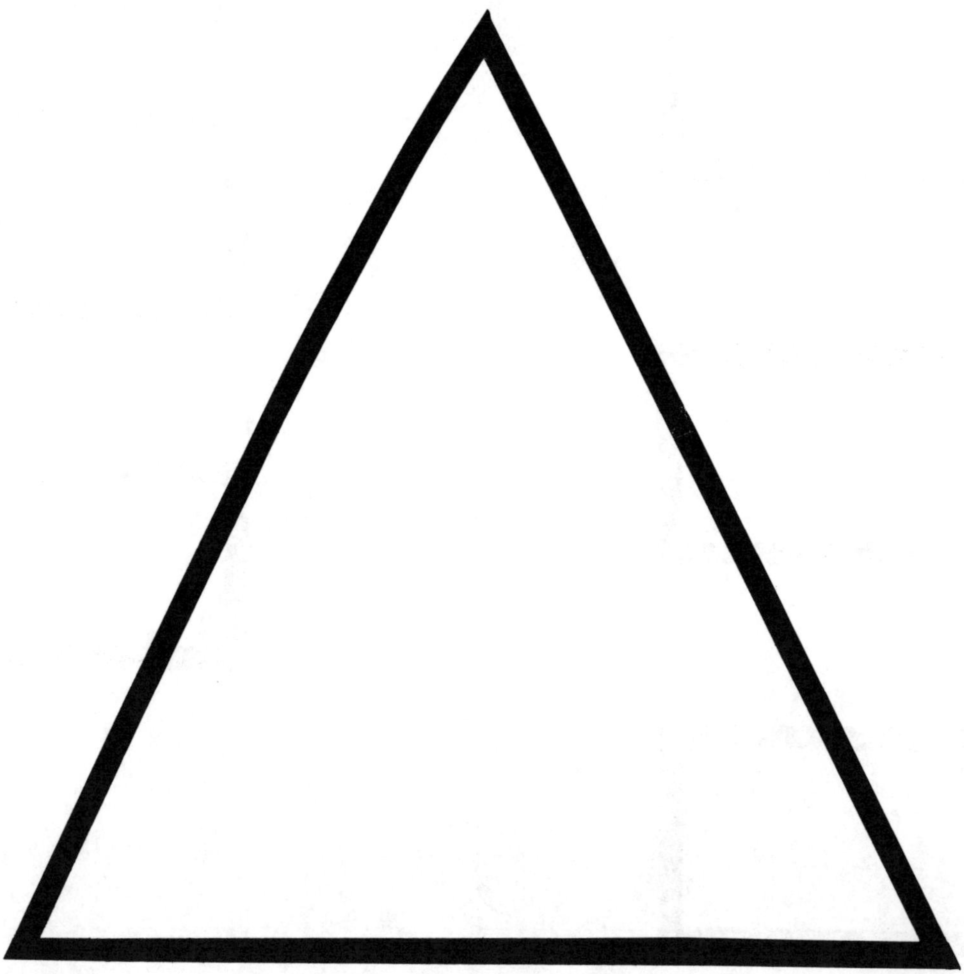

Skill 4
Step 4—Level #1 Worksheet (tepee)

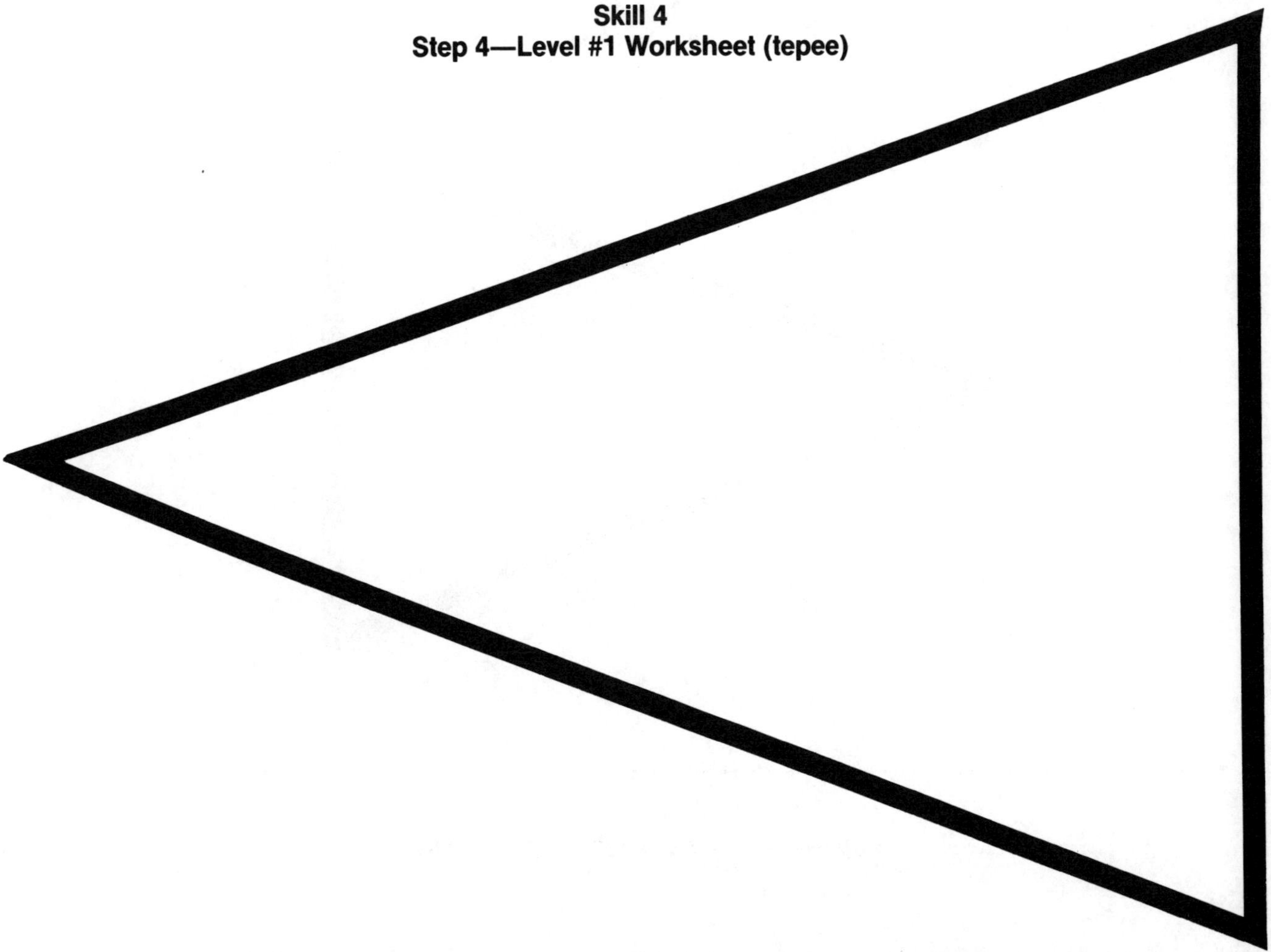

Skill 4
Step 4—Level #1 Worksheet (kite)

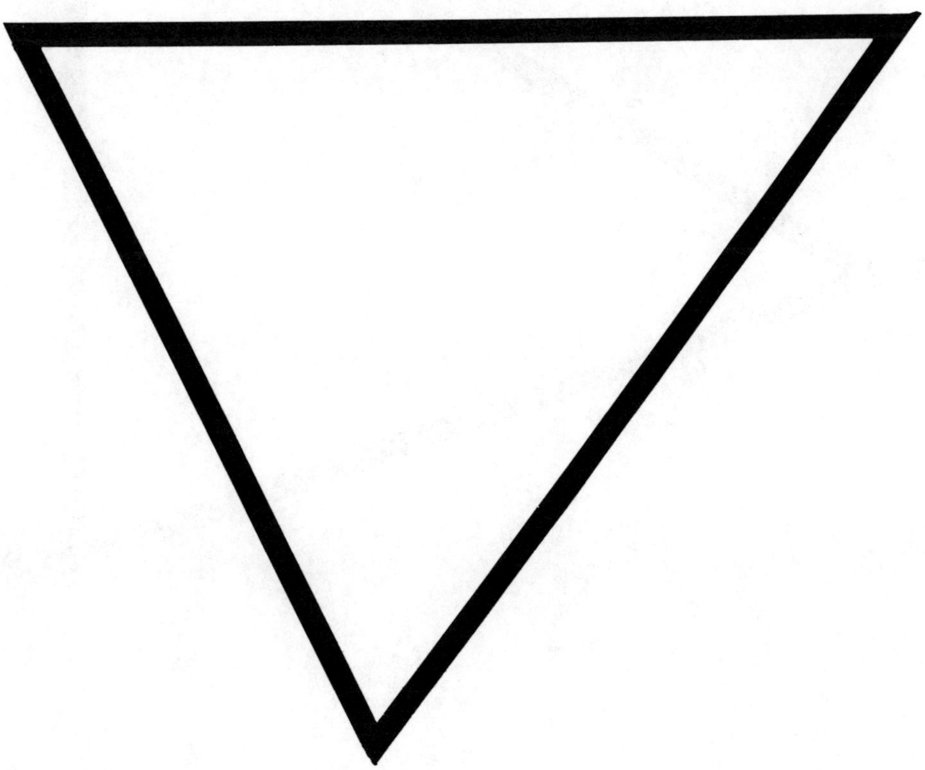

Skill 4
Step 4—Level #2 Pre/Posttest (drum)

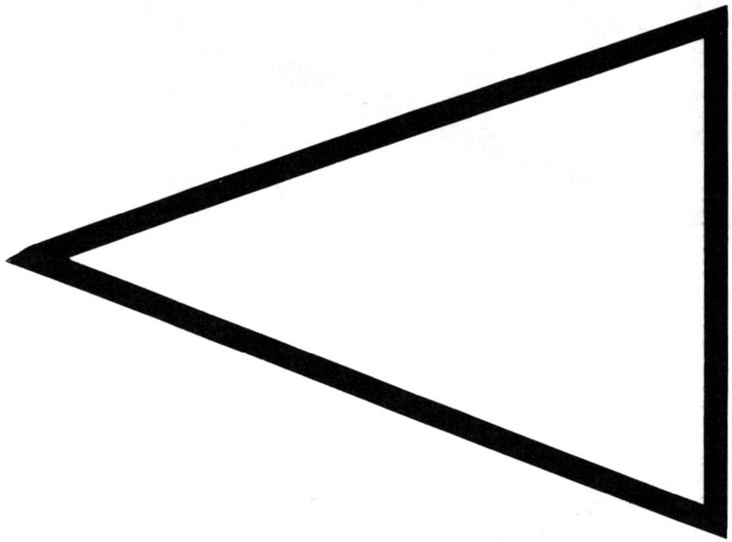

Skill 4
Step 4—Level #2 Worksheet (party hat)

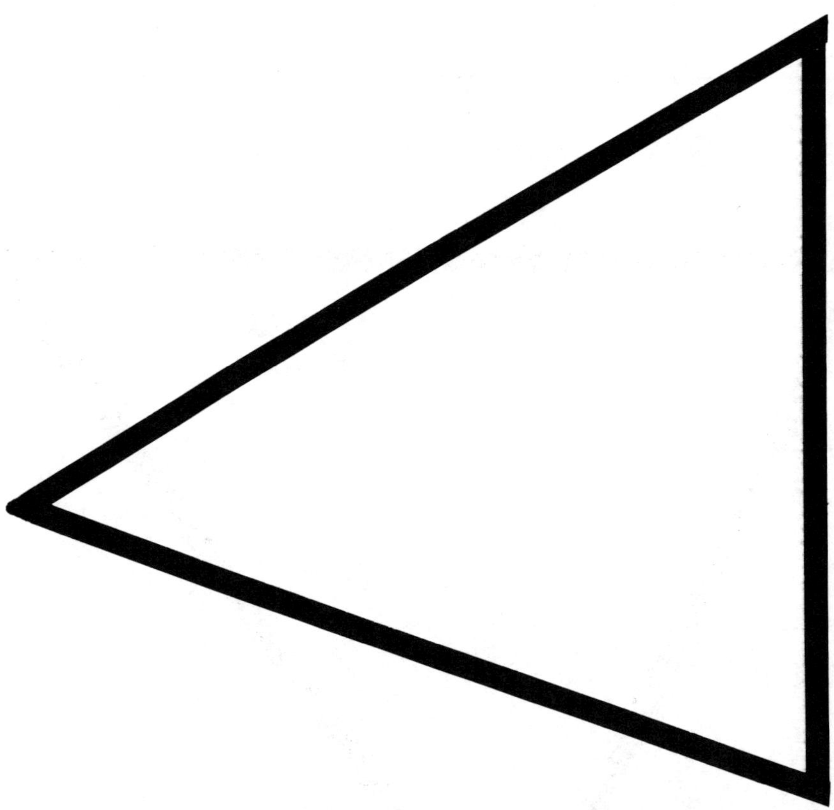

Skill 4
Step 4—Level #2 Worksheet (carrot)

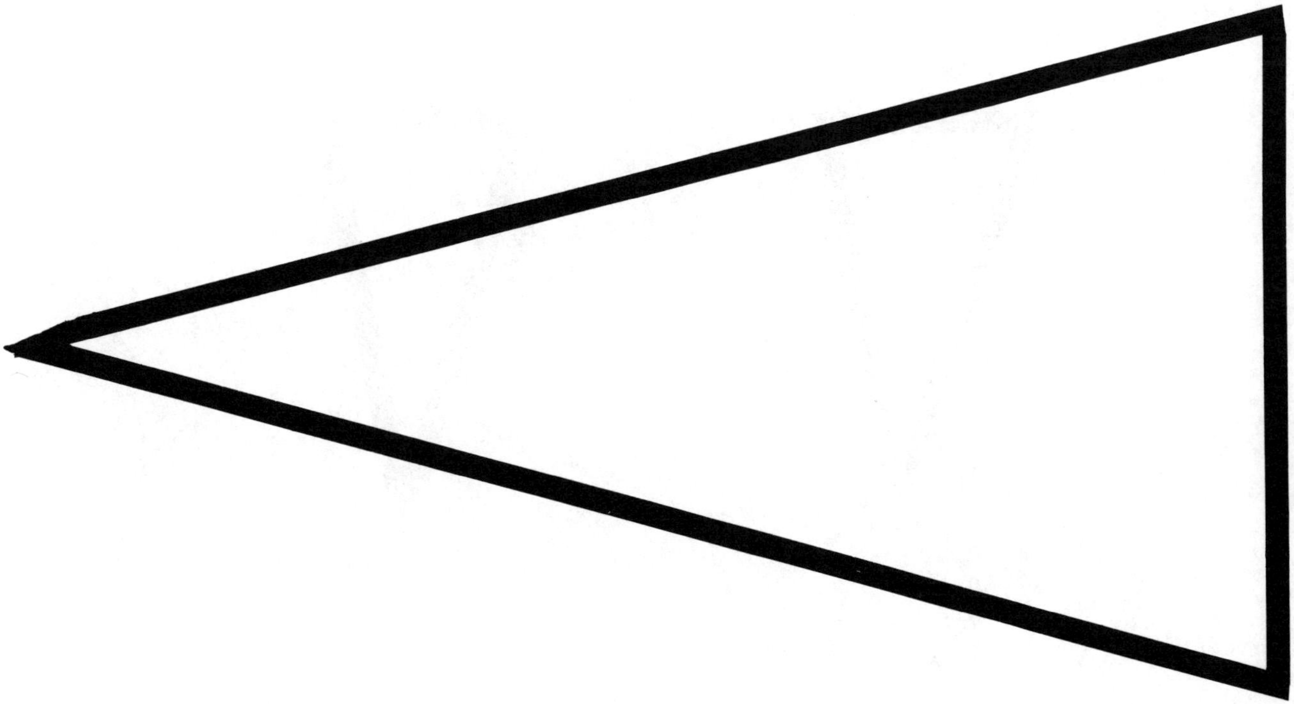

Skill 4
Step 4—Level #2 Worksheet (clown's hat)

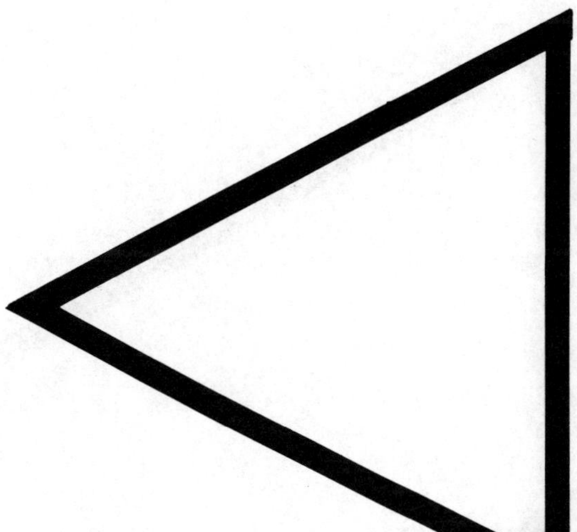

Skill 4
Step 4—Level #3 Pre/Posttest (walrus)

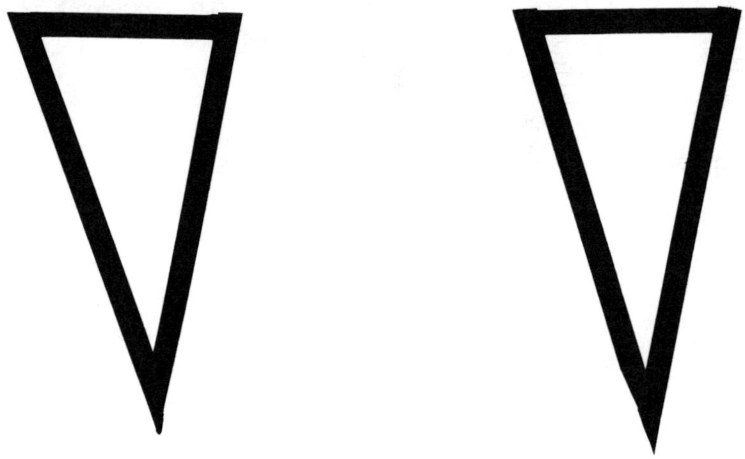

Skill 4
Step 4—Level #3 Worksheet (sailboat)

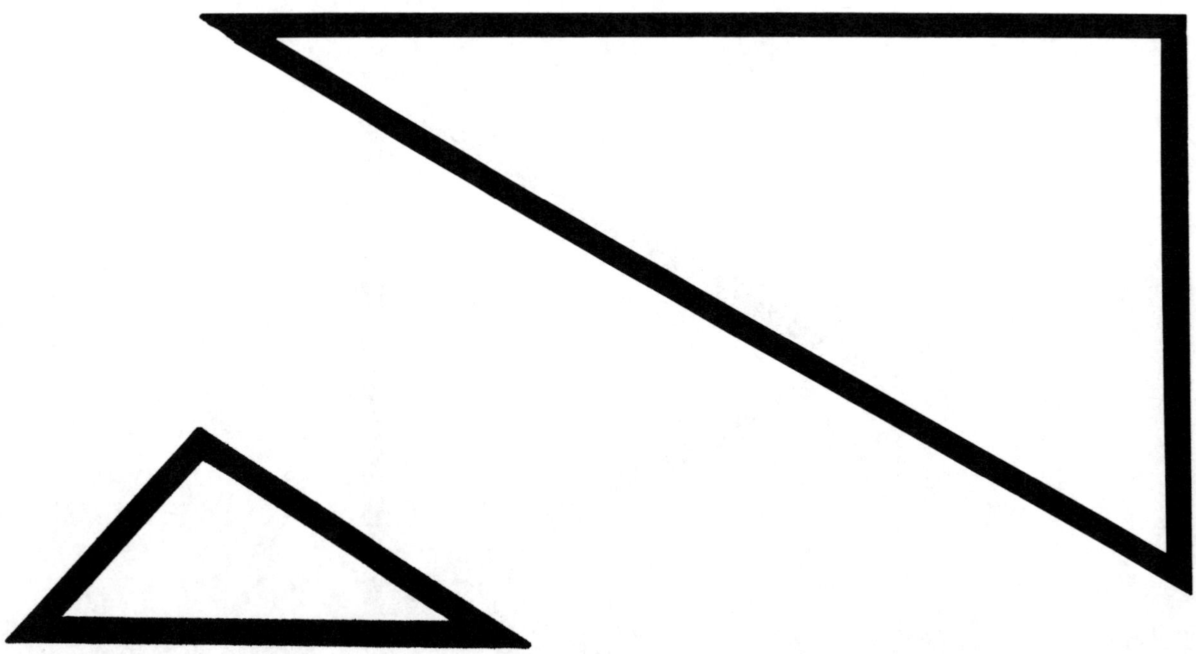

Skill 4
Step 5—Level #1 Pre/Posttest (door)

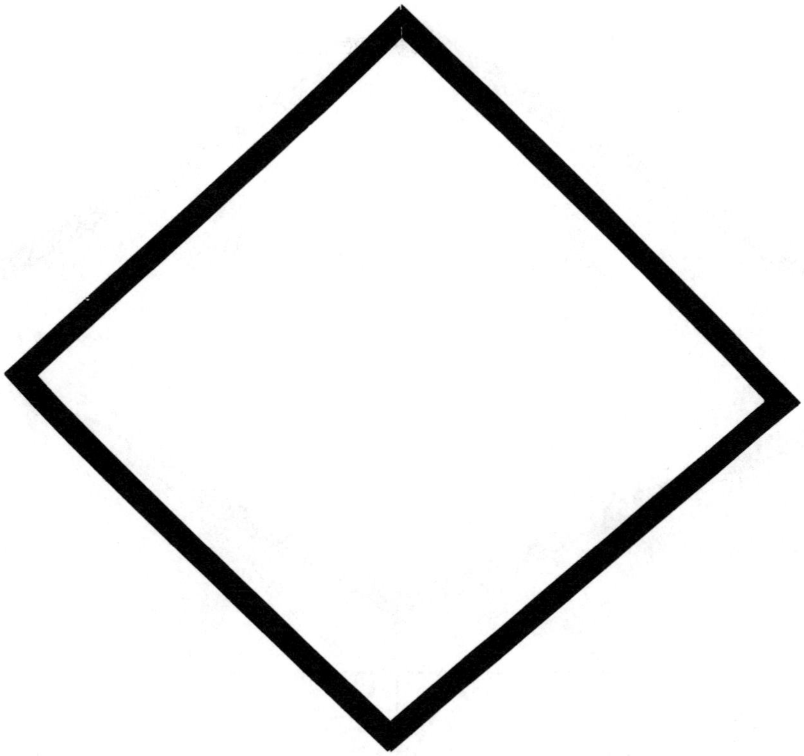

Skill 4
Step 5—Level #1 Worksheet (kite)

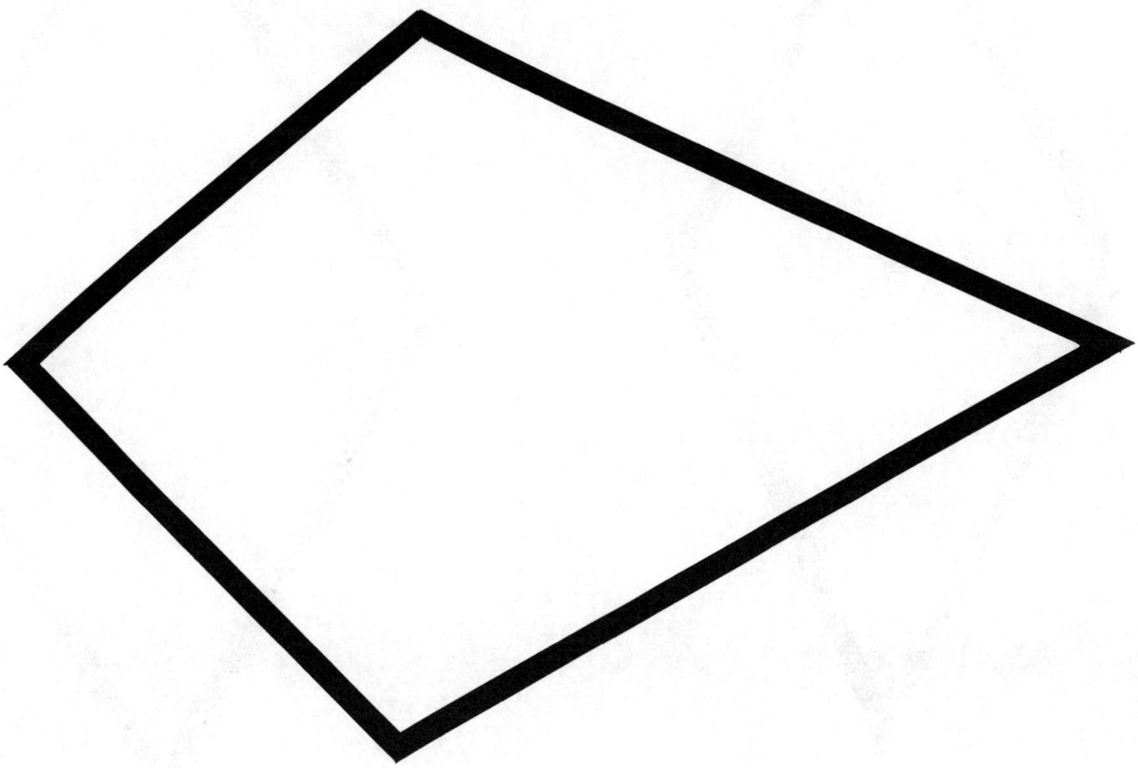

Skill 4
Step 5—Level #1 Worksheet (wishing well)

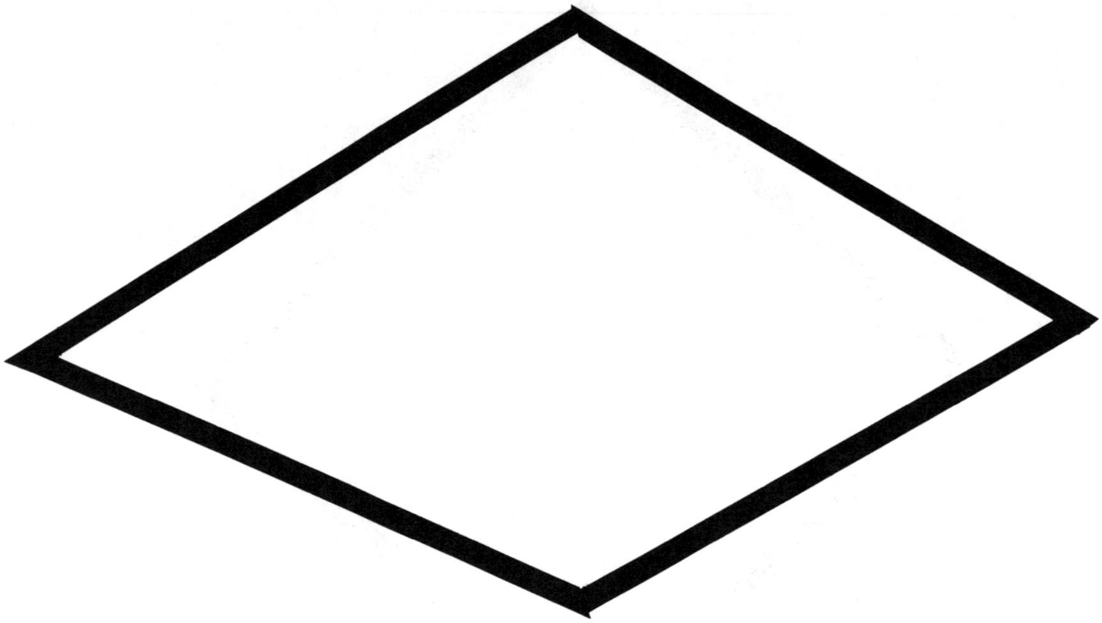

Skill 4
Step 5—Level #1 Worksheet (cookie in sundae)

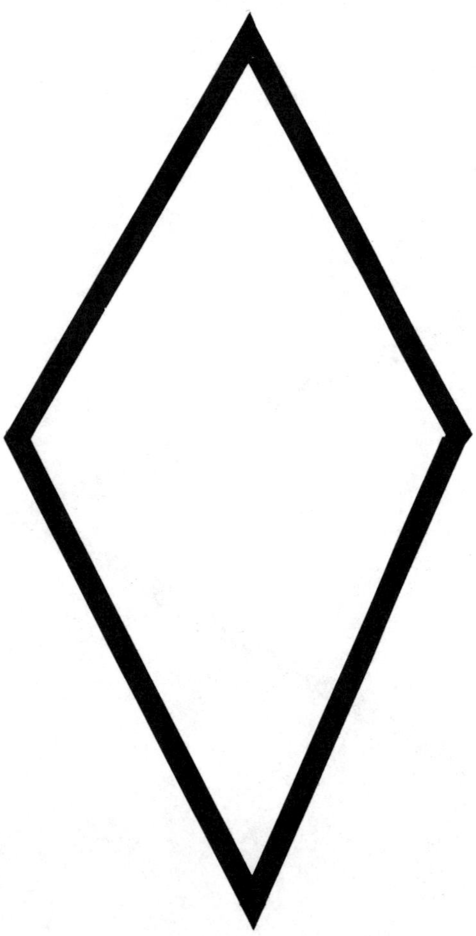

Skill 4
Step 5—Level #1 Worksheet (shape man)

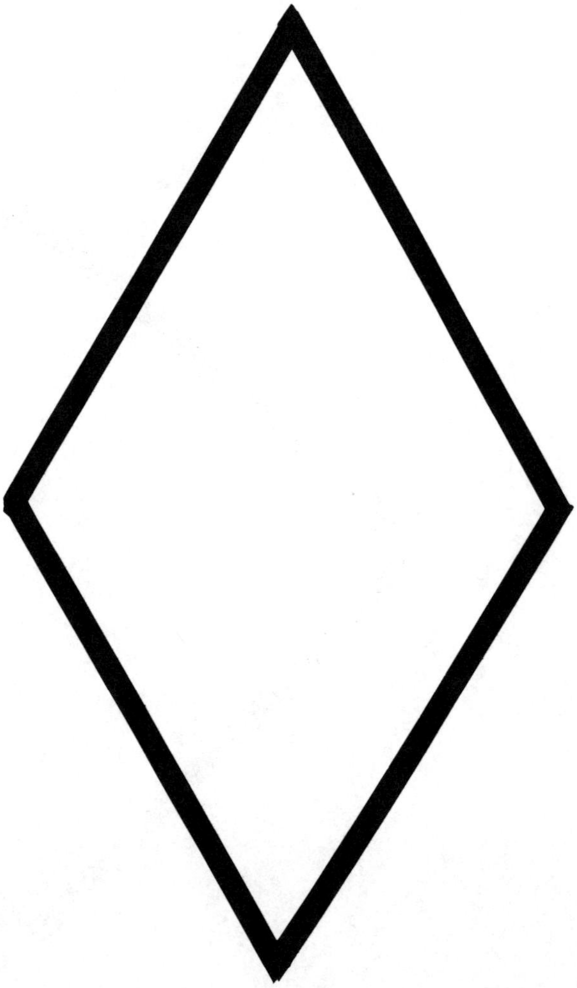

Skill 4
Step 5—Level #2 Pre/Posttest (candle)

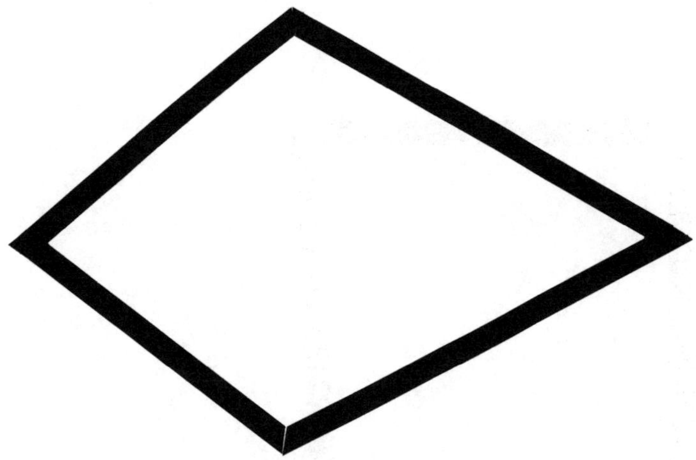

Skill 4
Step 5—Level #2 Worksheet (bird)

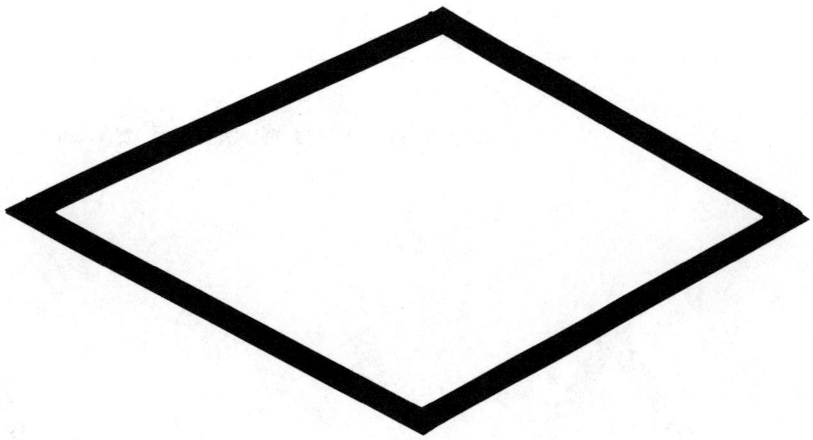

Skill 3
Step 5—Level #2 Worksheet (donkey)

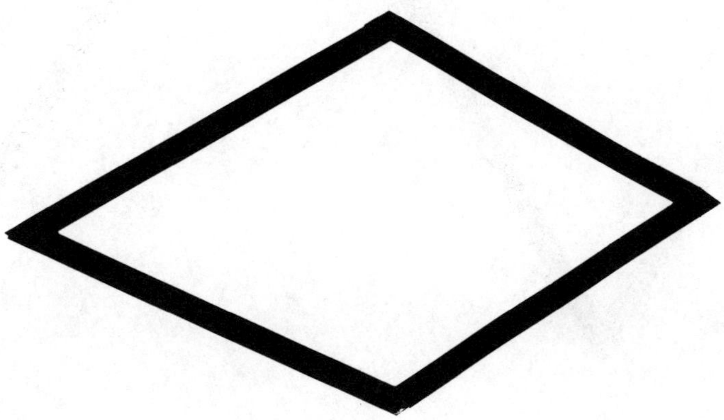

Skill 4
Step 5—Level #3 Pre/Posttest (overalls)

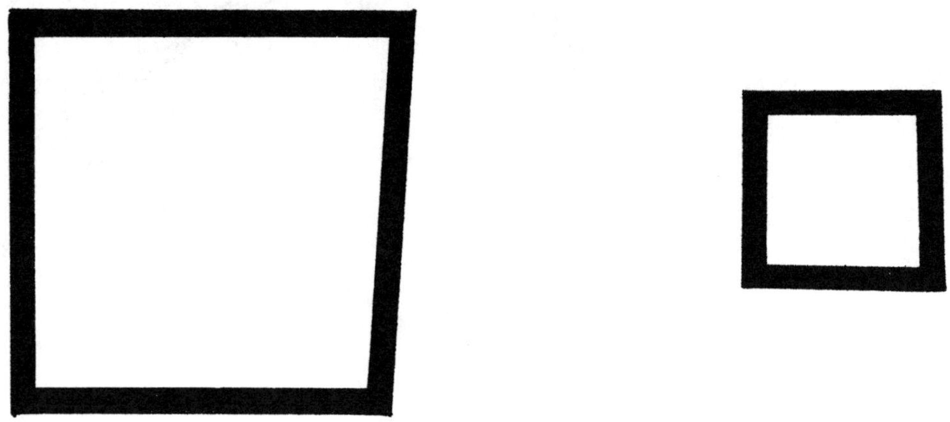

Skill 4
Step 5—Level #3 Worksheet (flower)

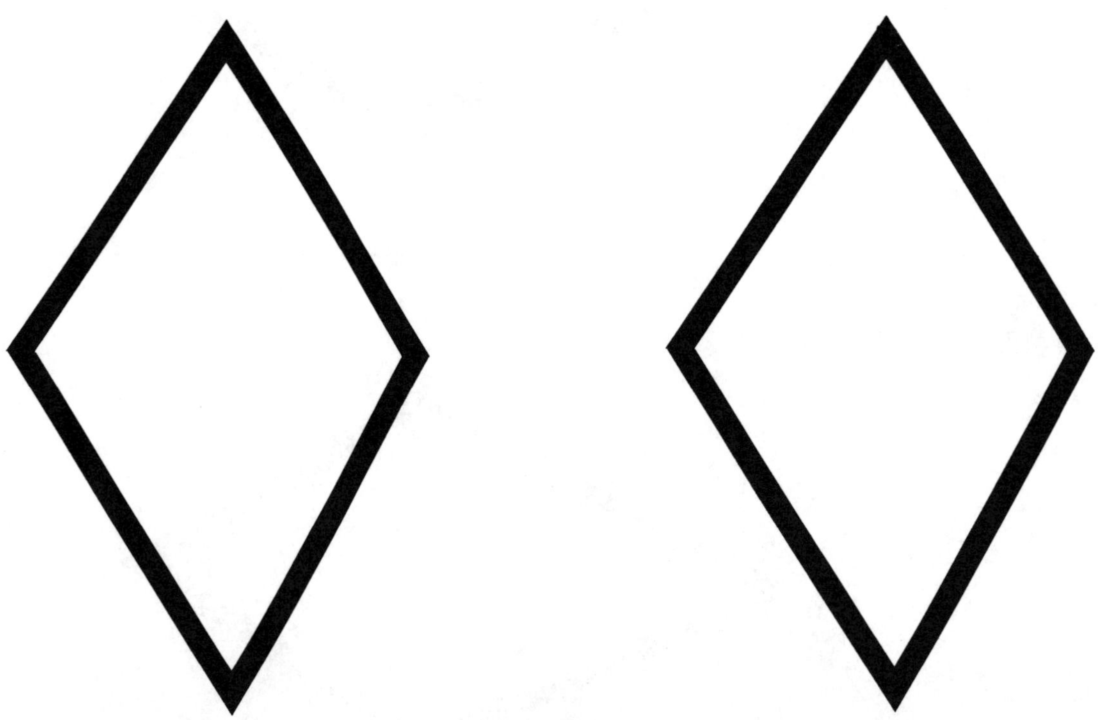

Skill 5—Cutting Combined Simple Shapes—1/8″ Line

Objective: Student cuts out two familiar shapes with a line 1/8″ wide, and pastes them on the corresponding fixed outlines, with 80% accuracy.

STEP 1—COMBINED SHAPES

Pretest: Student takes Step 1 Pretest (mailbox—strip and rectangle).

If criterion met: Student advances to Step 2.

If criterion not met:

1. Student cuts Step 1 worksheets:
   elephant—square and triangle
   turtle—strip and square
   balloons—square and triangle
   shape people—square and triangle
2. Student takes Step 1 Posttest (mailbox).

   If criterion met: Student advances to Step 2.

   If criterion not met: Student repeats Step 1 worksheets and Posttest.

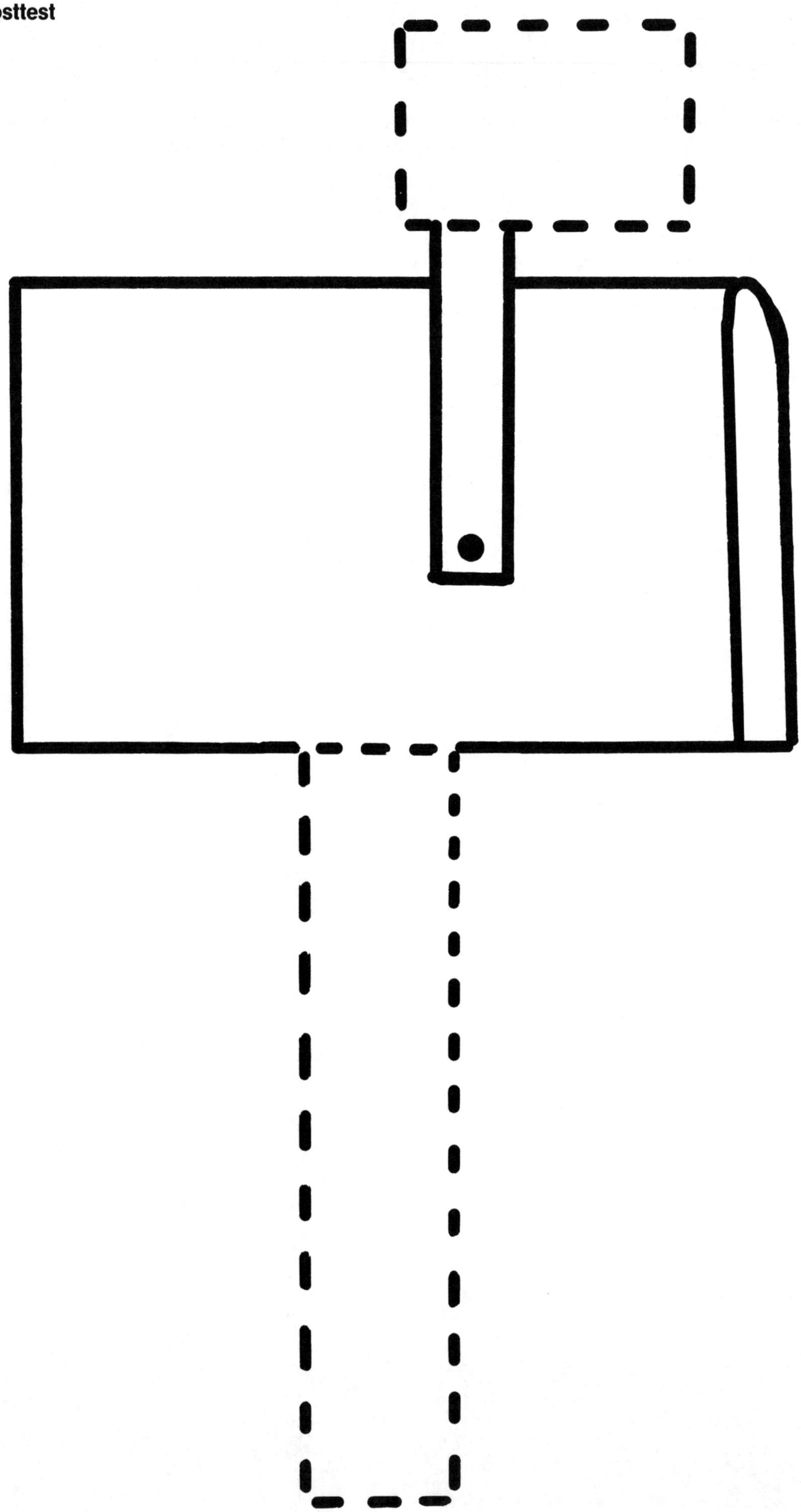

Skill 5
Step 1 Worksheet

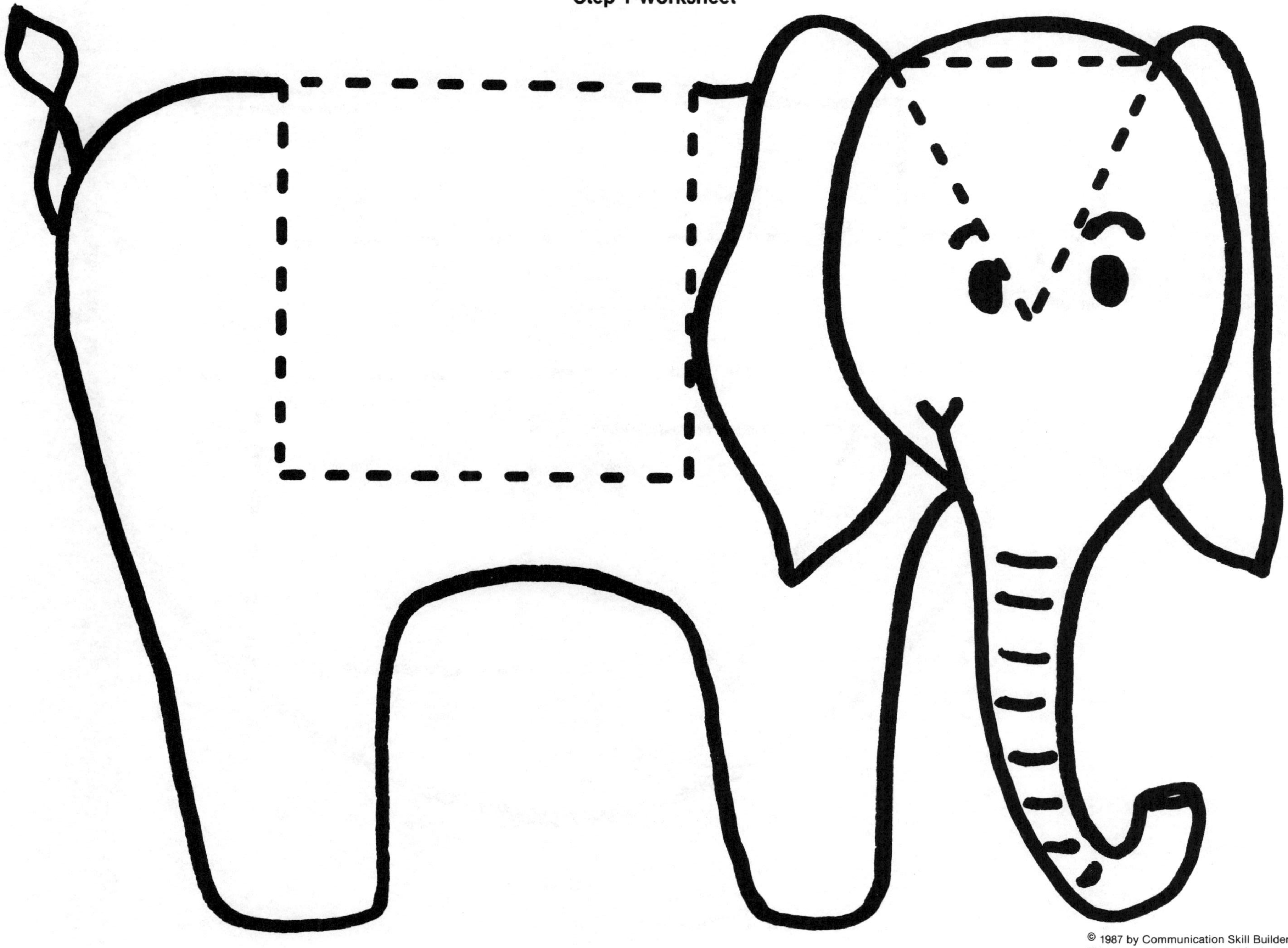

Skill 5
Step 1 Worksheet

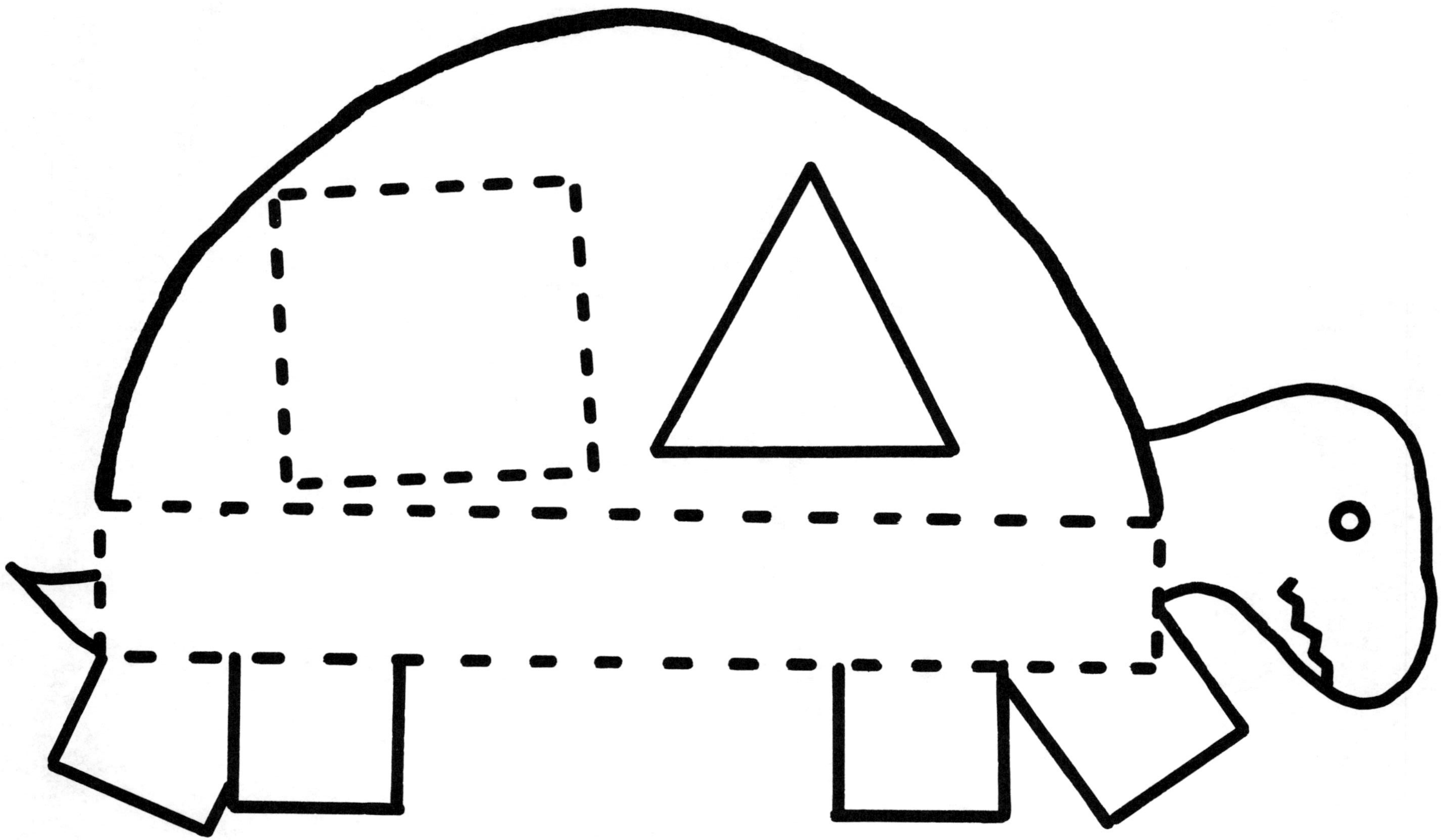

Skill 5
Step 1 Worksheet

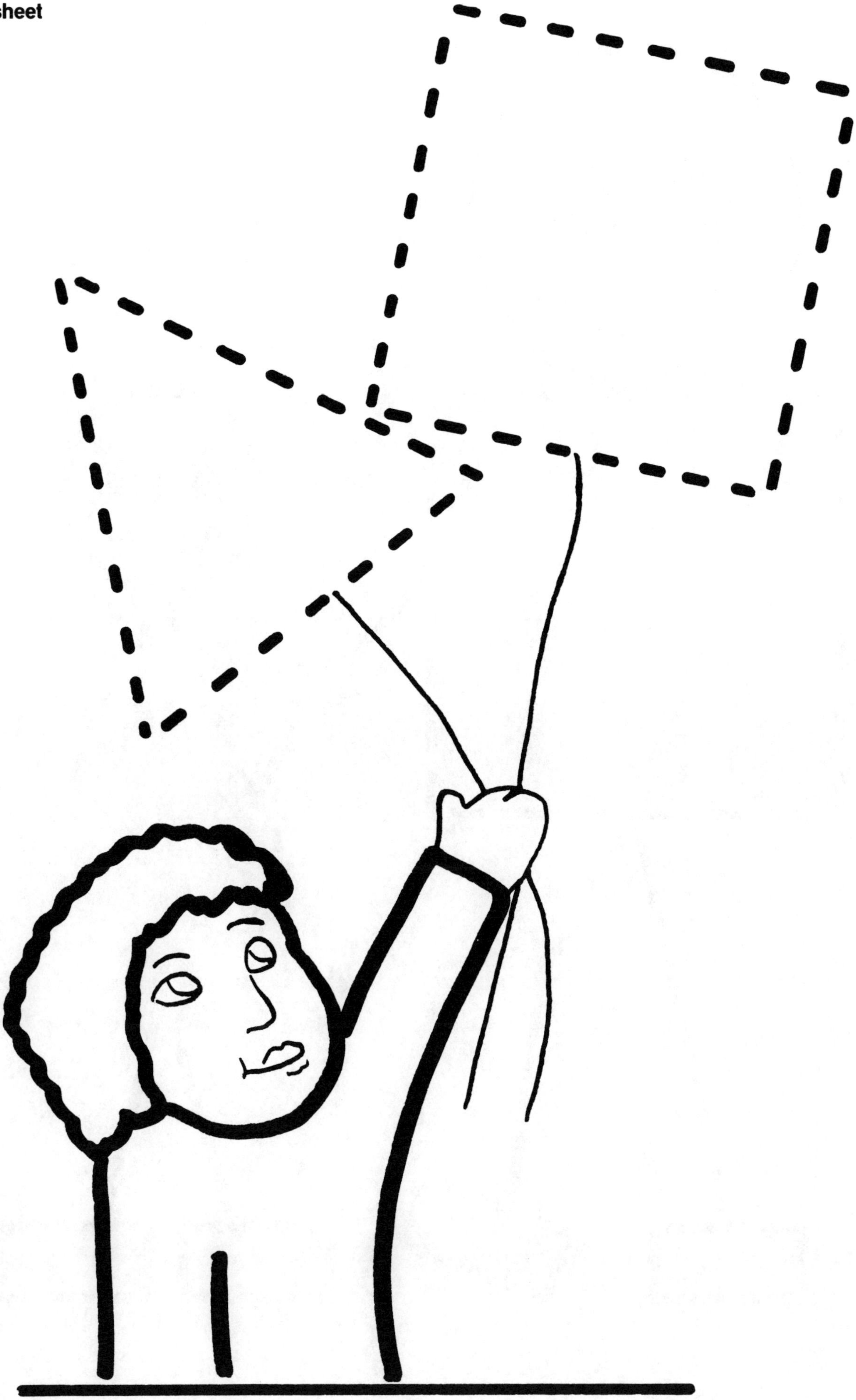

Skill 5
Step 1 Worksheet

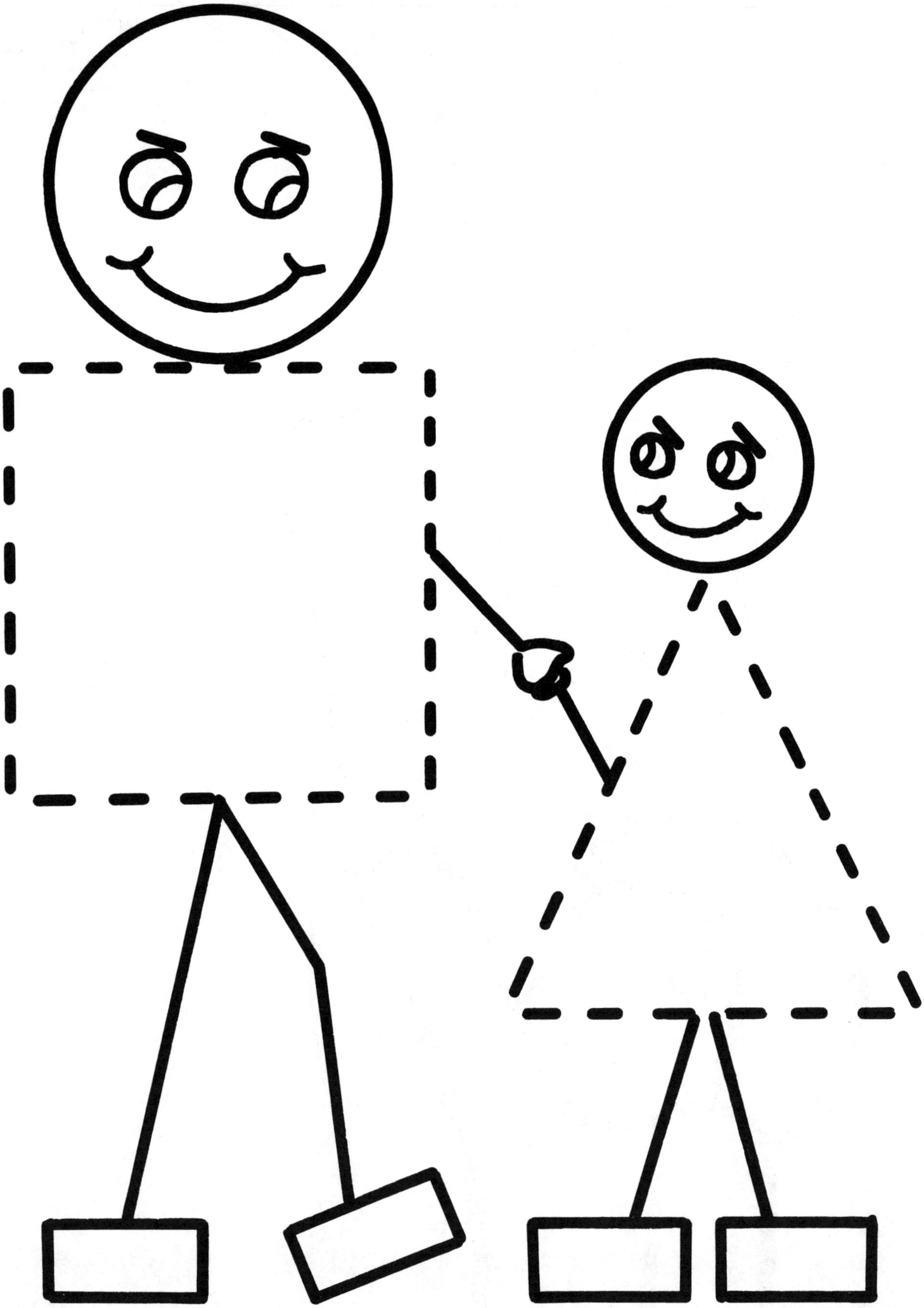

Skill 5
Step 1 Pre/Posttest (mailbox)

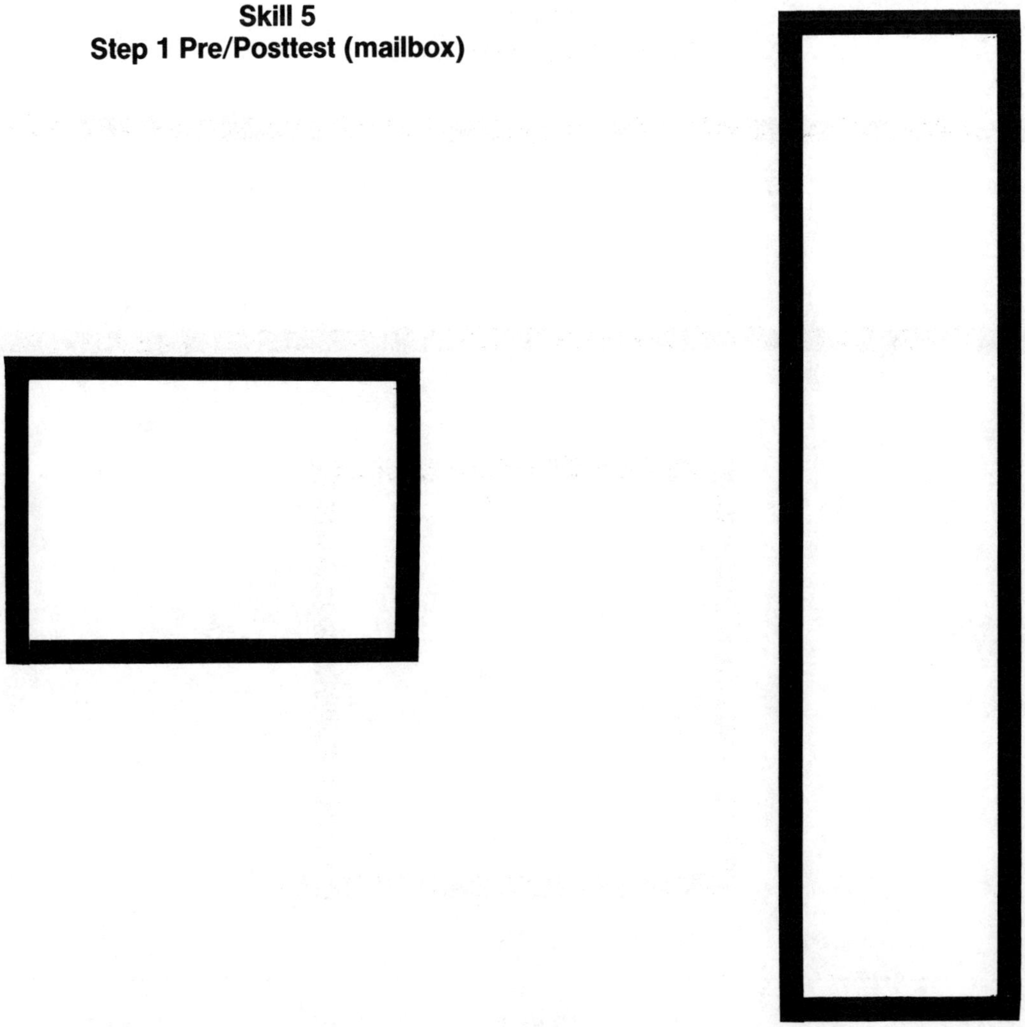

Skill 5
Step 1 Worksheet (elephant)

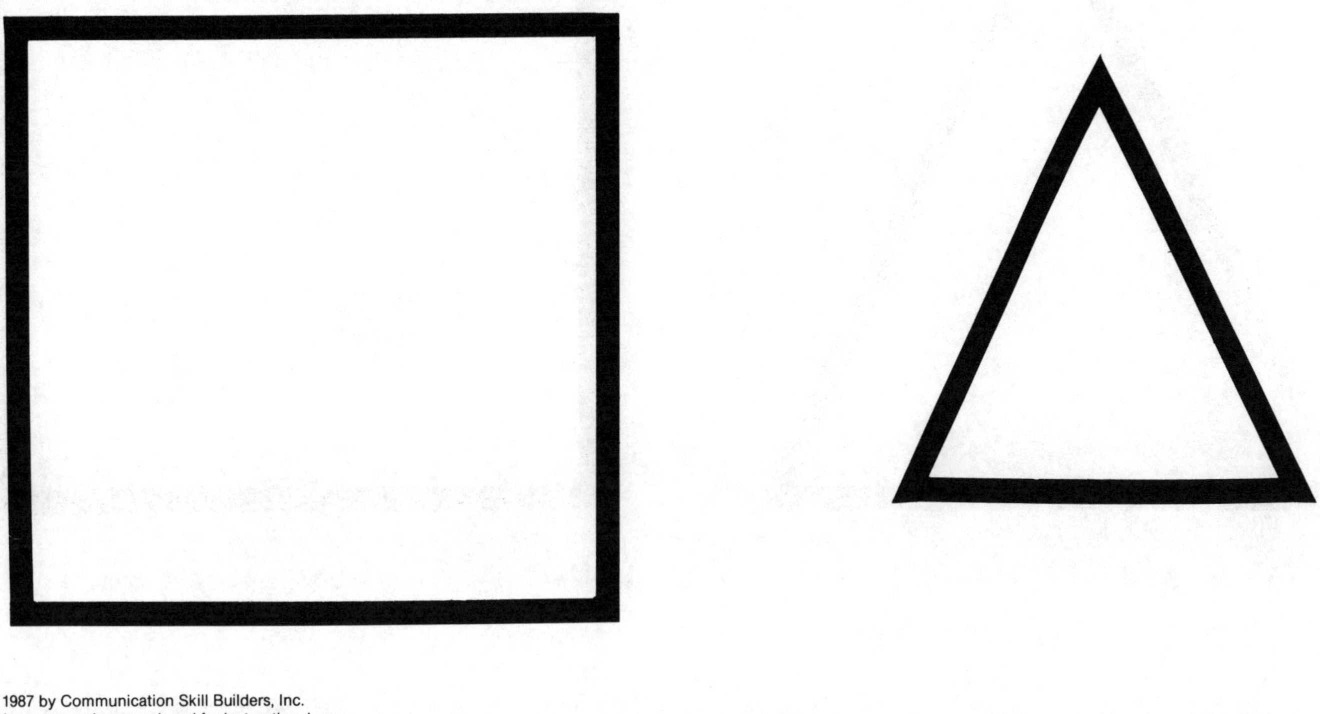

Skill 5
Step 1 Worksheet (turtle)

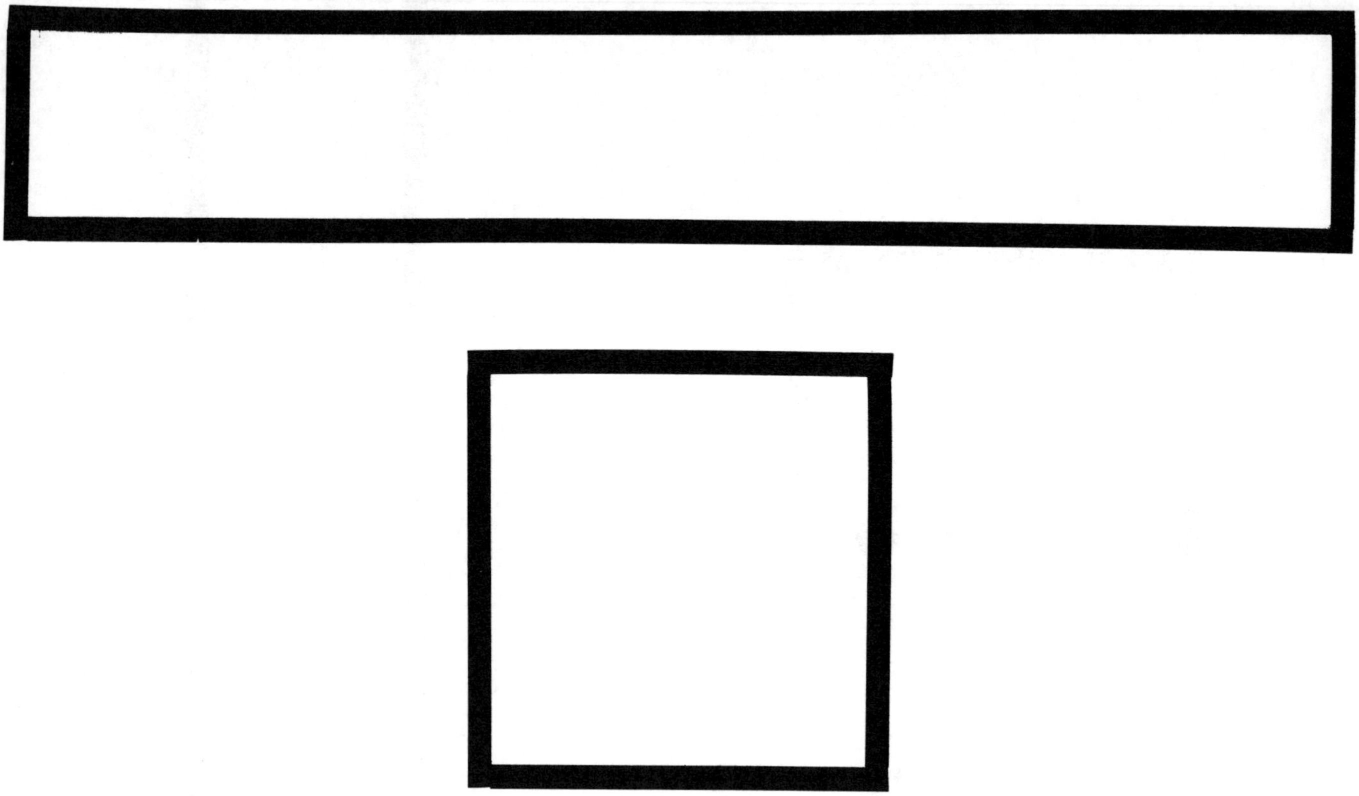

Skill 5
Step 1 Worksheet (balloons)

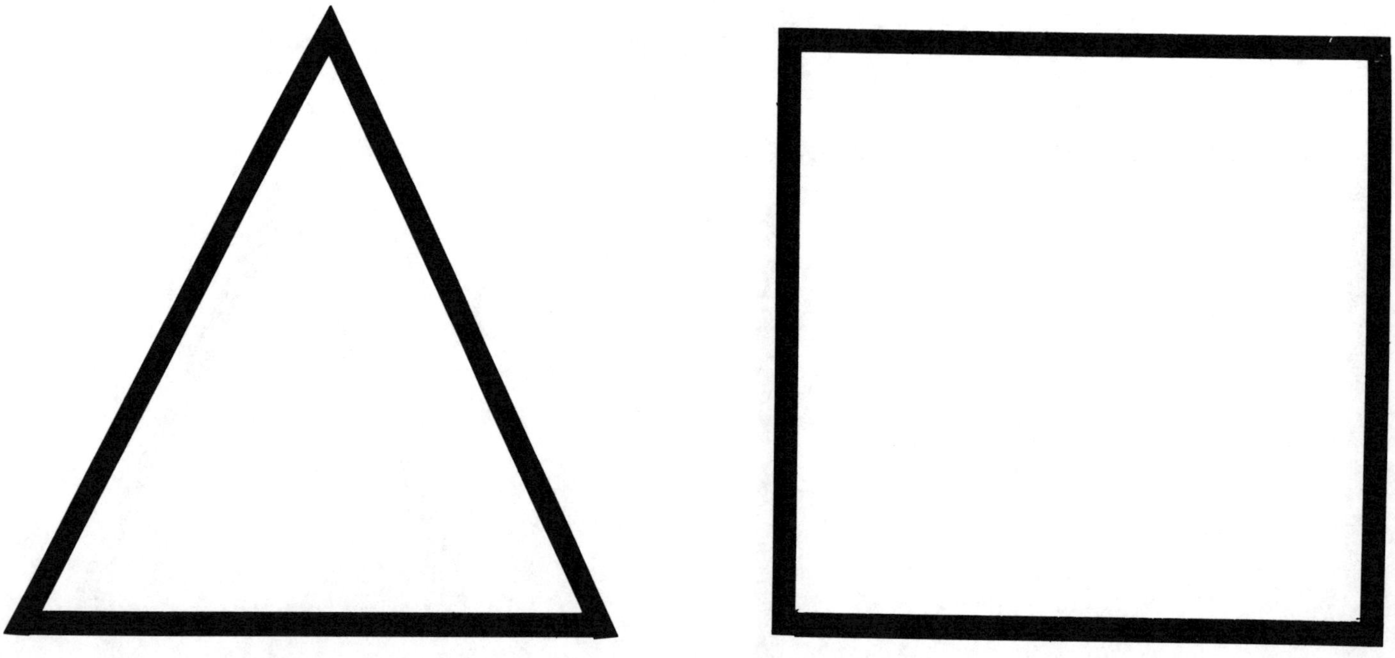

Skill 5
Step 1 Worksheet (shape people)

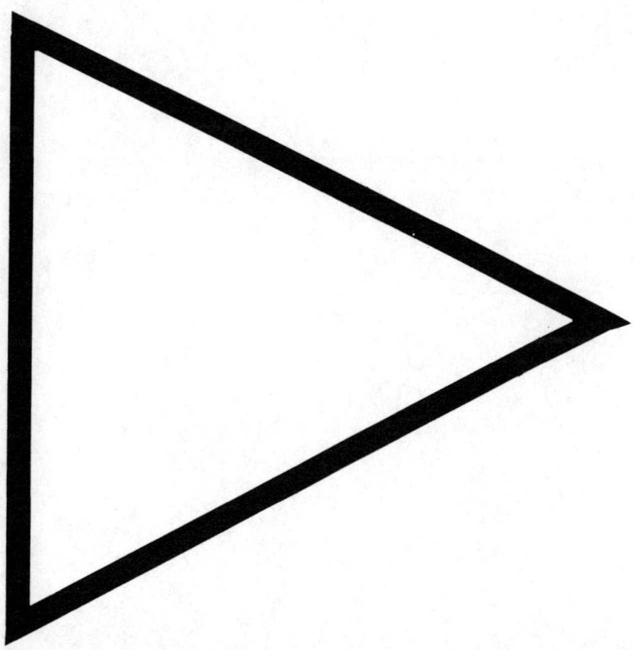

SKILL 5—STEP 2—SMALLER COMBINED SHAPES

Pretest: Student takes Step 2 Pretest (castle—square and triangle).

If criterion met: Student advances to Skill 6.

If criterion not met:

1. Student cuts Step 2 worksheets:
   house—two rectangles
   mittens—strip and triangle
   soldier—strip and triangle
   mask—large and small triangles

2. Student takes Step 2 Posttest (castle).

   If criterion met: Student advances to Skill 6.

   If criterion not met: Student repeats Step 2 worksheets and Posttest.

Skill 5
Step 2 Pre/Posttest

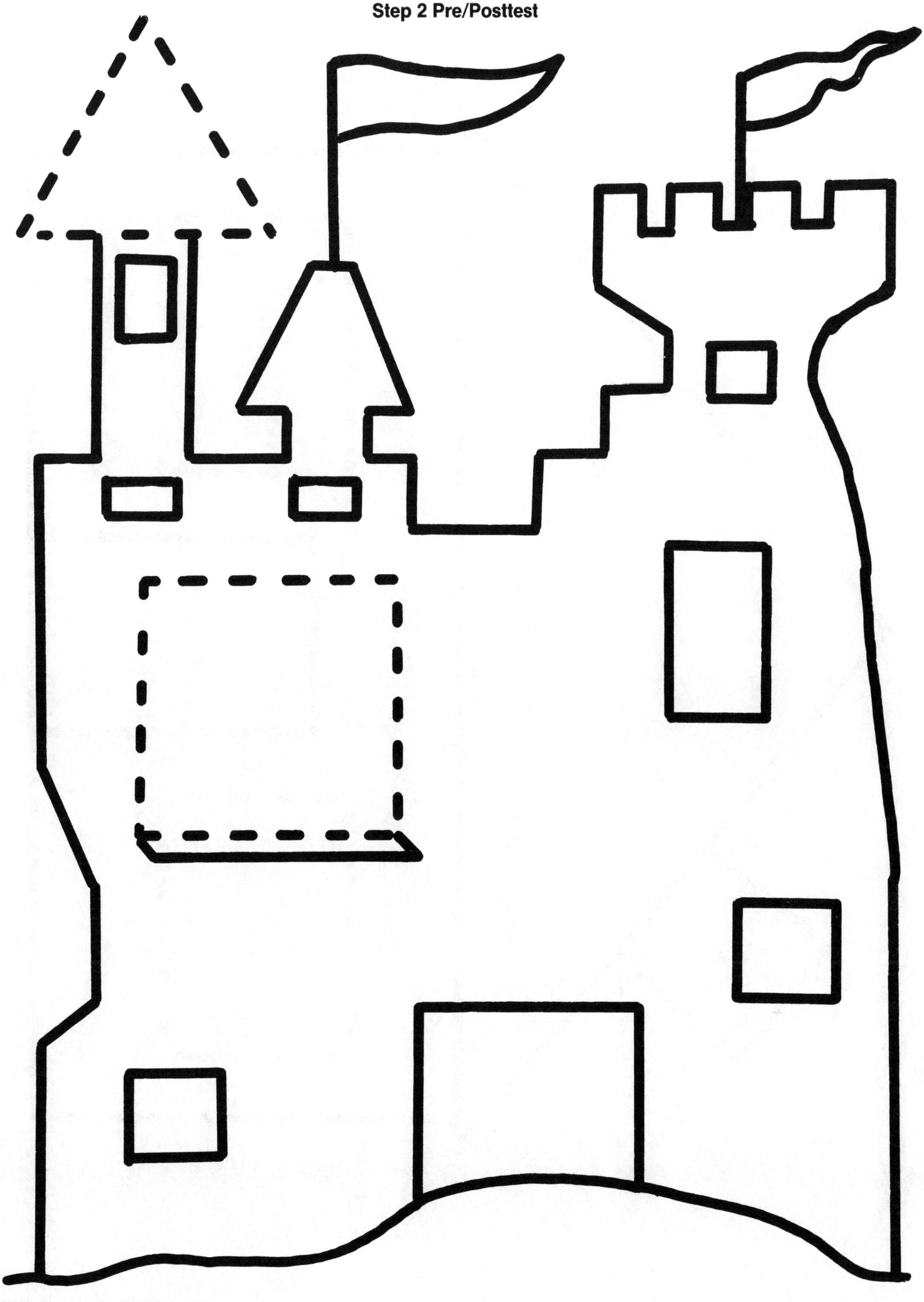

Skill 5
Step 2 Worksheet

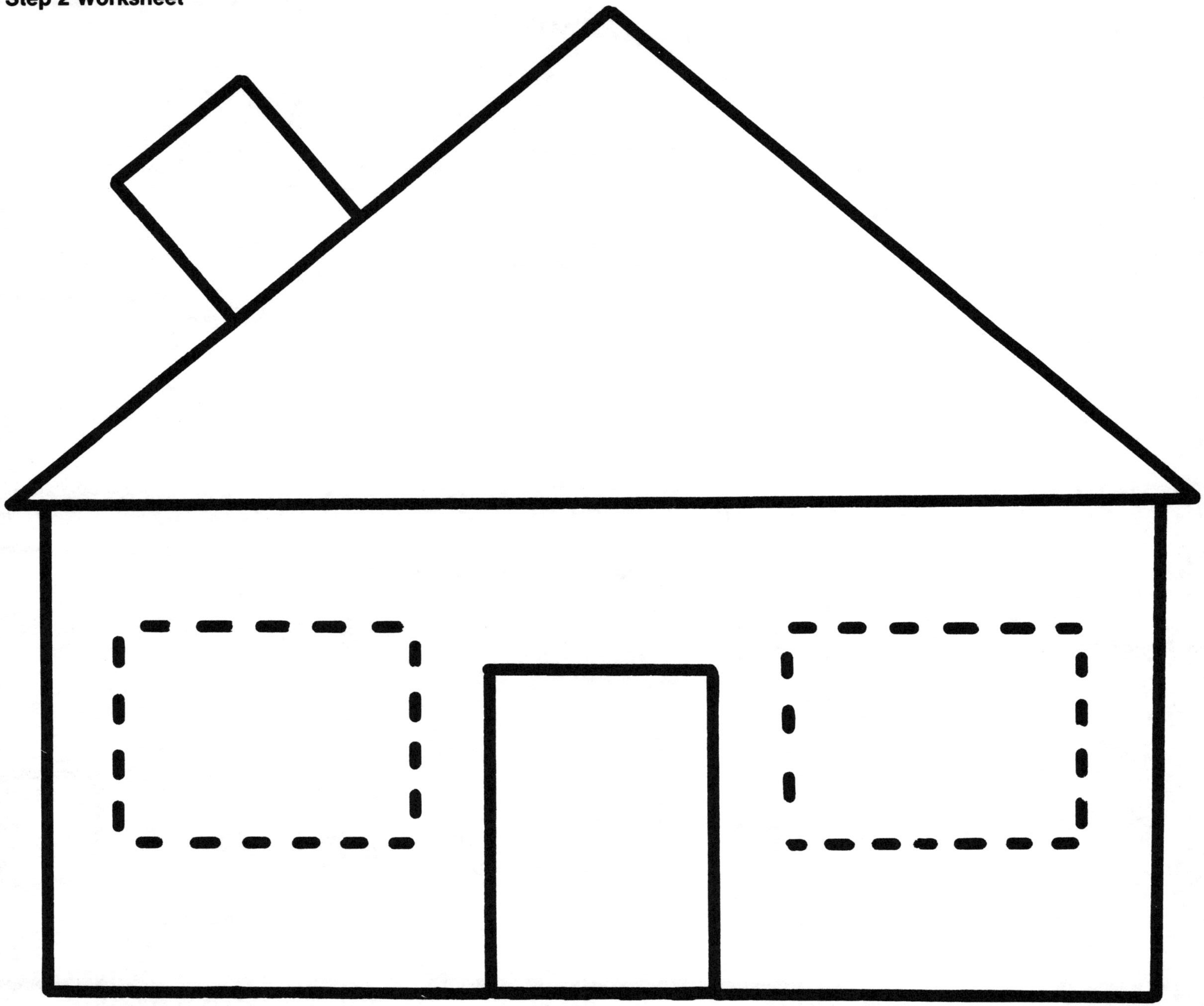

Skill 5
Step 2 Worksheet

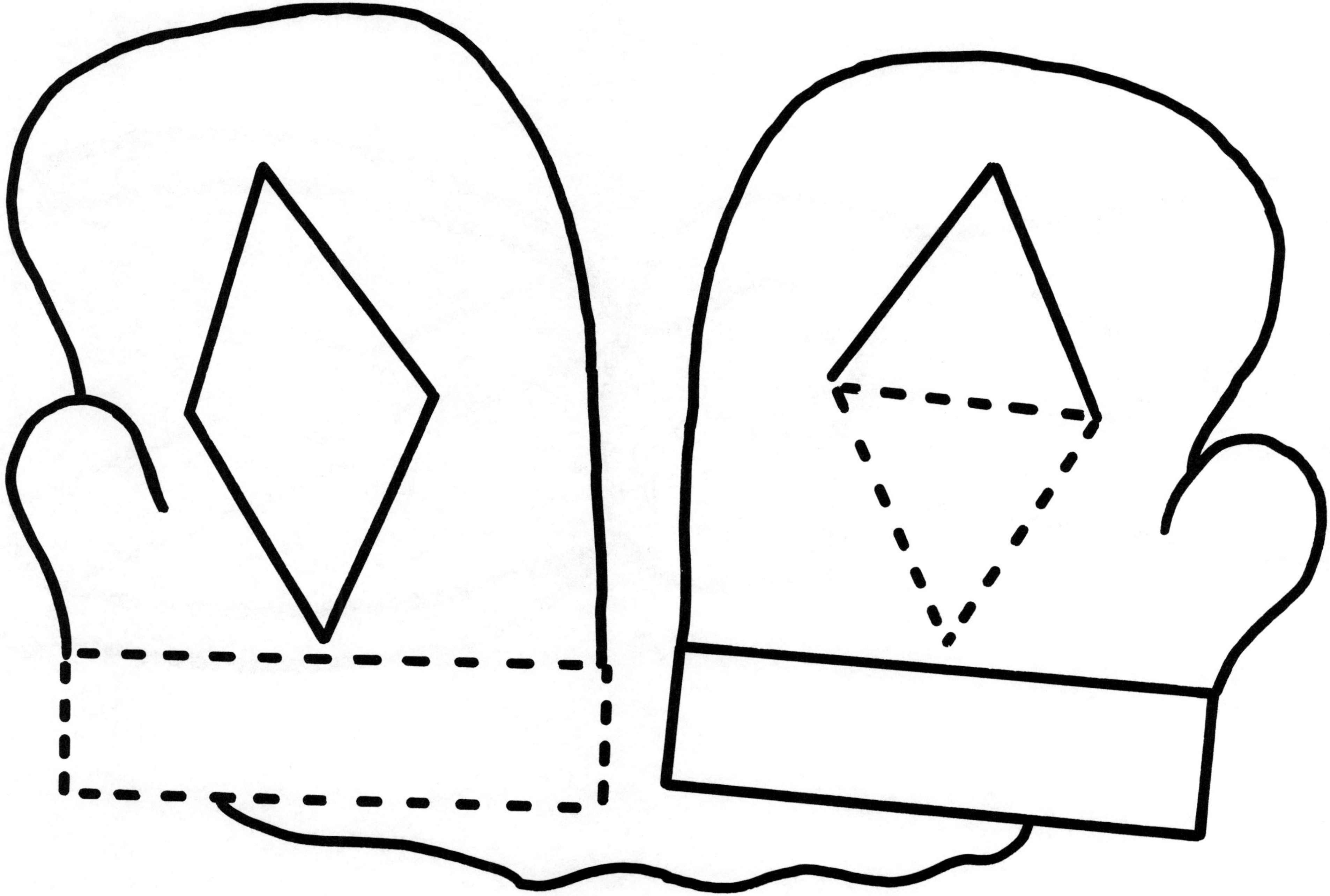

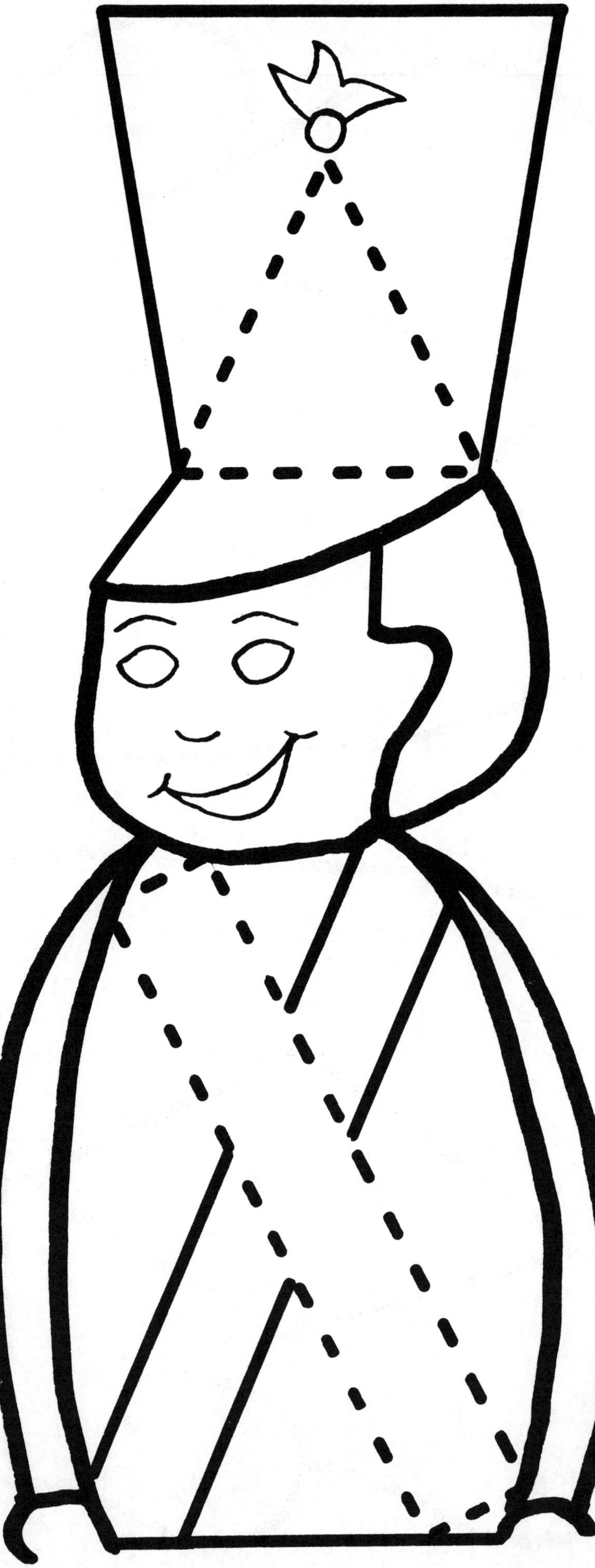

Skill 5
Step 2 Worksheet

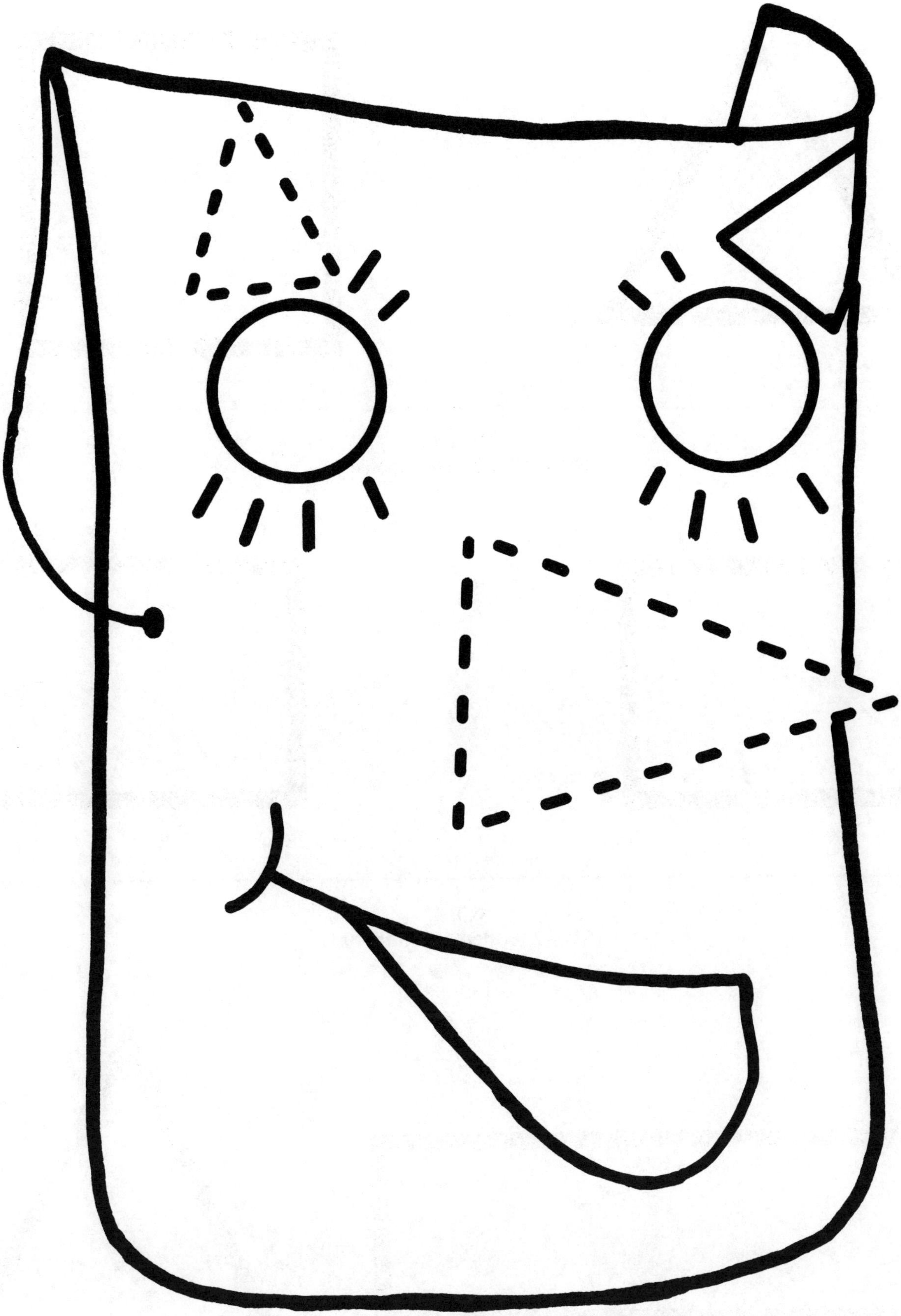

Skill 5
Step 2 Pre/Posttest (castle)

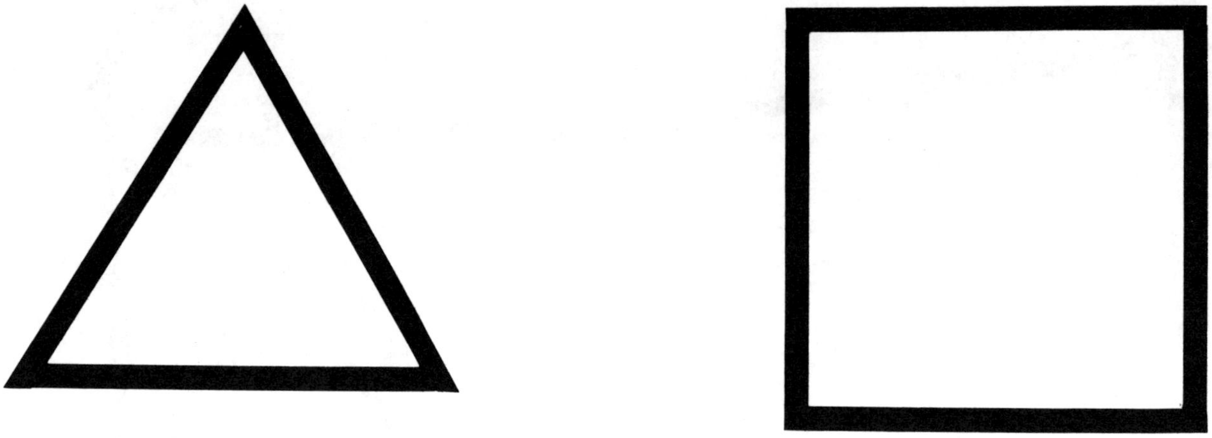

Skill 5
Step 2 Worksheet (house)

Skill 5
Step 2 Worksheet (mittens)

Skill 5
Step 2 Worksheet (soldier)

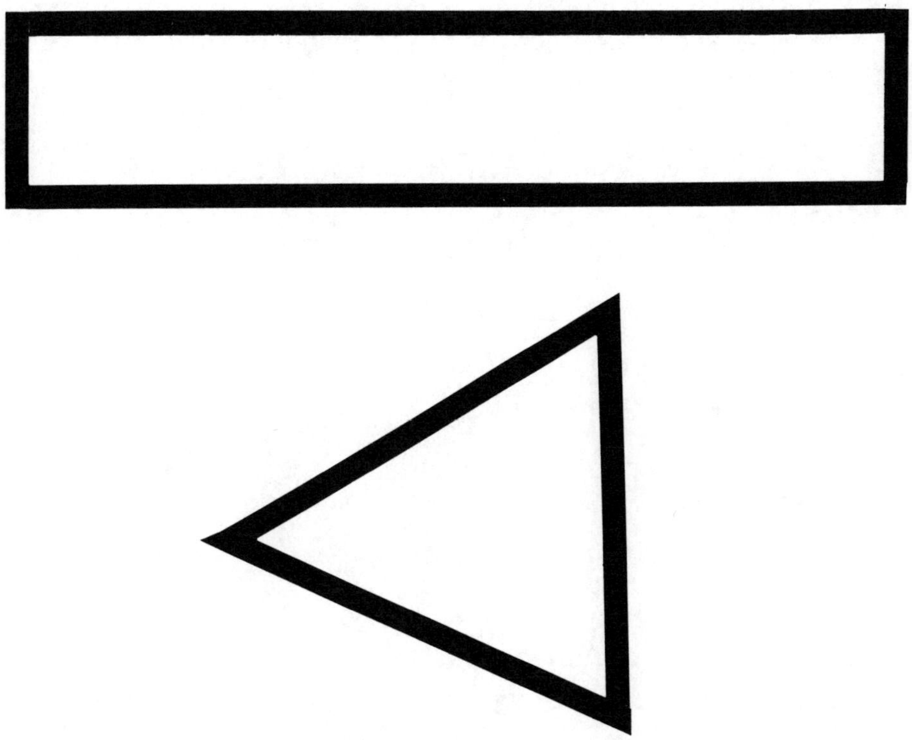

Skill 5
Step 2 Worksheet (mask)

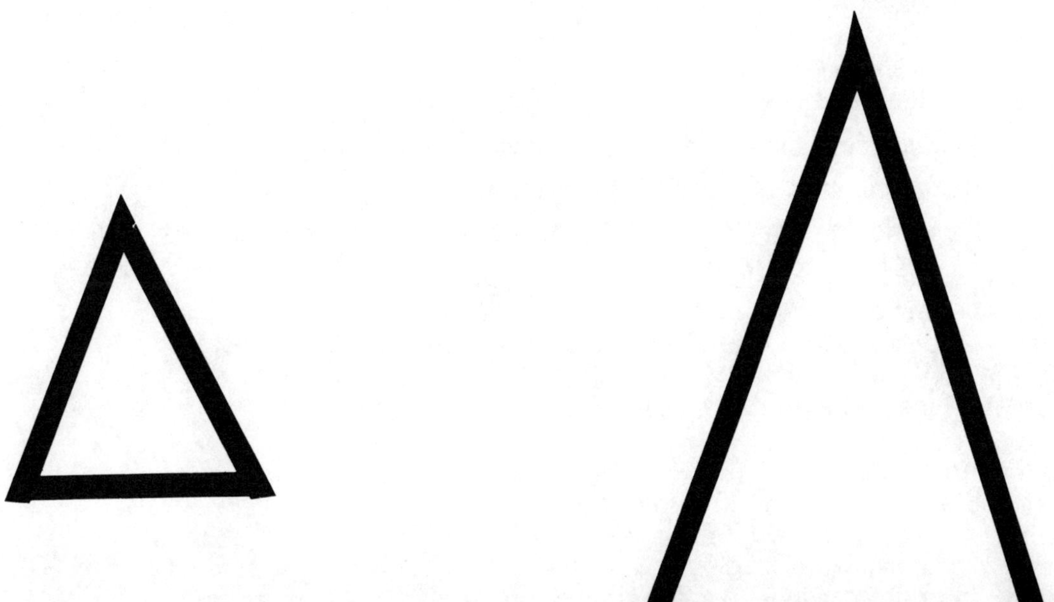

Skill 6—Cutting Circles and Complex Shapes—¼″ Line

Objective: Student cuts out circles and complex shapes of varying sizes with a line ¼″ wide, and pastes them on the corresponding fixed outlines, with 80% accuracy.

SKILL 6—STEP 1—CIRCLES

Level #1—Circles
Pretest: Student takes Level #1 Pretest (shape person—3″ circle).

If criterion met: Student advances to Level #2.

If criterion not met:

1. Student cuts Level #1 worksheets:
   snail—6″
   clock—5½″
   baseball—3½″
   tricycle—3½″
   sun—3½″
2. Student takes Level #1 Posttest (shape person).
   If criterion met: Student advances to Level #2.
   If criterion not met: Student repeats Level #1 worksheets and Posttest.

Level #2—Circles
Pretest: Student takes Level #2 Pretest (fish with air bubble—1½″).

If criterion met: Student advances to Level #3.

If criterion not met:

1. Student cuts Level #2 worksheets:
   balloon—3″
   soap bubble—2½″
   traffic signal—2½″
   flower—2″
2. Student takes Level #2 Posttest (fish with air bubble).
   If criterion met: Student advances to Level #3.
   If criterion not met: Student repeats Level #2 worksheets and Posttest.

Level #3—Circles
Pretest: Student takes Level #3 Pretest (sunglasses—two 1½″ circles).

If criterion met: Student advances to Step 2—Ovals.

If criterion not met:

1. Student cuts Level #3 worksheets:
   golf cart—two 2½″ circles
   car—two 2″ circles
   baby carriage—two 2″ circles
2. Student takes Level #3 Posttest (sunglasses).
   If criterion met: Student advances to Step 2—Ovals.
   If criterion not met: Student repeats Level #3 worksheets and Posttest.

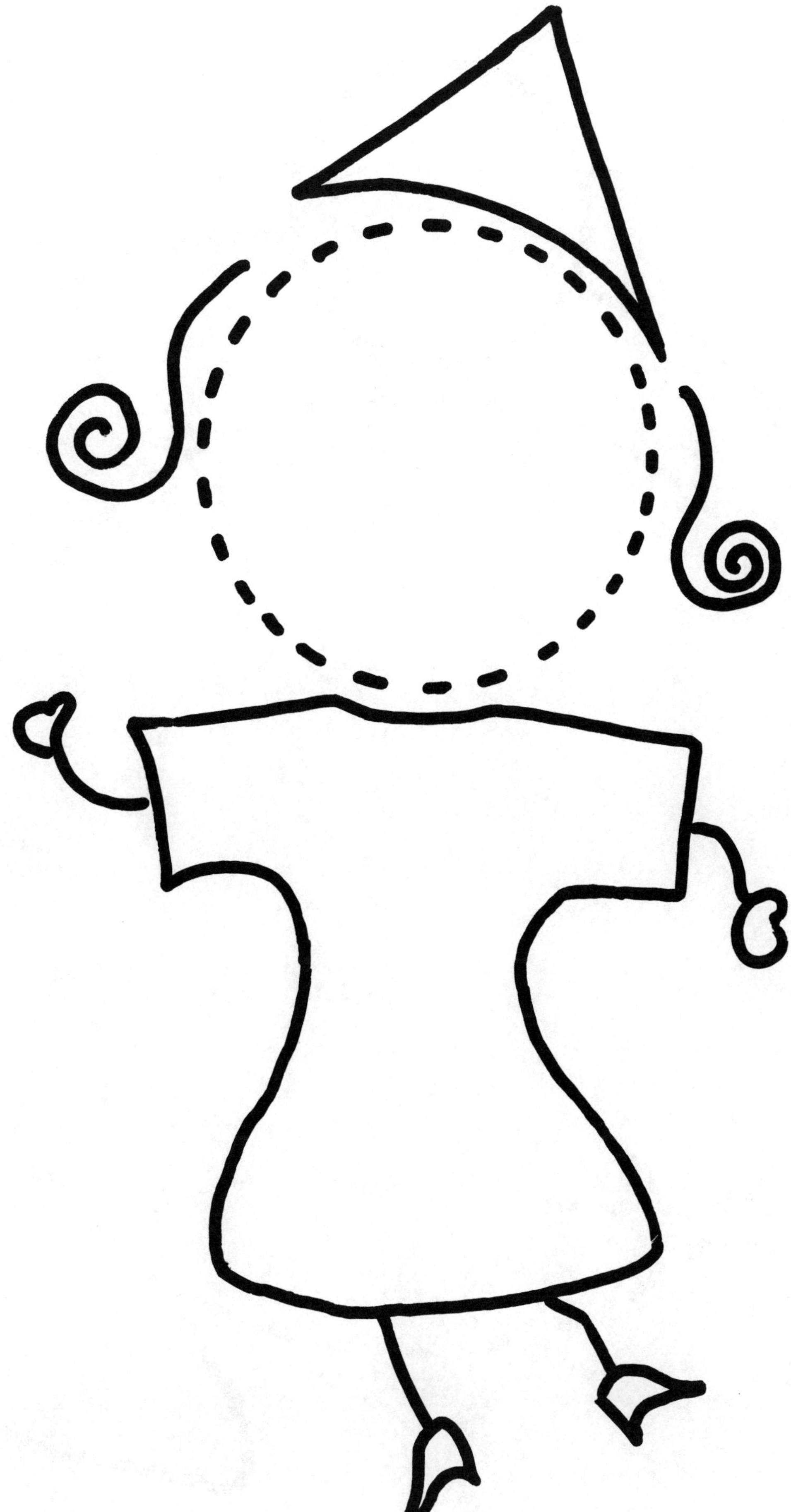

Step 1—Level #1 Worksheet

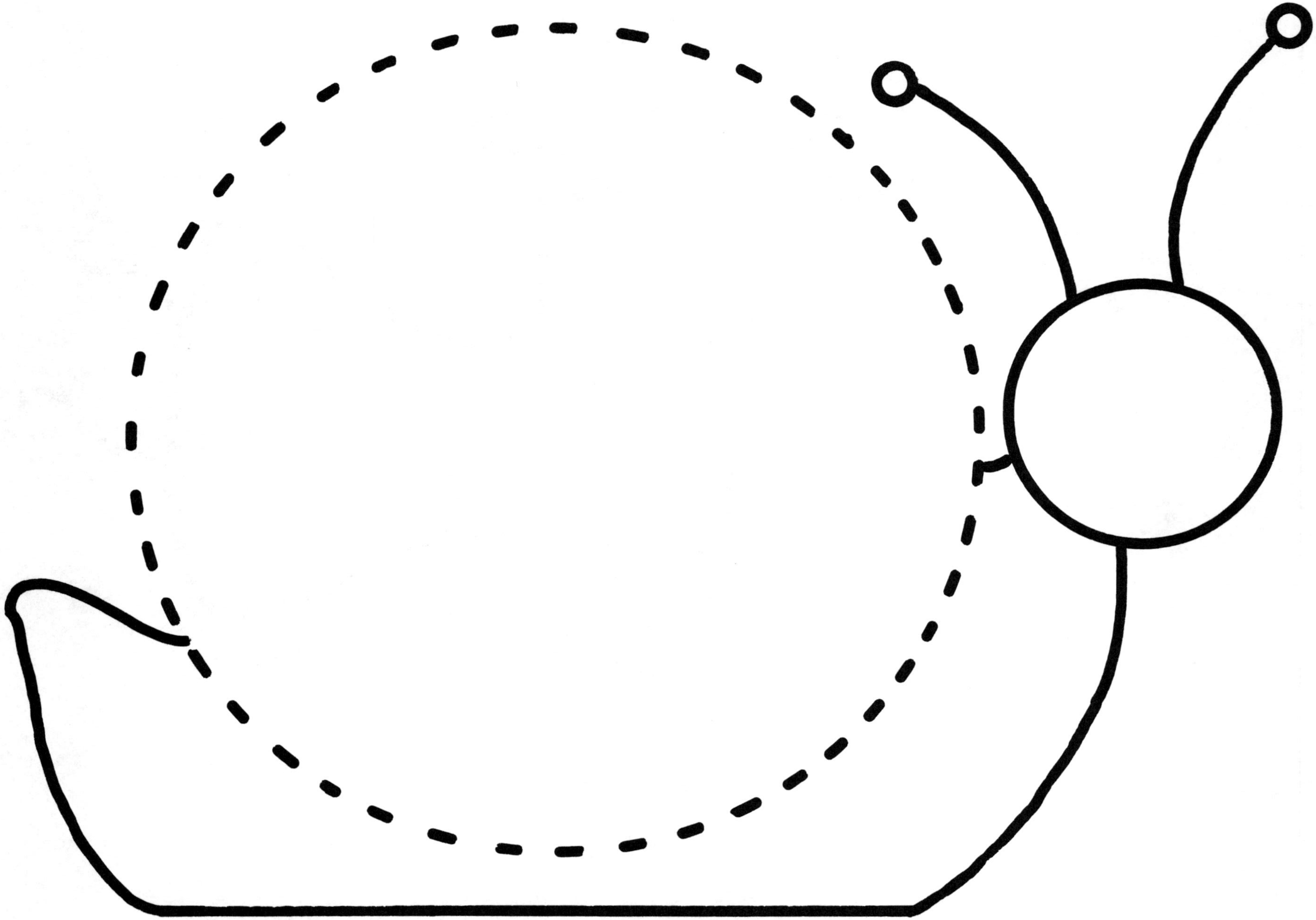

Step 1—Level #1 Worksheet

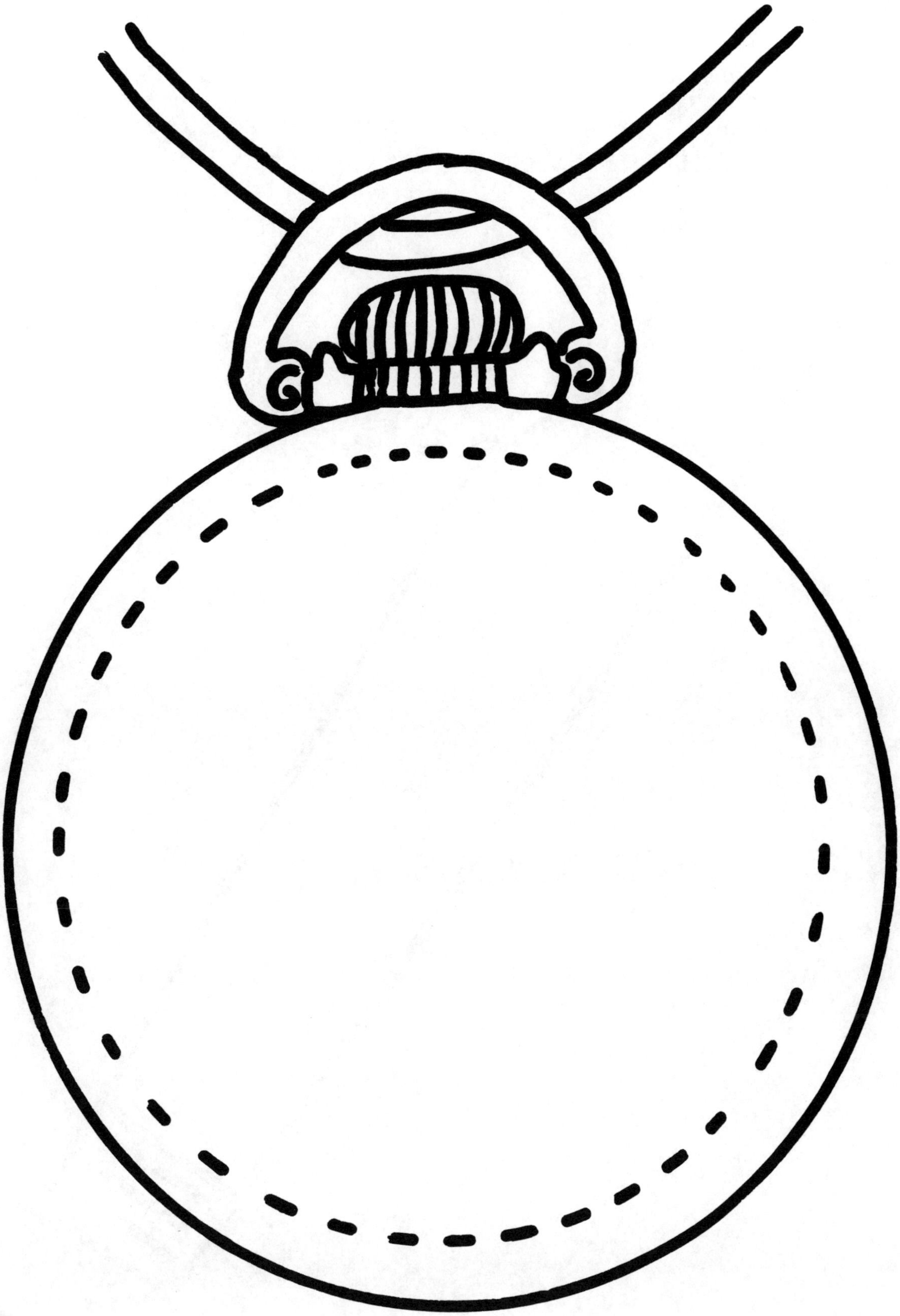

Step 1—Level #1 Worksheet

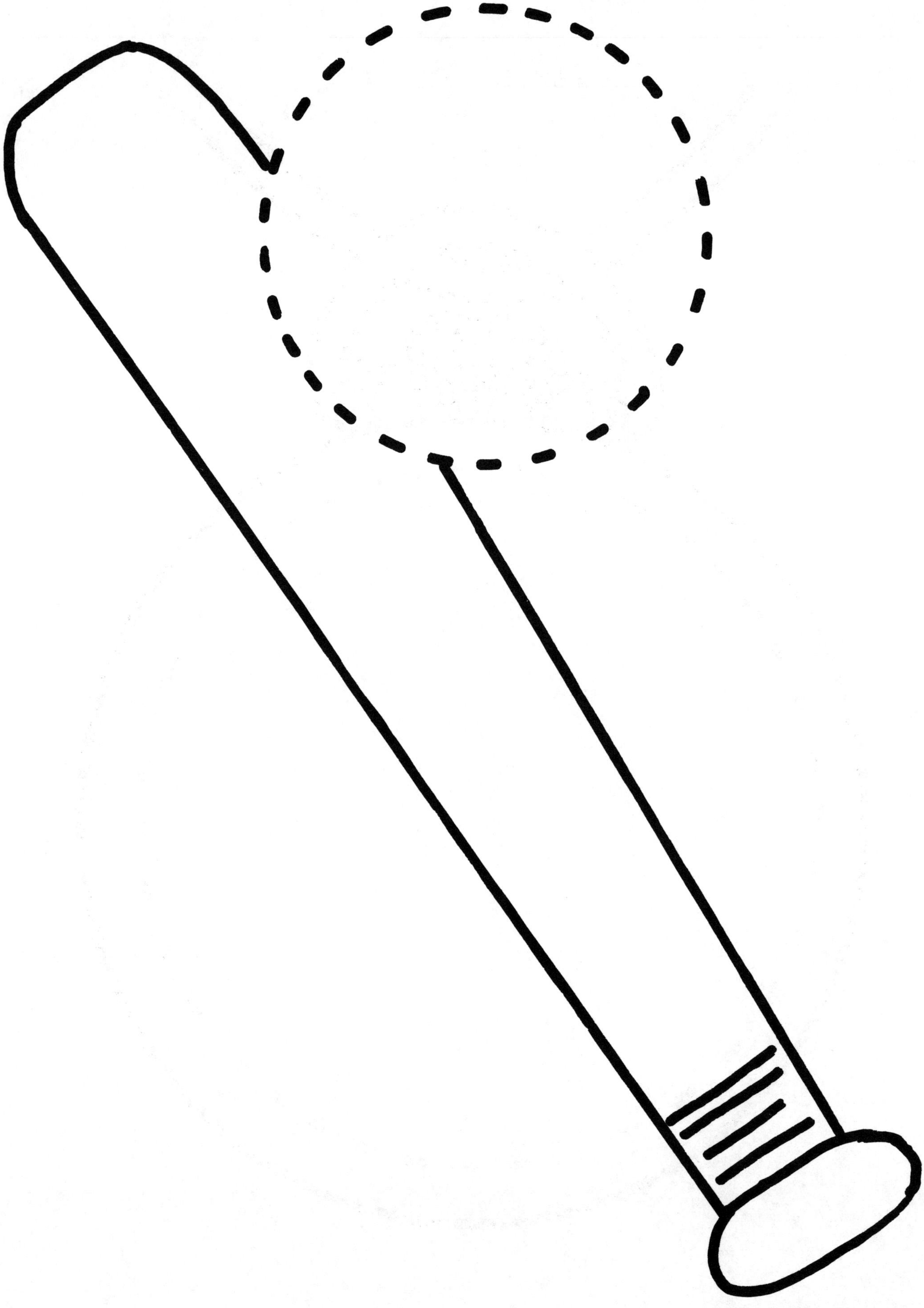

Step 1—Level #1 Worksheet

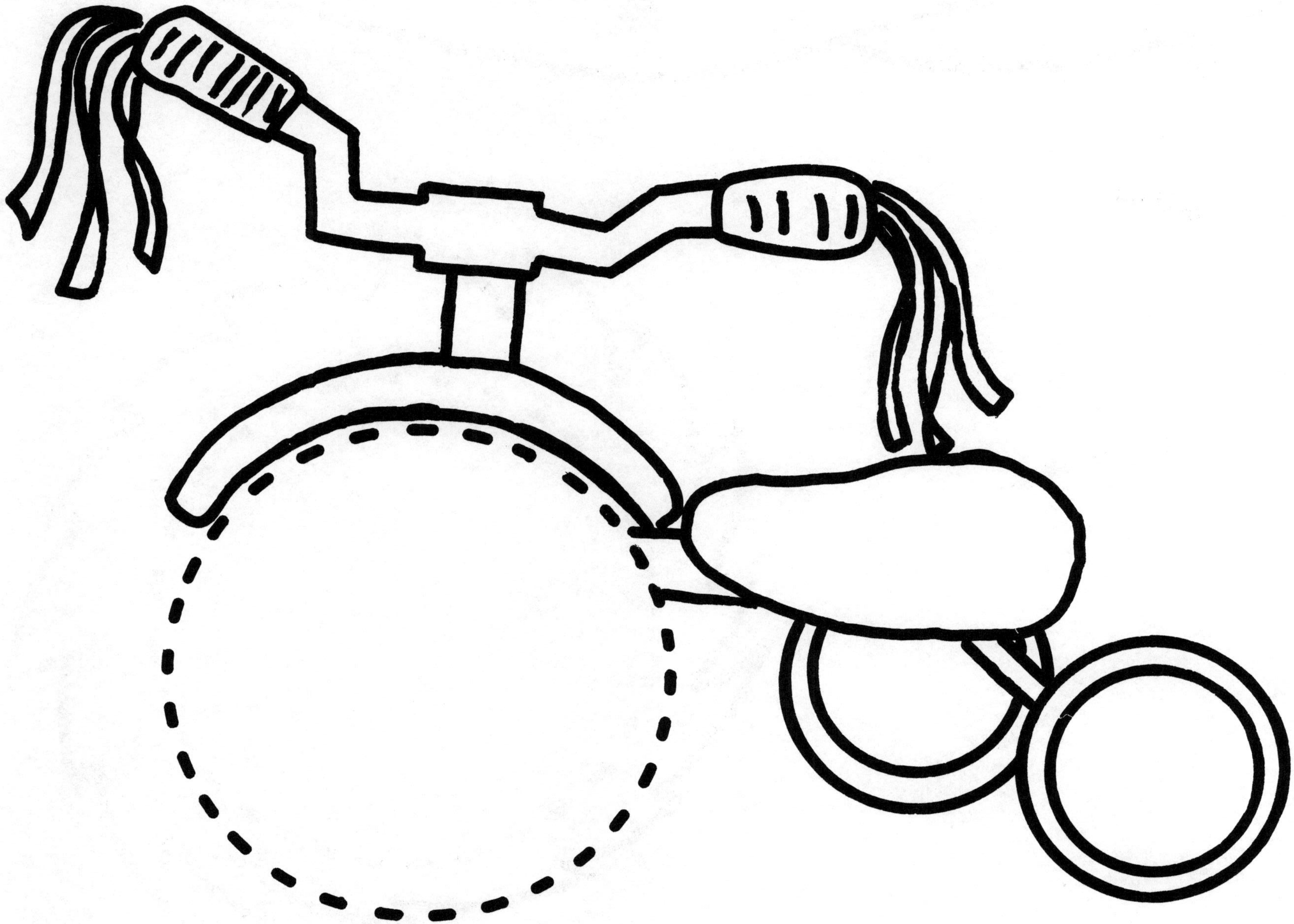

Step 1—Level #1 Worksheet

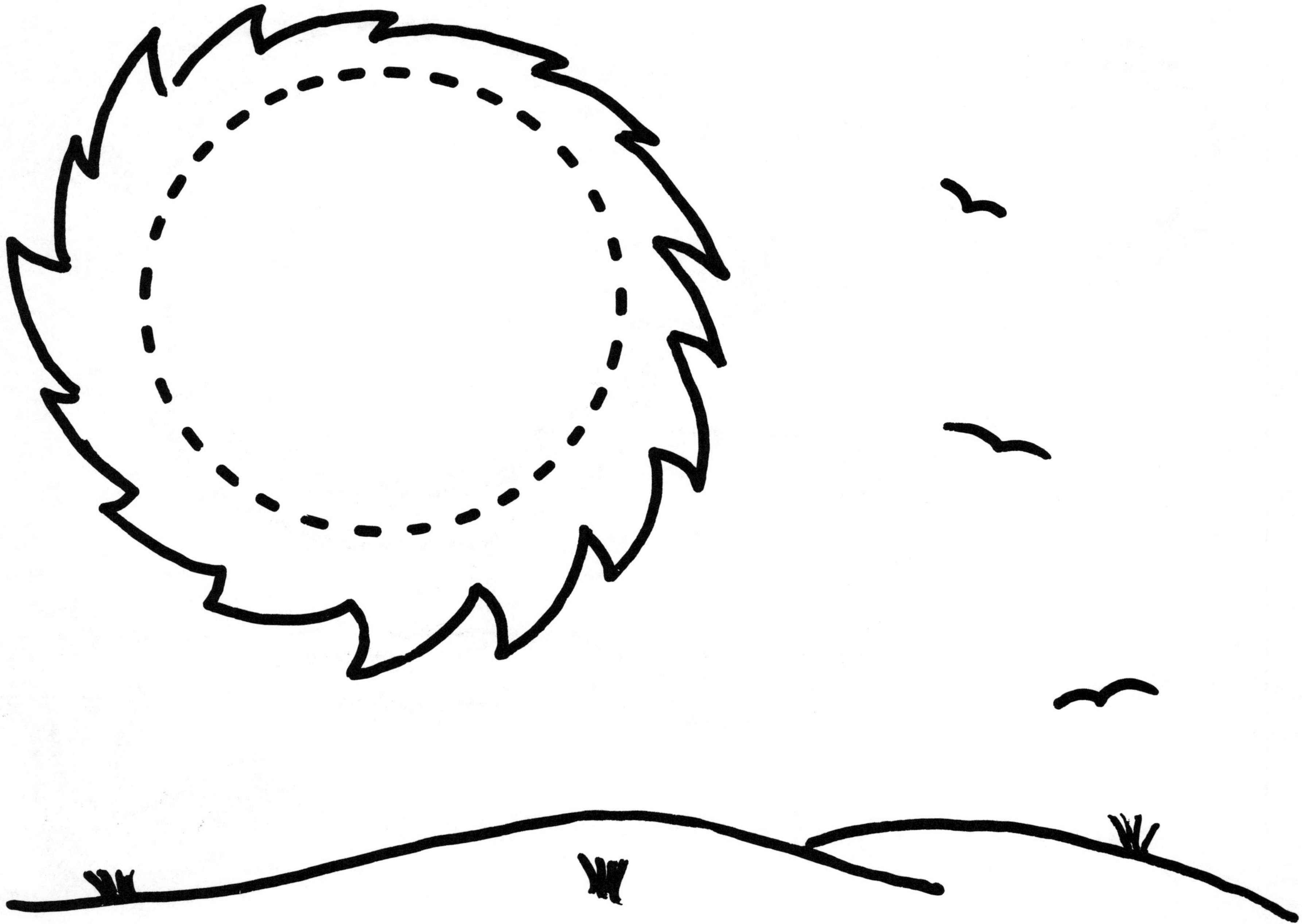

Skill 6
Step 1—Level #1 Pre/Posttest (shape person)

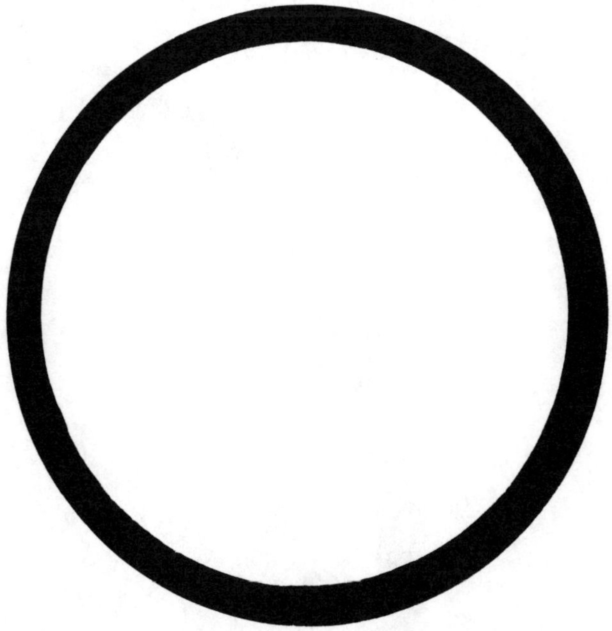

Skill 6
Step 1—Level #1 Worksheet (snail)

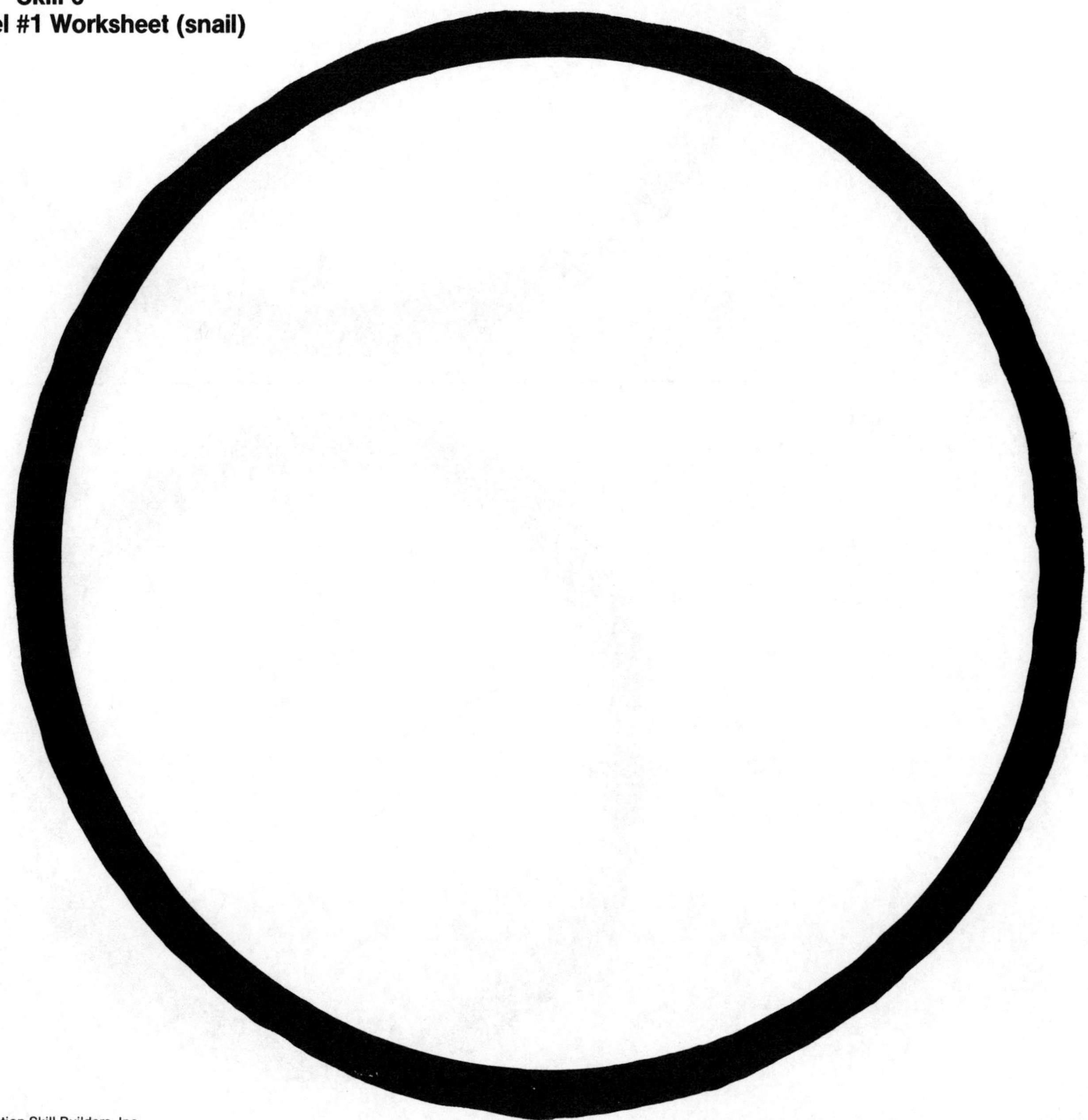

Skill 6
Step 1—Level #1 Worksheet (clock)

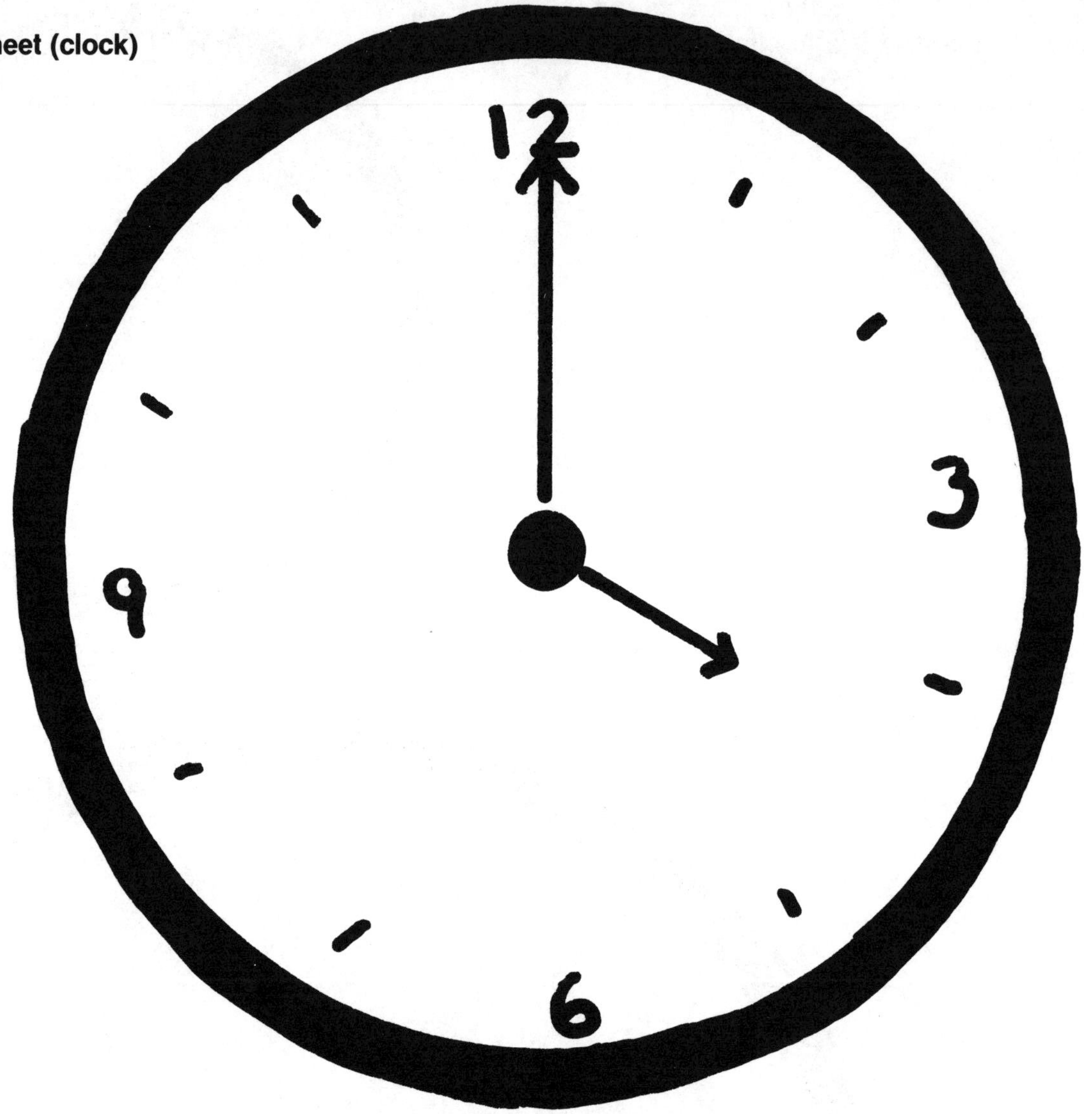

Skill 6
Step 1—Level #1 Worksheet (baseball)

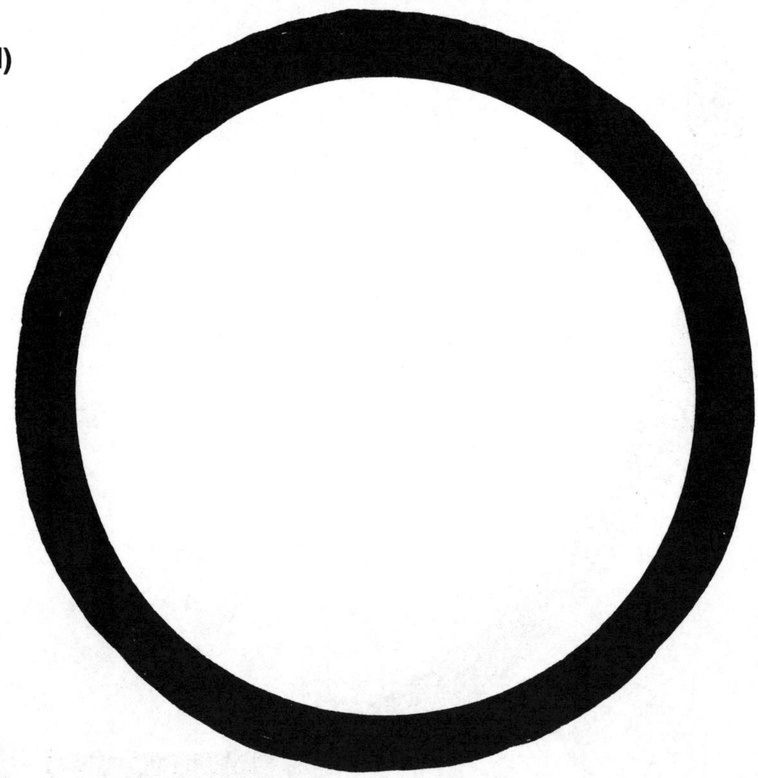

Skill 6
Step 1—Level #1 Worksheet (tricycle)

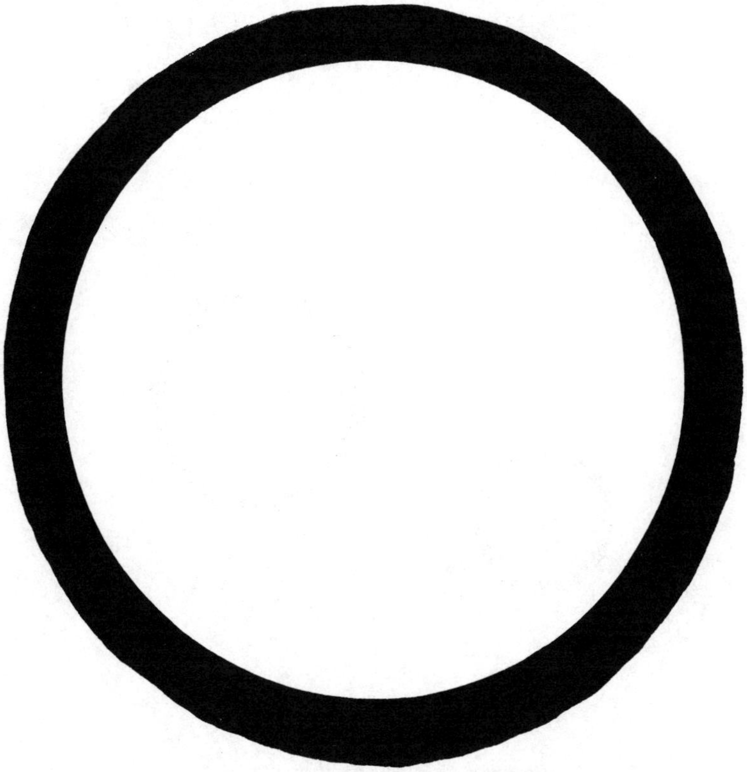

Skill 6
Step 1—Level #1 Worksheet (sun)

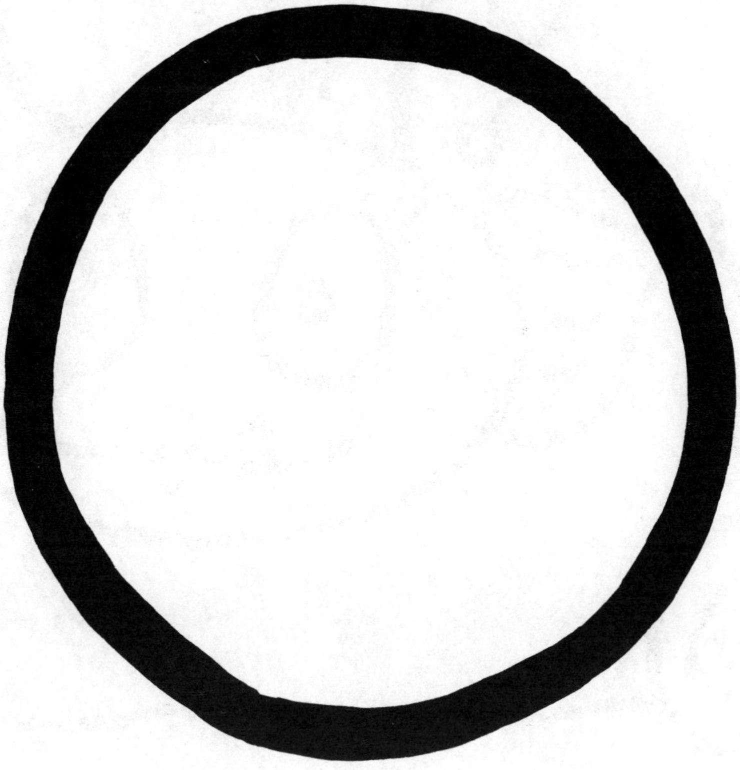

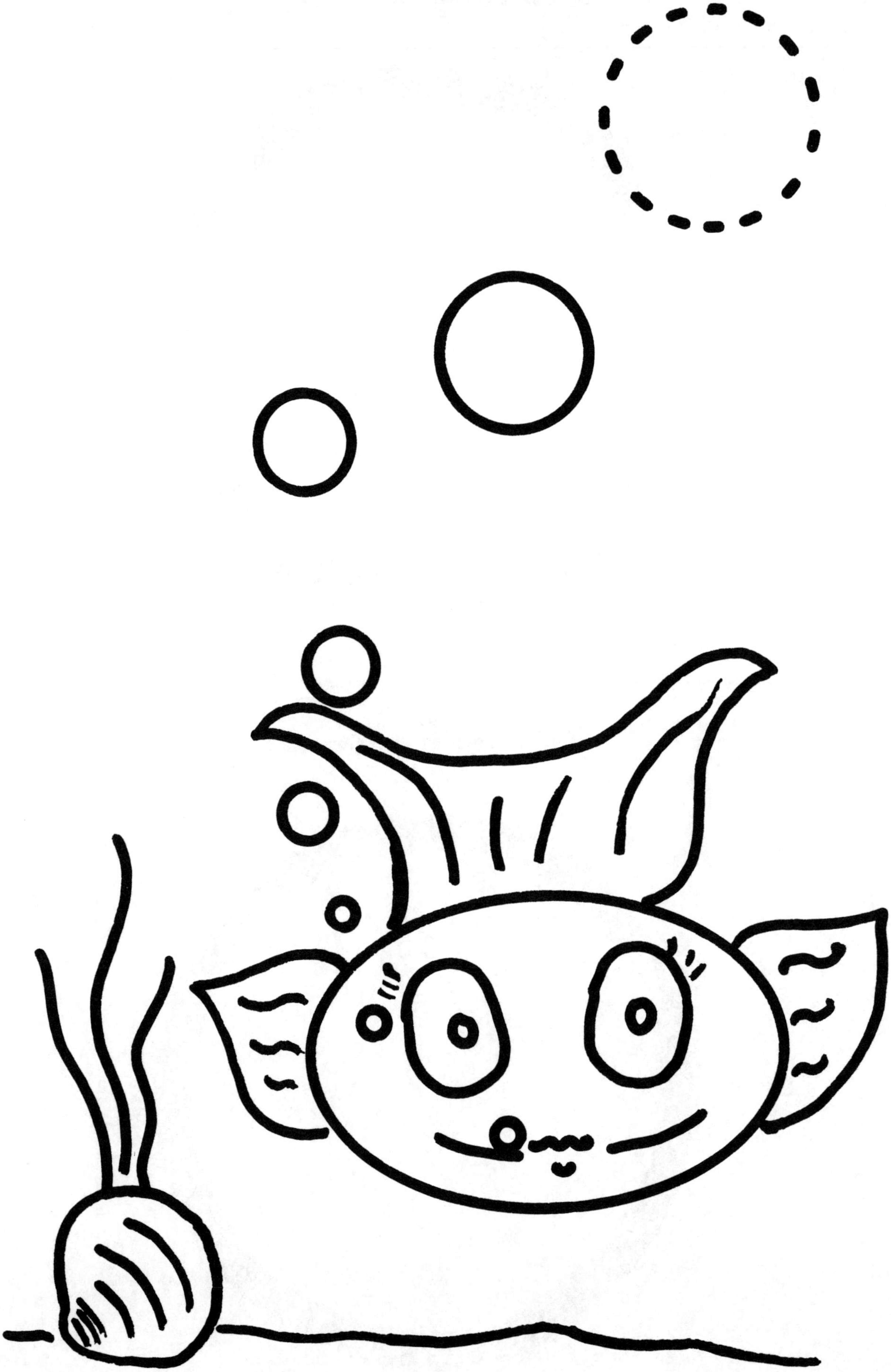

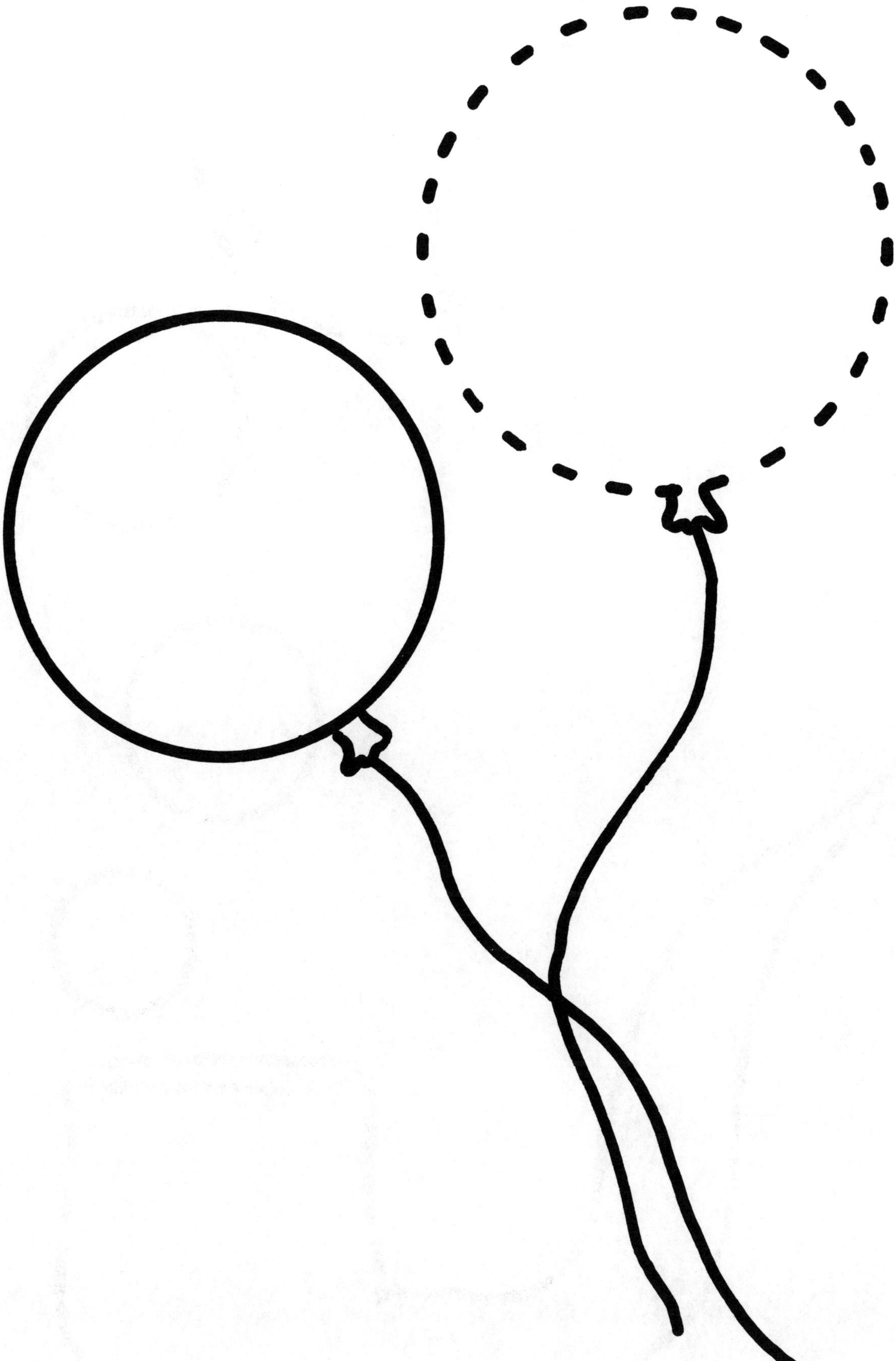

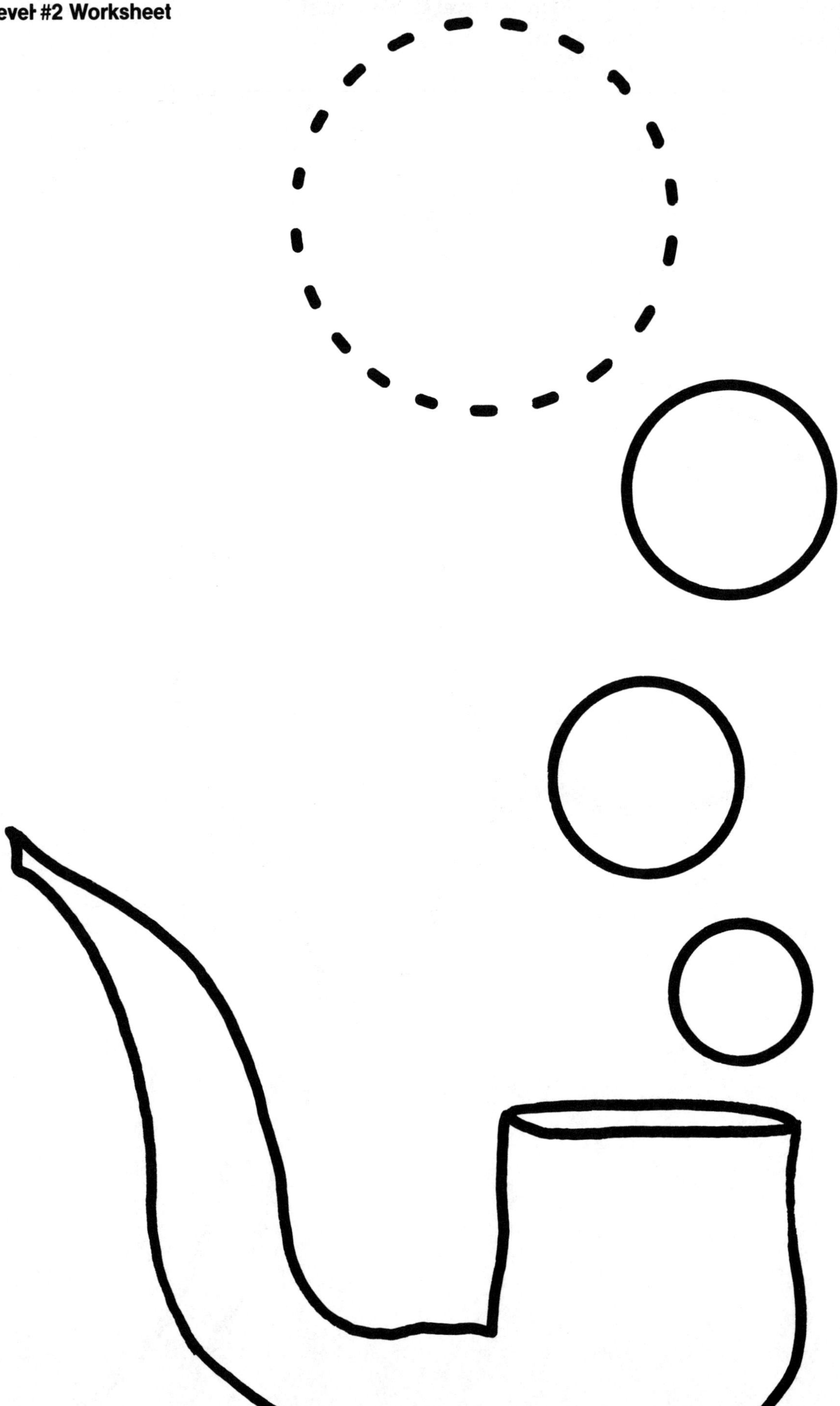

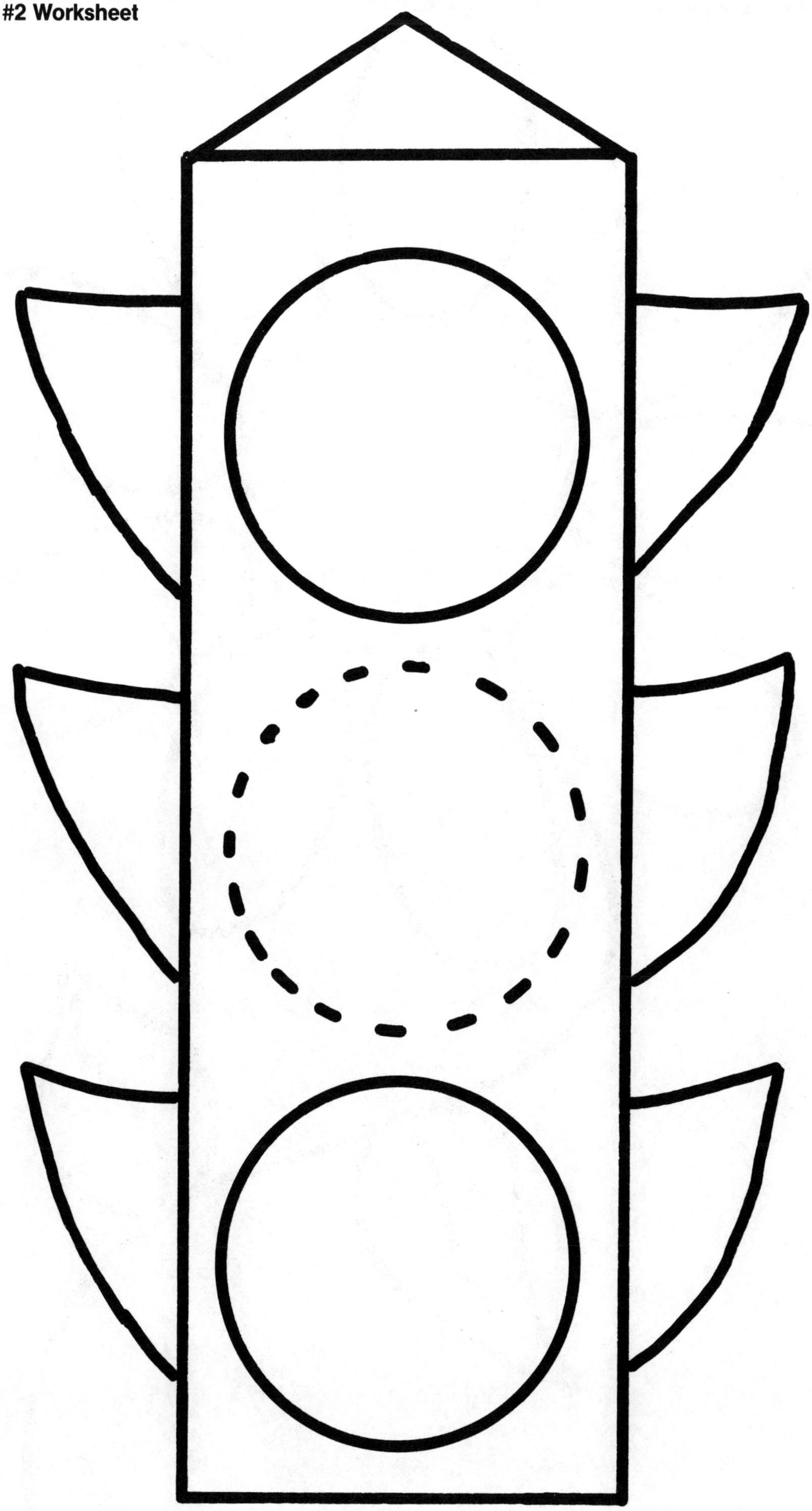

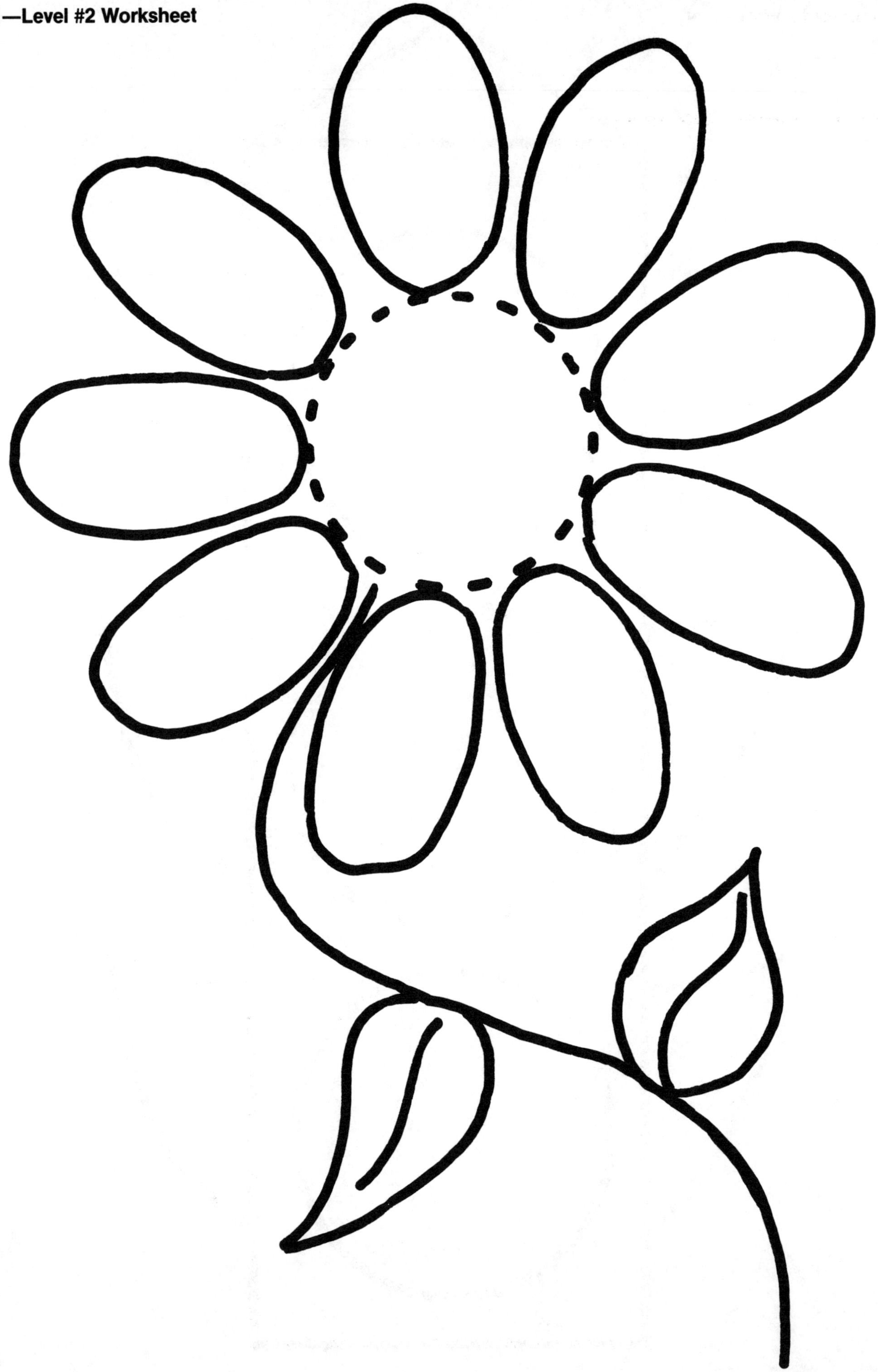

Skill 6
Step 1—Level #2 Pre/Posttest (fish with air bubble)

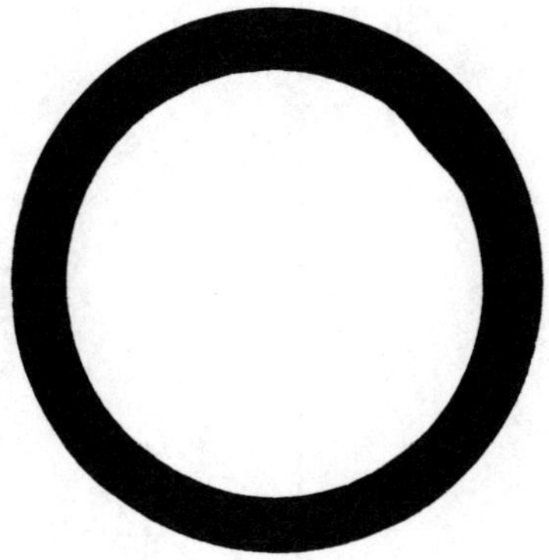

Skill 6
Step 1—Level #2 Worksheet (balloon)

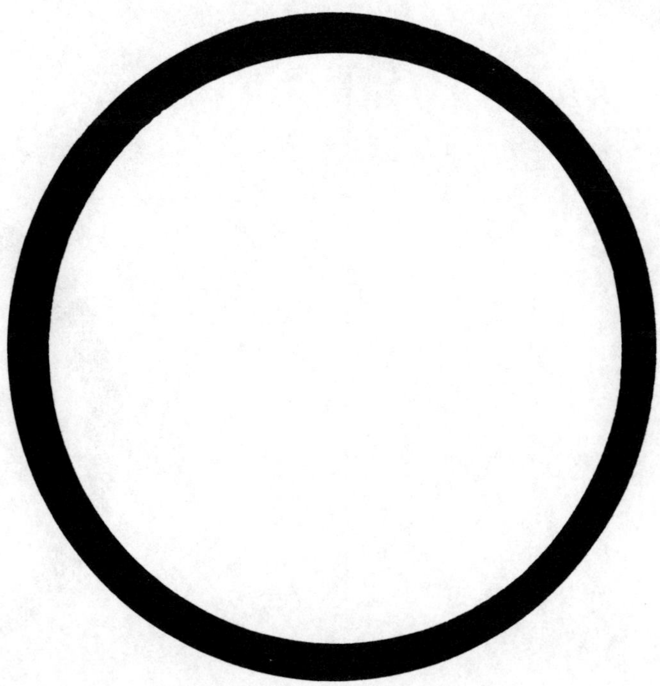

Skill 6
Step 1—Level #2 Worksheet (soap bubble)

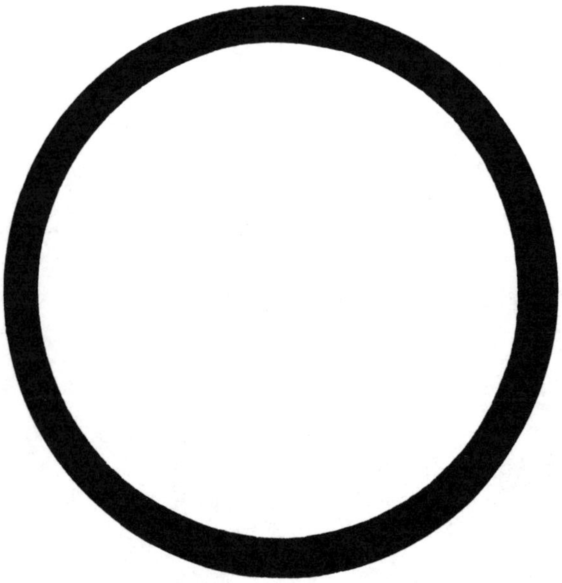

Skill 6
Step 1—Level #2 Worksheet (traffic signal)

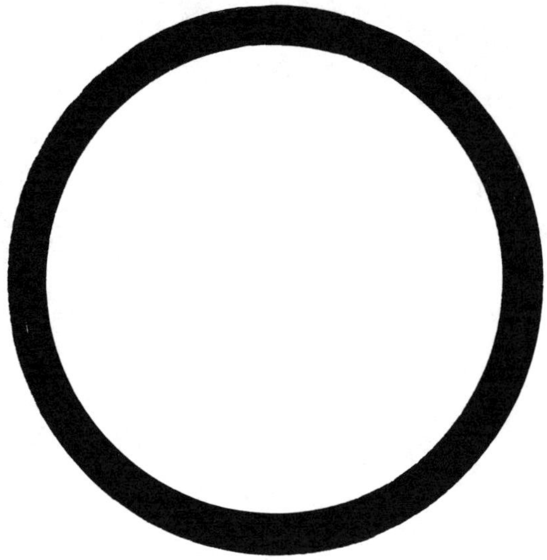

Skill 6
Step 1—Level #2 Worksheet (flower)

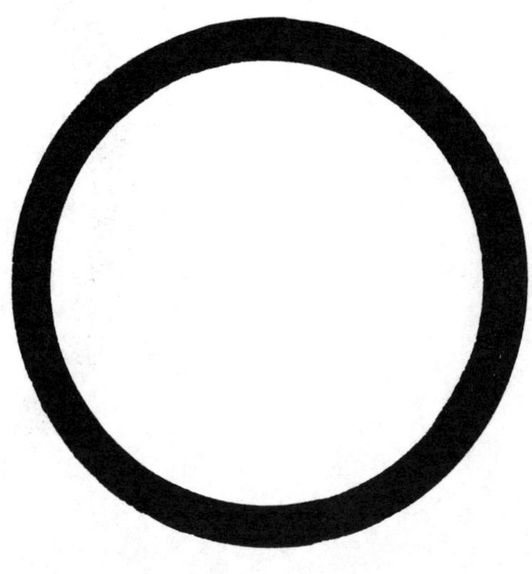

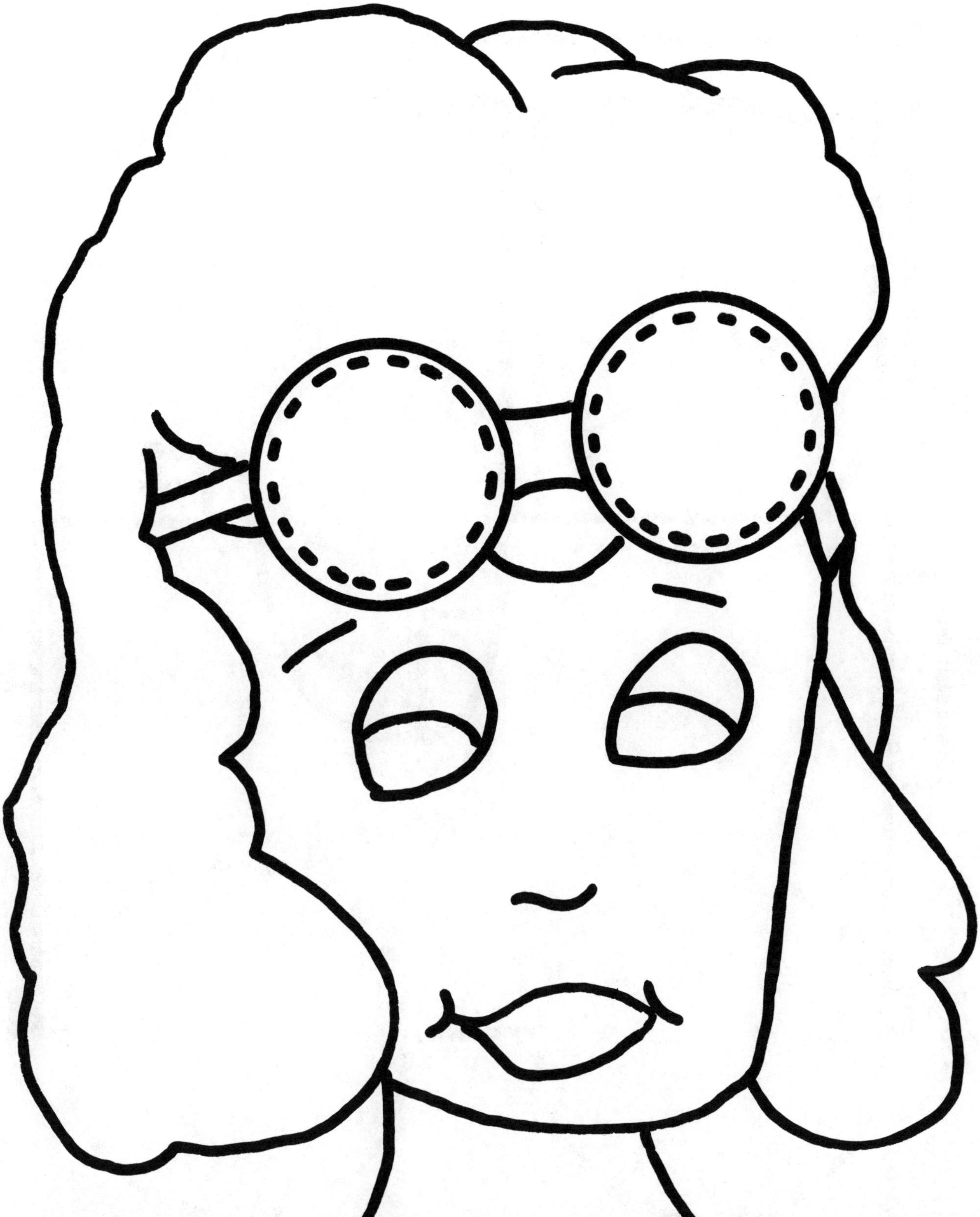

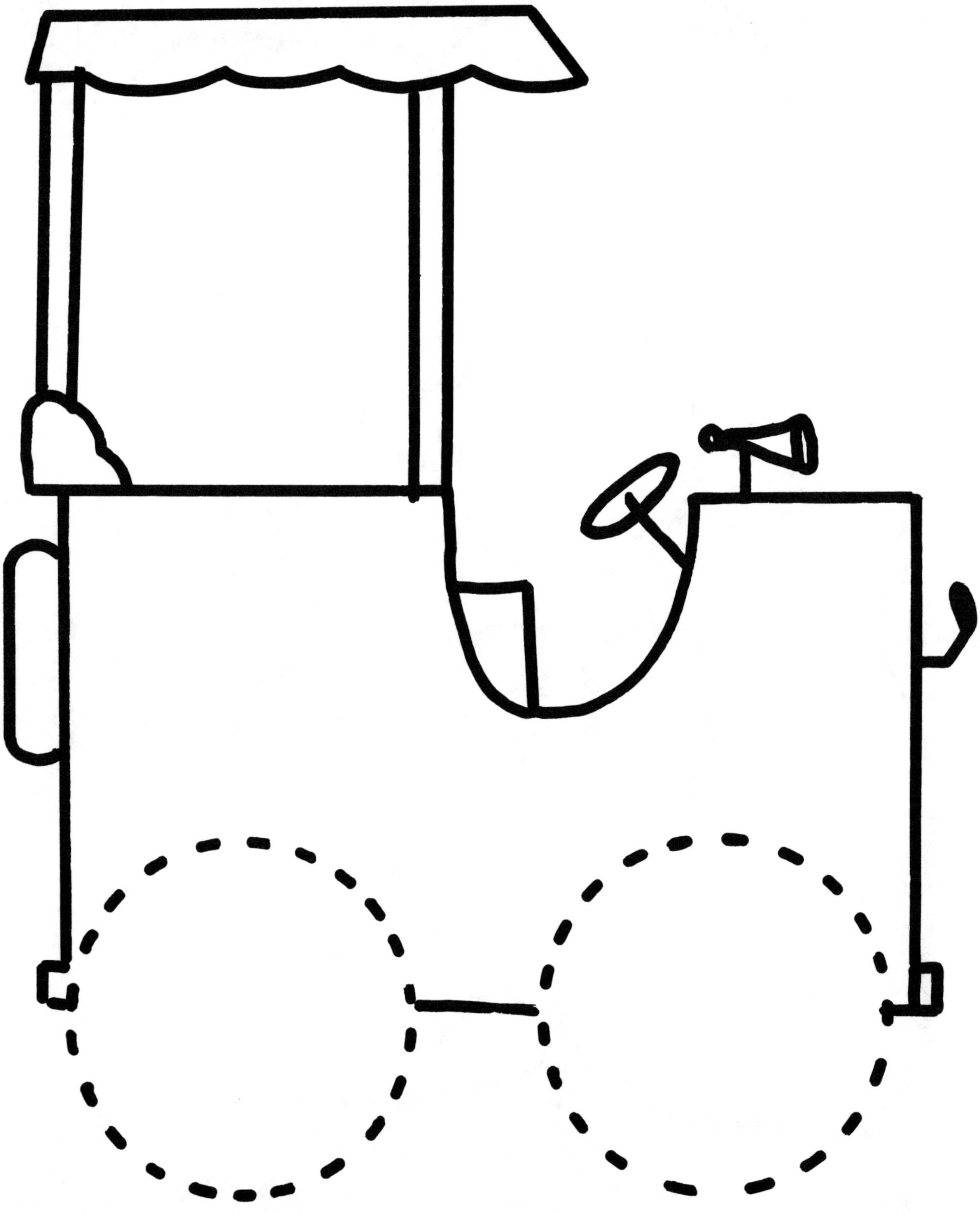

Step 1—Level #3 Worksheet

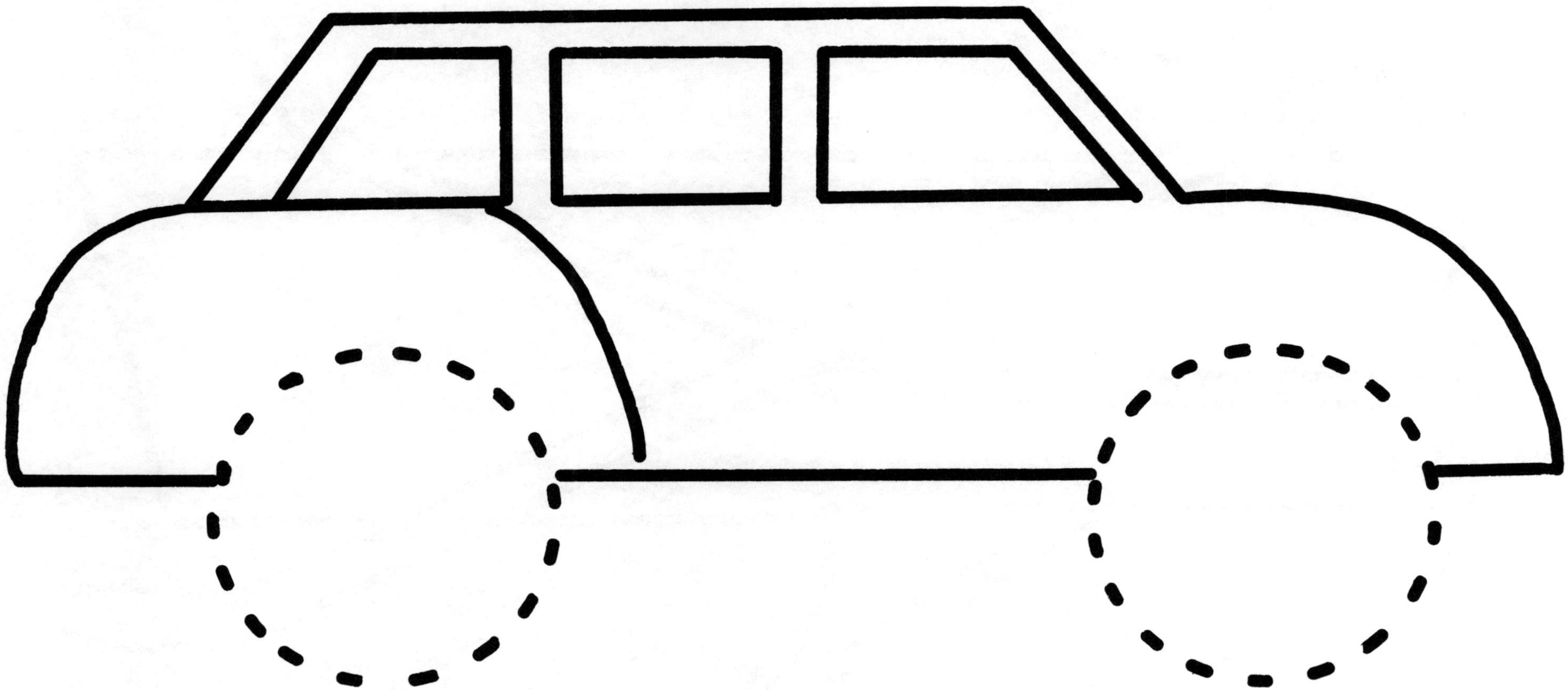

Step 1—Level #3 Worksheet

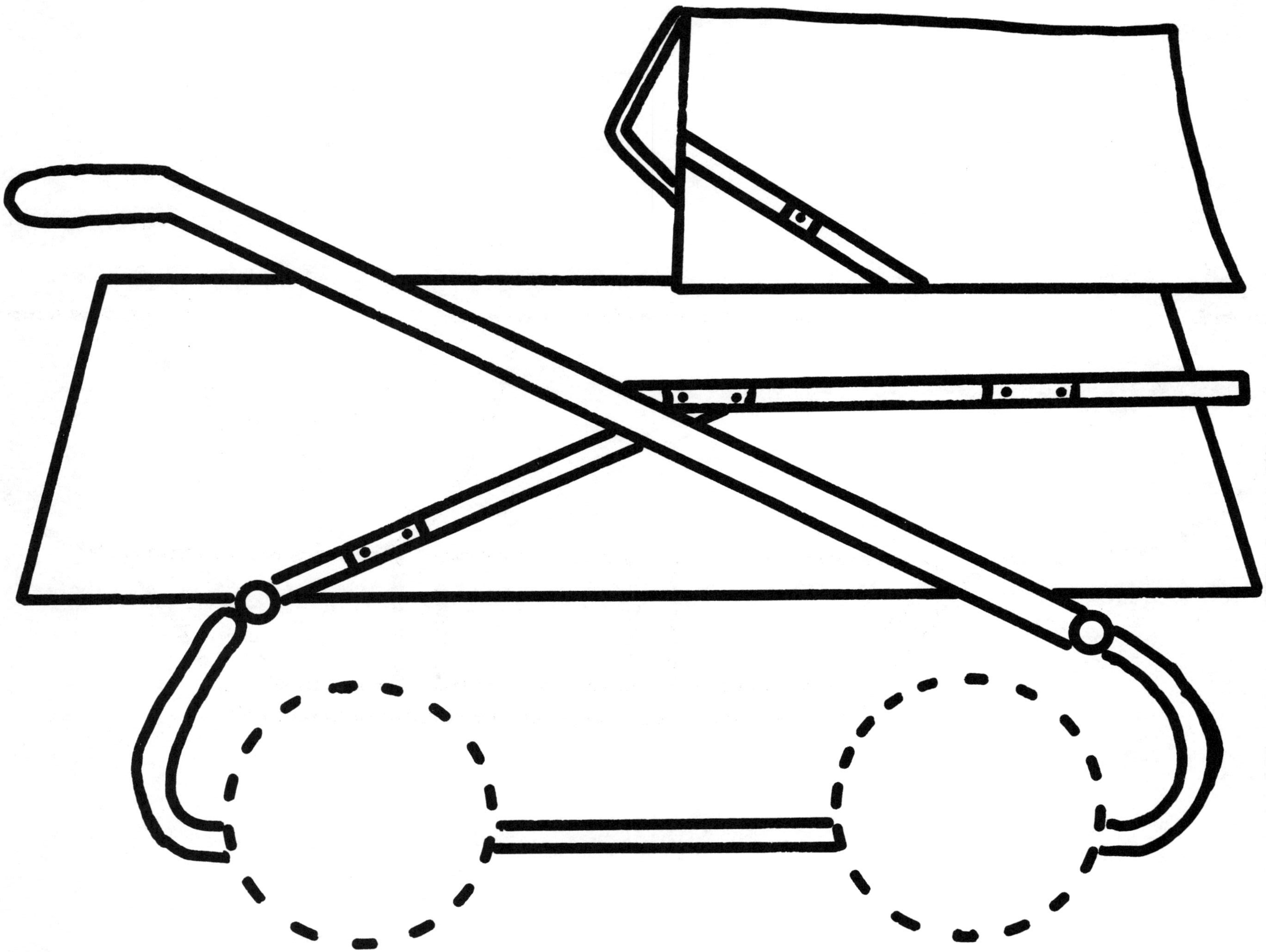

Skill 6
Step 1—Level #3 Pre/Posttest (sunglasses)

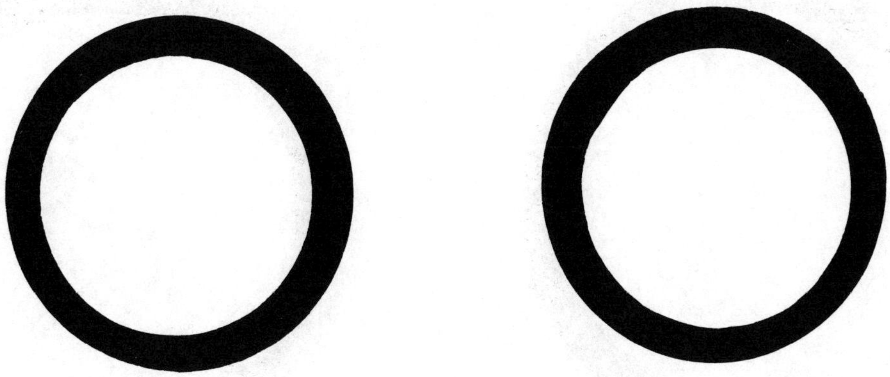

Skill 6
Step 1—Level #3 Worksheet (golf cart)

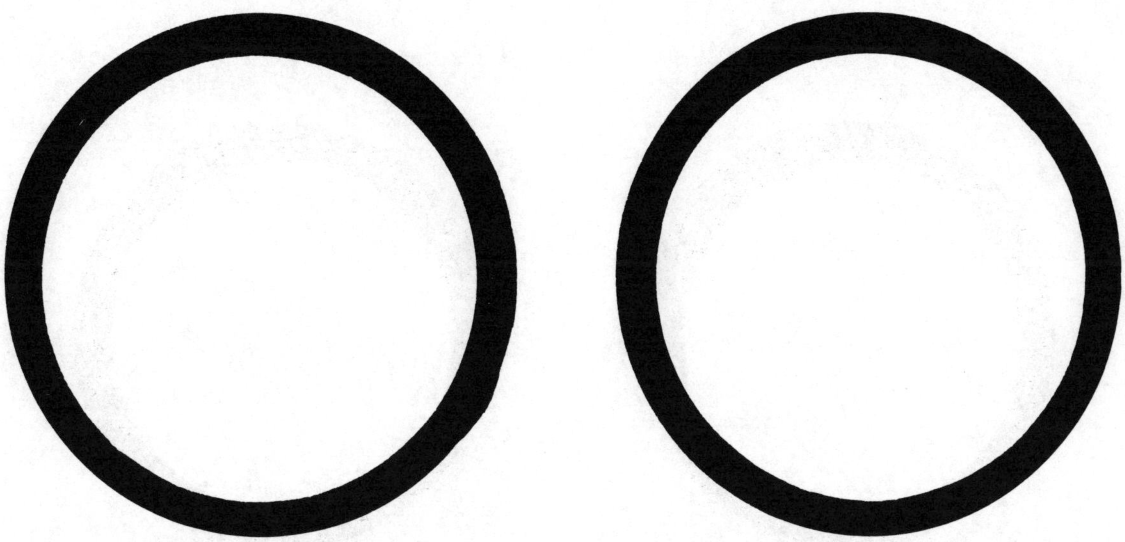

Skill 6
Step 1—Level #3 Worksheet (car)

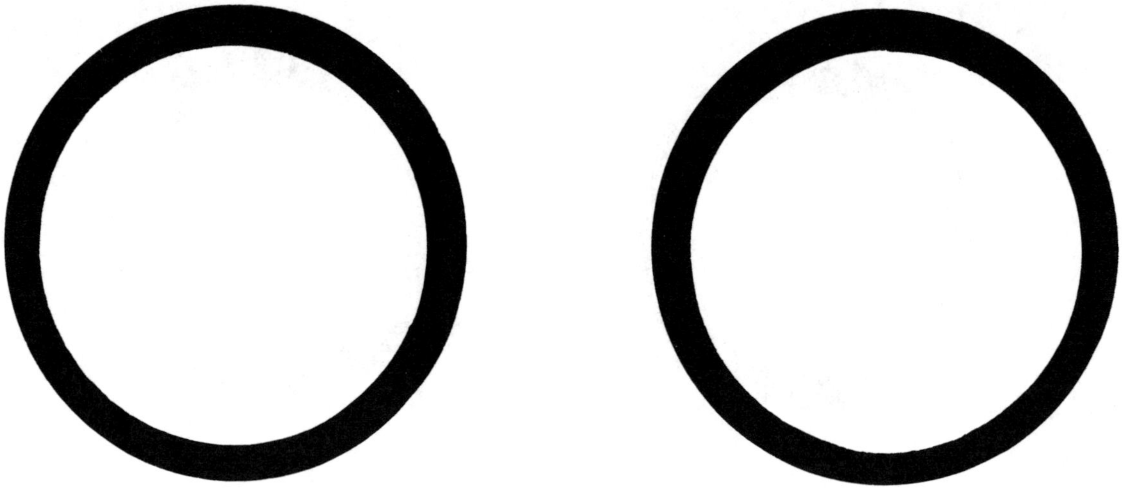

Skill 6
Step 1—Level #3 Worksheet (baby carriage)

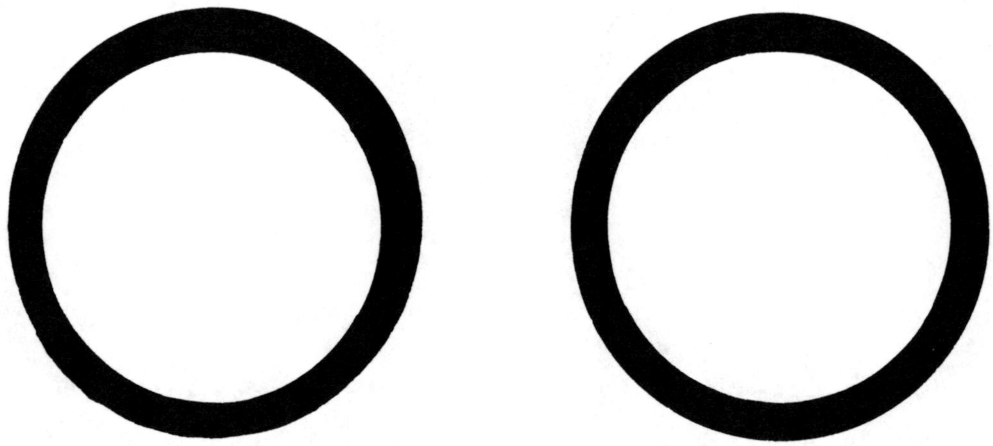

SKILL 6—STEP 2—OVALS

Level #1—Ovals
Pretest: Student takes Level #1 Pretest (cattail plant—3″ oval).

If criterion met: Student advances to Level #2.

If criterion not met:

1. Student cuts Level #1 worksheets:
   clown with balloon—4″
   egg—4″
   mirror—4″
   garbage can cover—4″
2. Student takes Level #1 Posttest (cattail plant).
   If criterion met: Student advances to Level #2.
   If criterion not met: Student repeats Level #1 worksheets and Posttest.

Level #2—Smaller Ovals, 1/4″ wide line
Pretest: Student takes Level #1 Pretest (flower petal—2 1/4″ oval).

If criterion met: Student advances to Step 3—Crescents.

If criterion not met:

1. Student cuts Level #2 worksheets:
   paint palette—3″
   pig snout—3″
   apple leaf—2 1/2″
   teddy bear's foot—2 1/2″
2. Student takes Level #2 Posttest (flower petal).
   If criterion met: Student advances to Step 3—Crescents.
   If criterion not met: Student repeats Level #2 worksheets and Posttest.

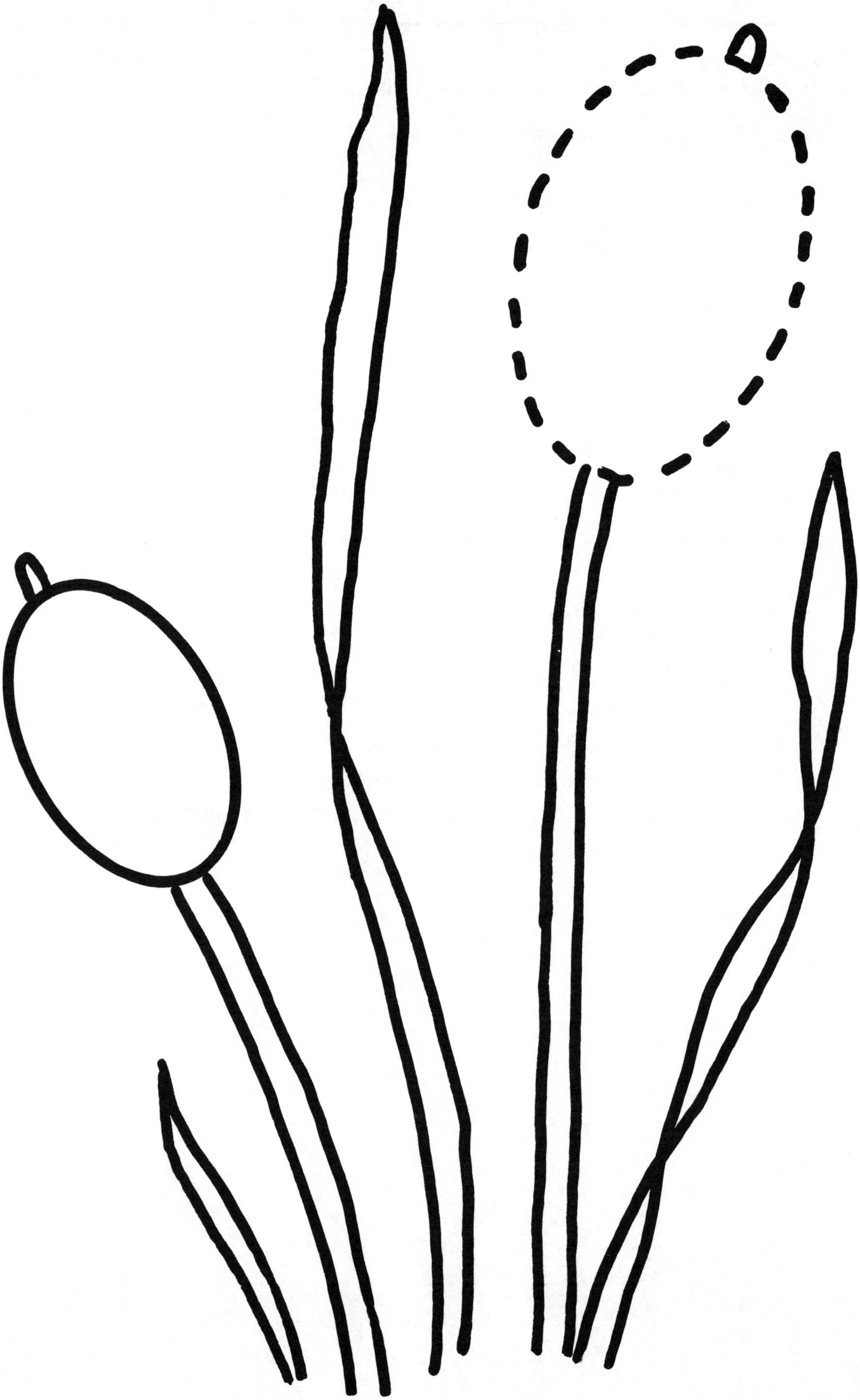

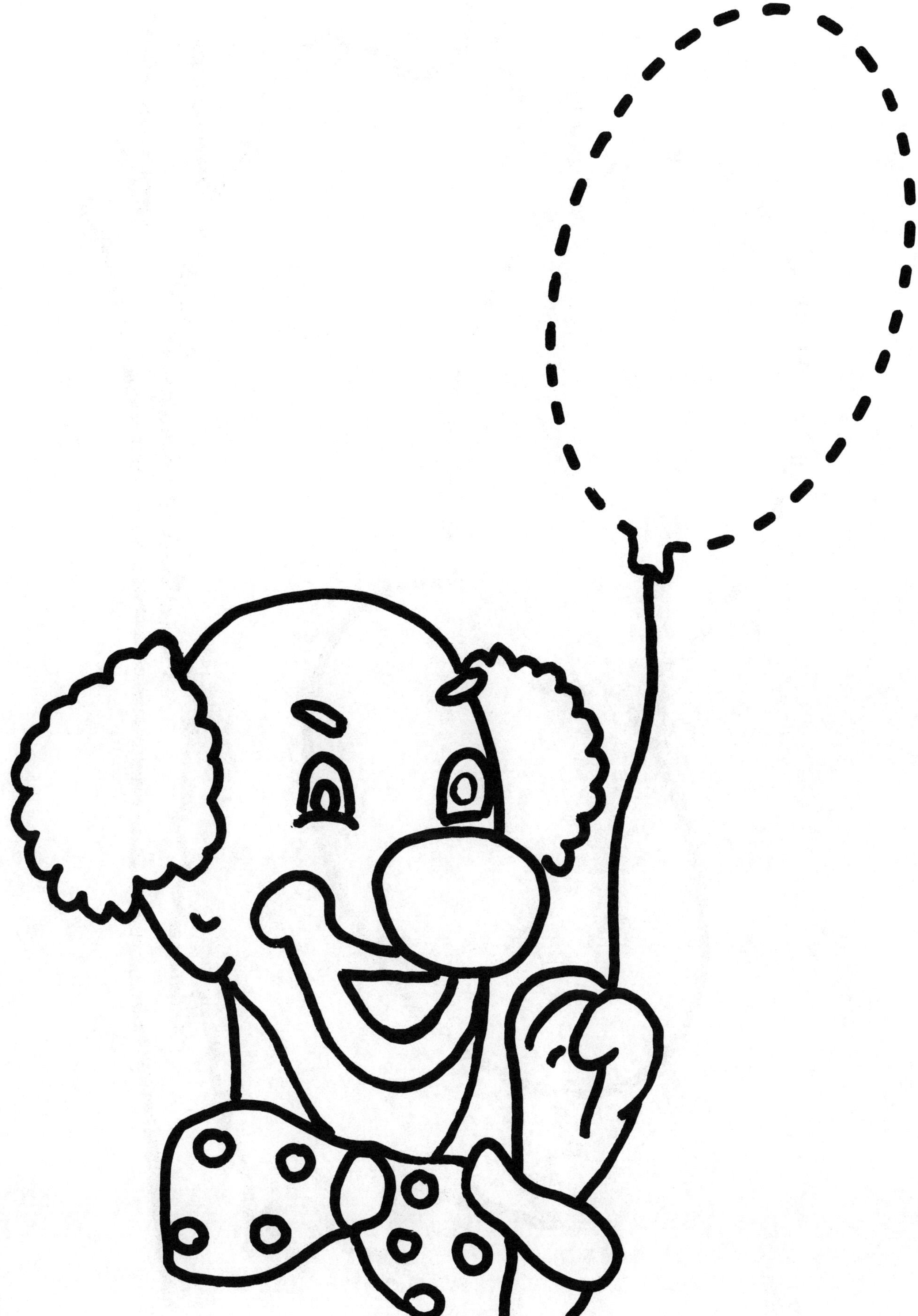

Step 2—Level #1 Worksheet

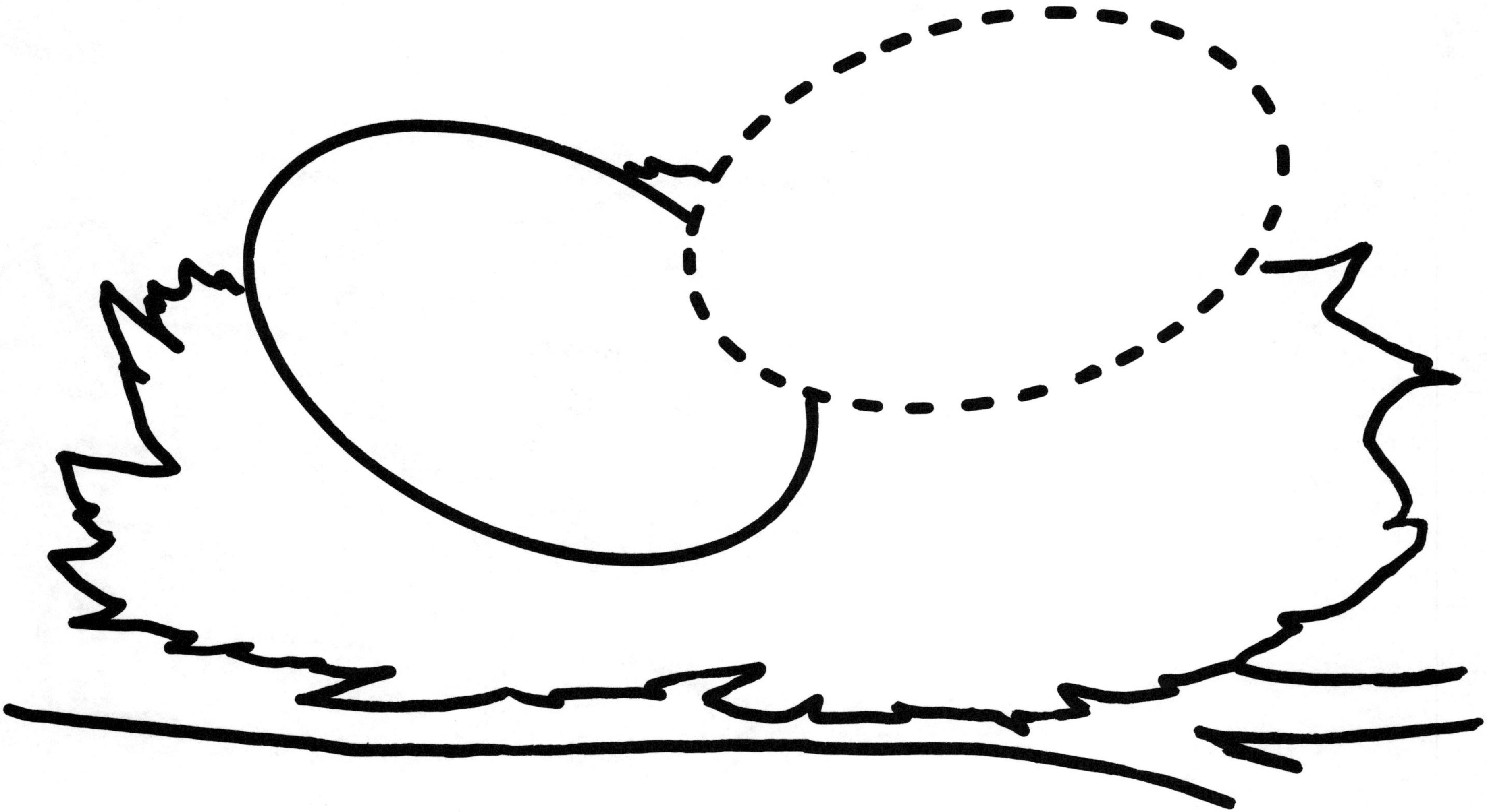

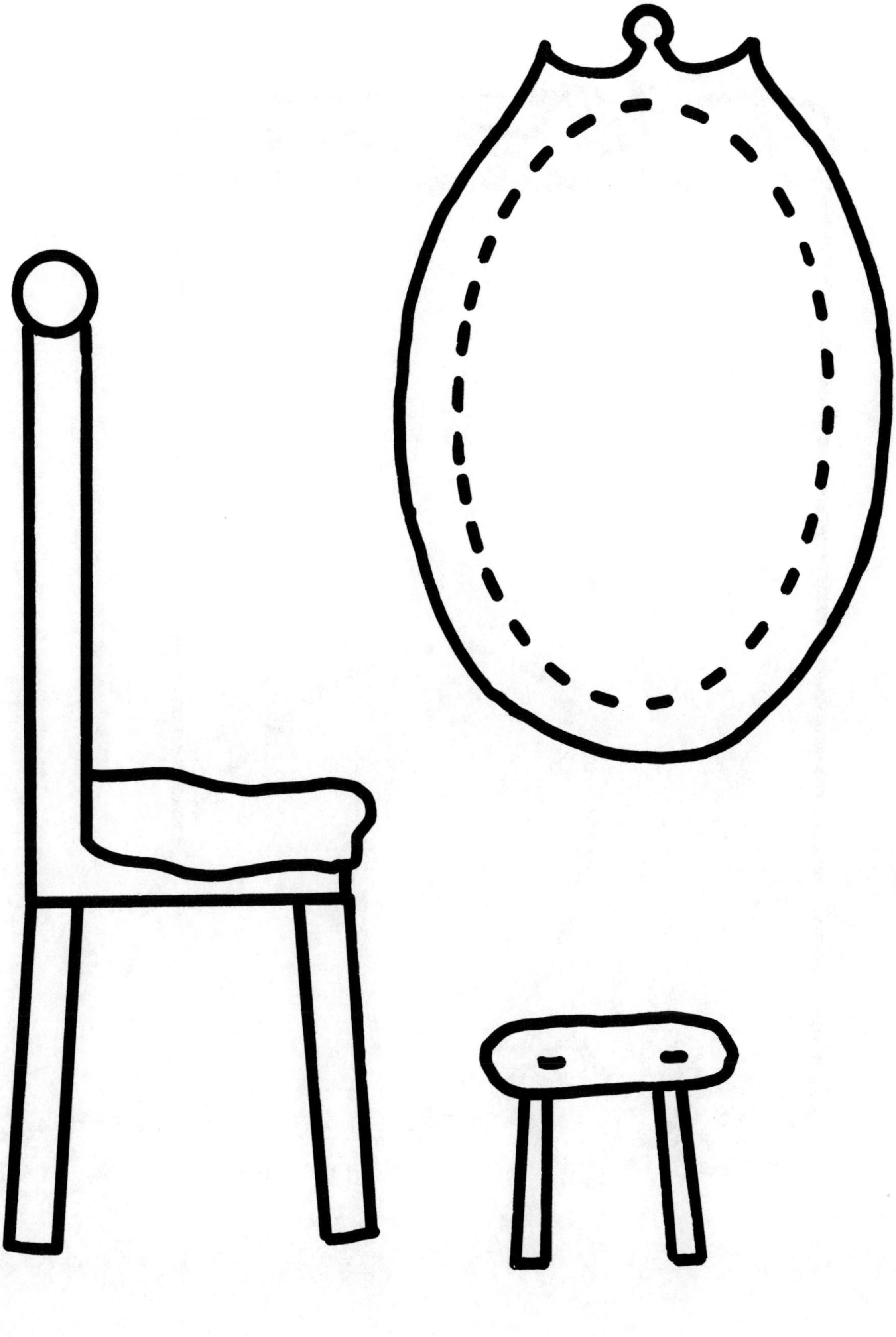

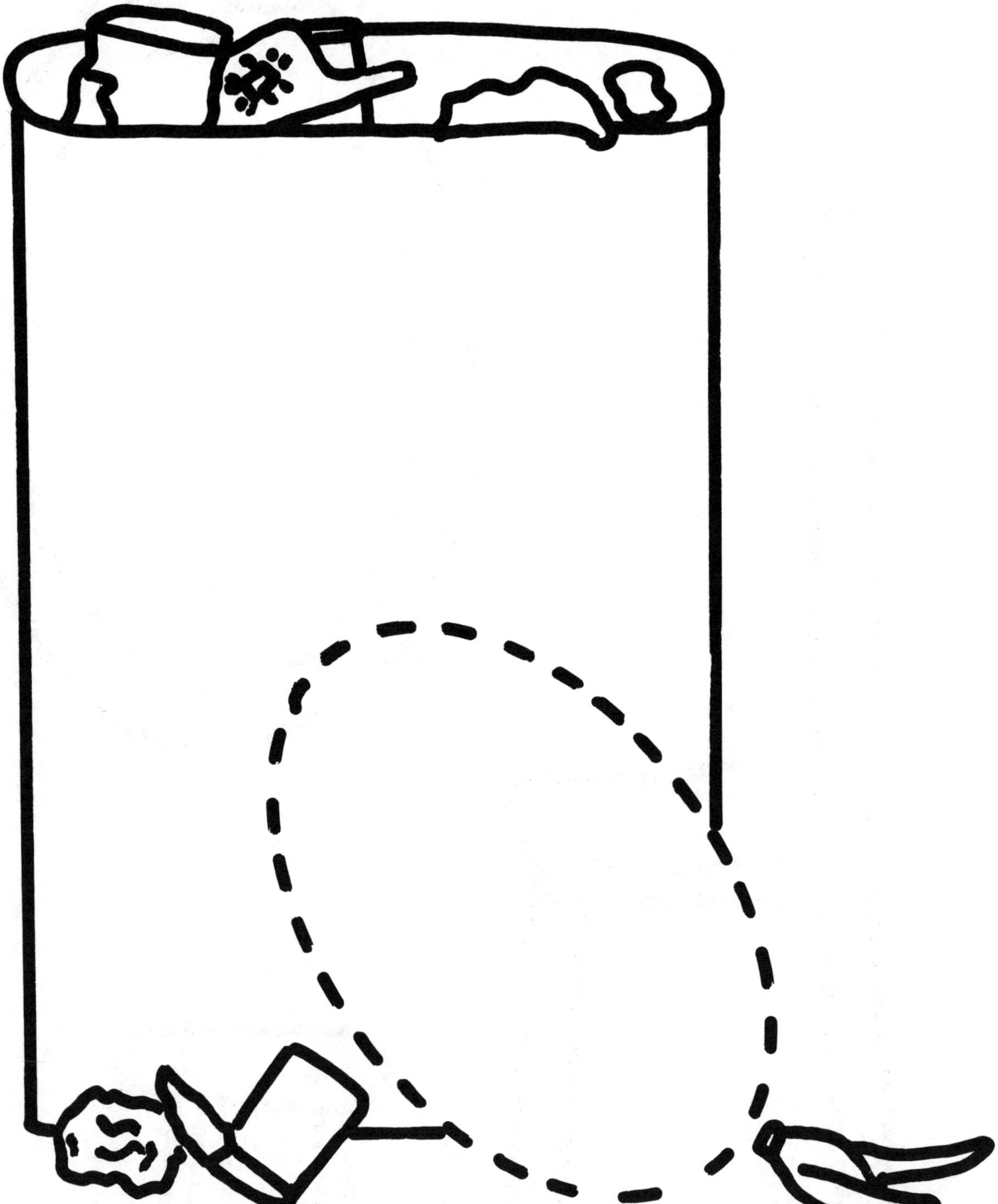

Skill 6
Step 2—Level #1 Pre/Posttest (cattail plant)

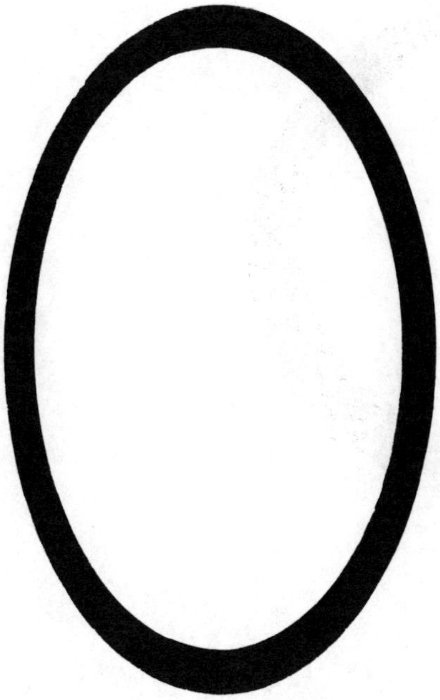

Skill 6
Step 2—Level #1 Worksheet (clown with balloon)

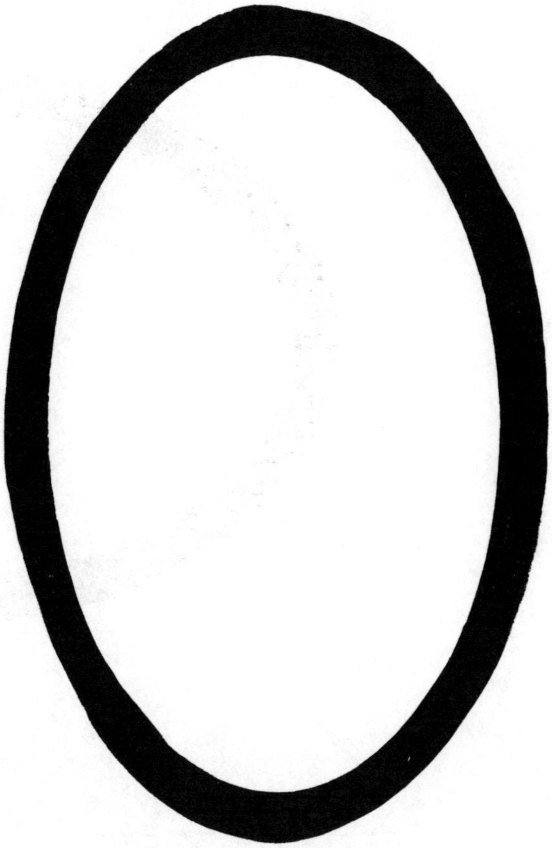

Skill 6
Step 2—Level #1 Worksheet (egg)

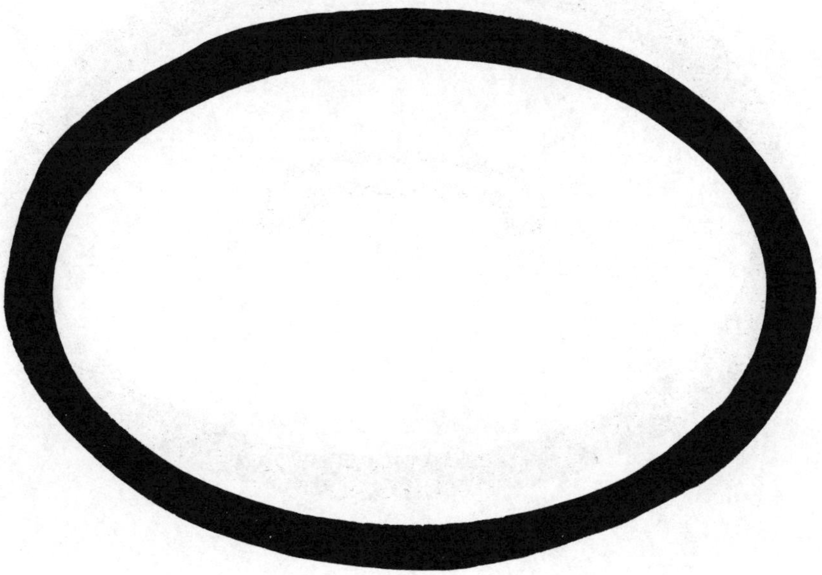

Skill 6
Step 2—Level #1 Worksheet (mirror)

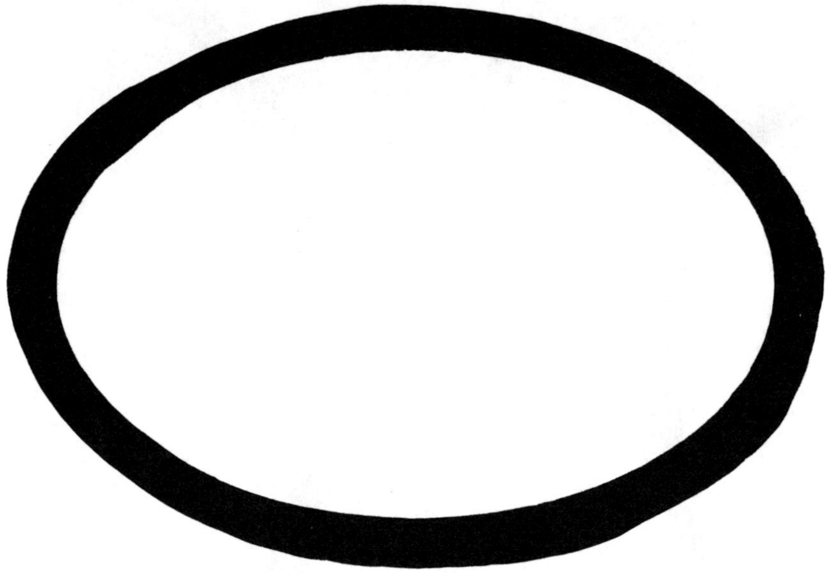

Skill 6
Step 2—Level #1 Worksheet (garbage can cover)

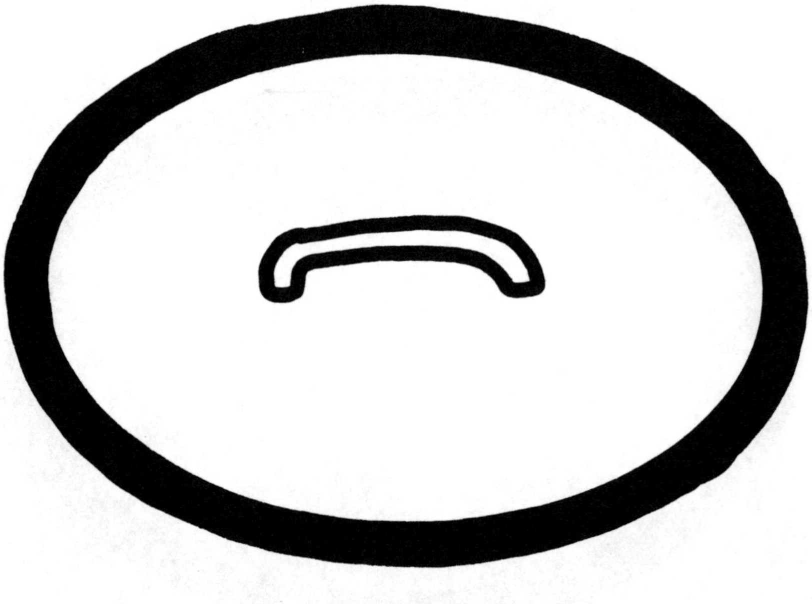

Step 2—Level #2 Pre/Posttest

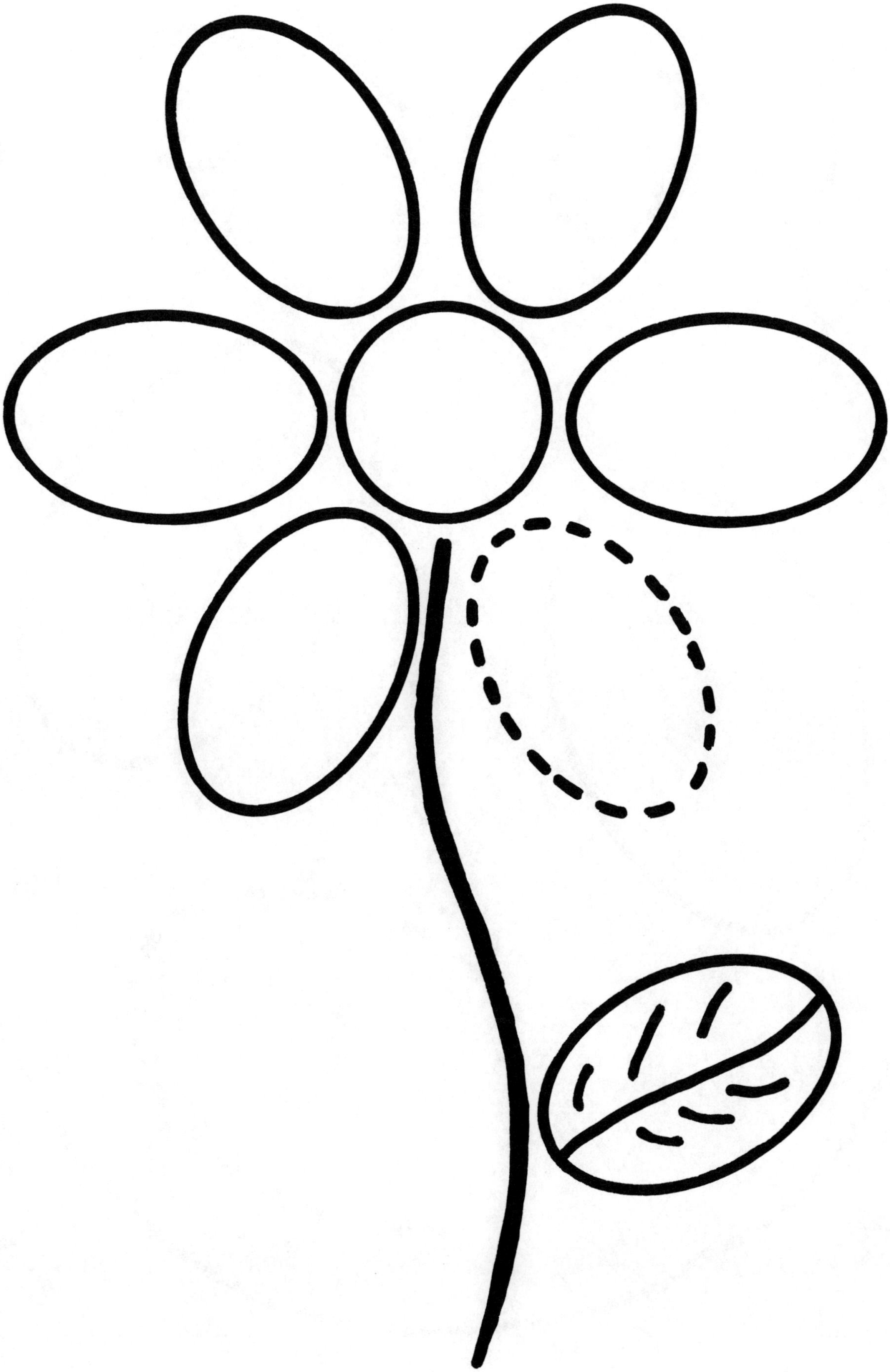

Step 2—Level #2 Worksheet

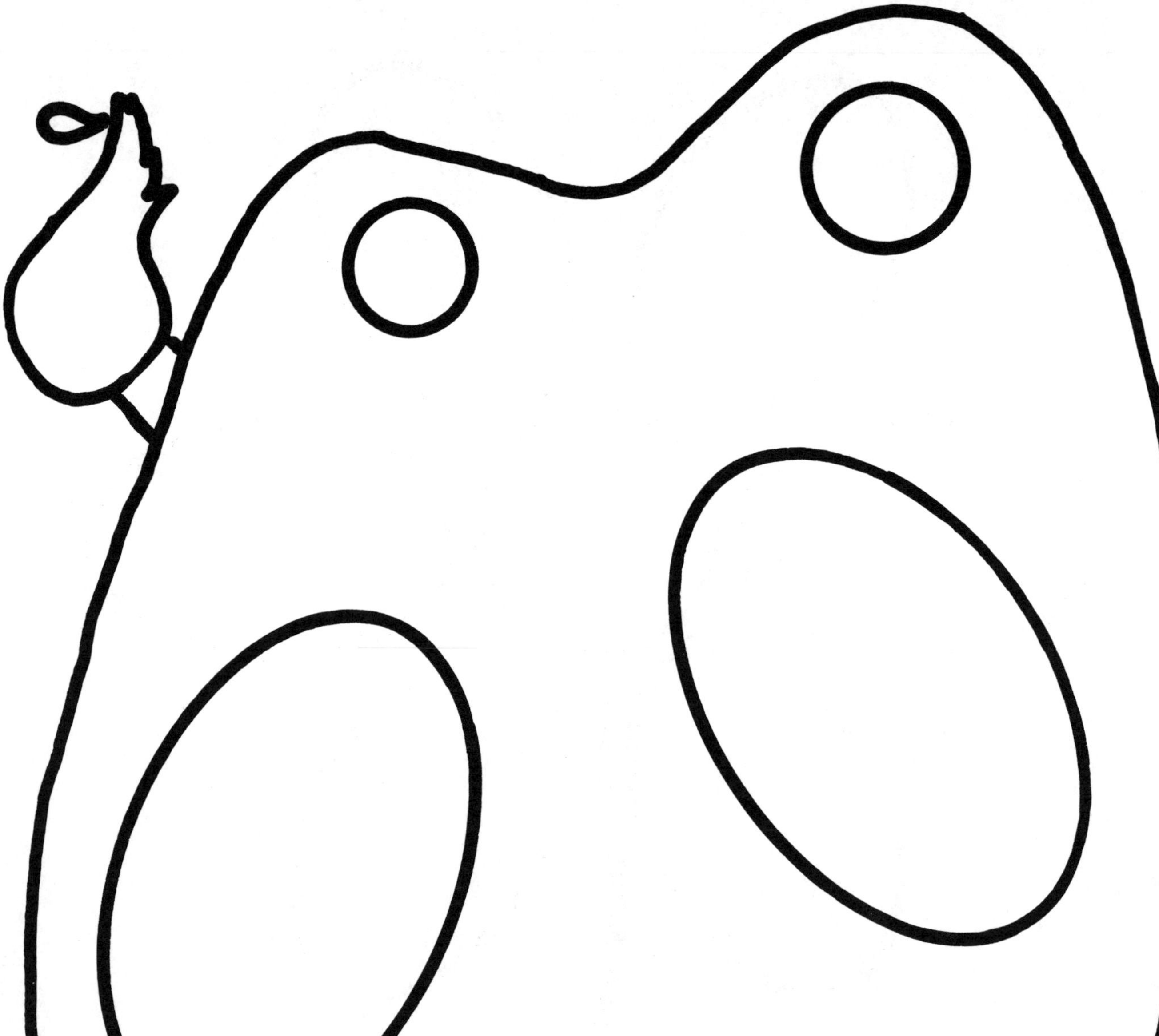

Step 2—Level #2 Worksheet

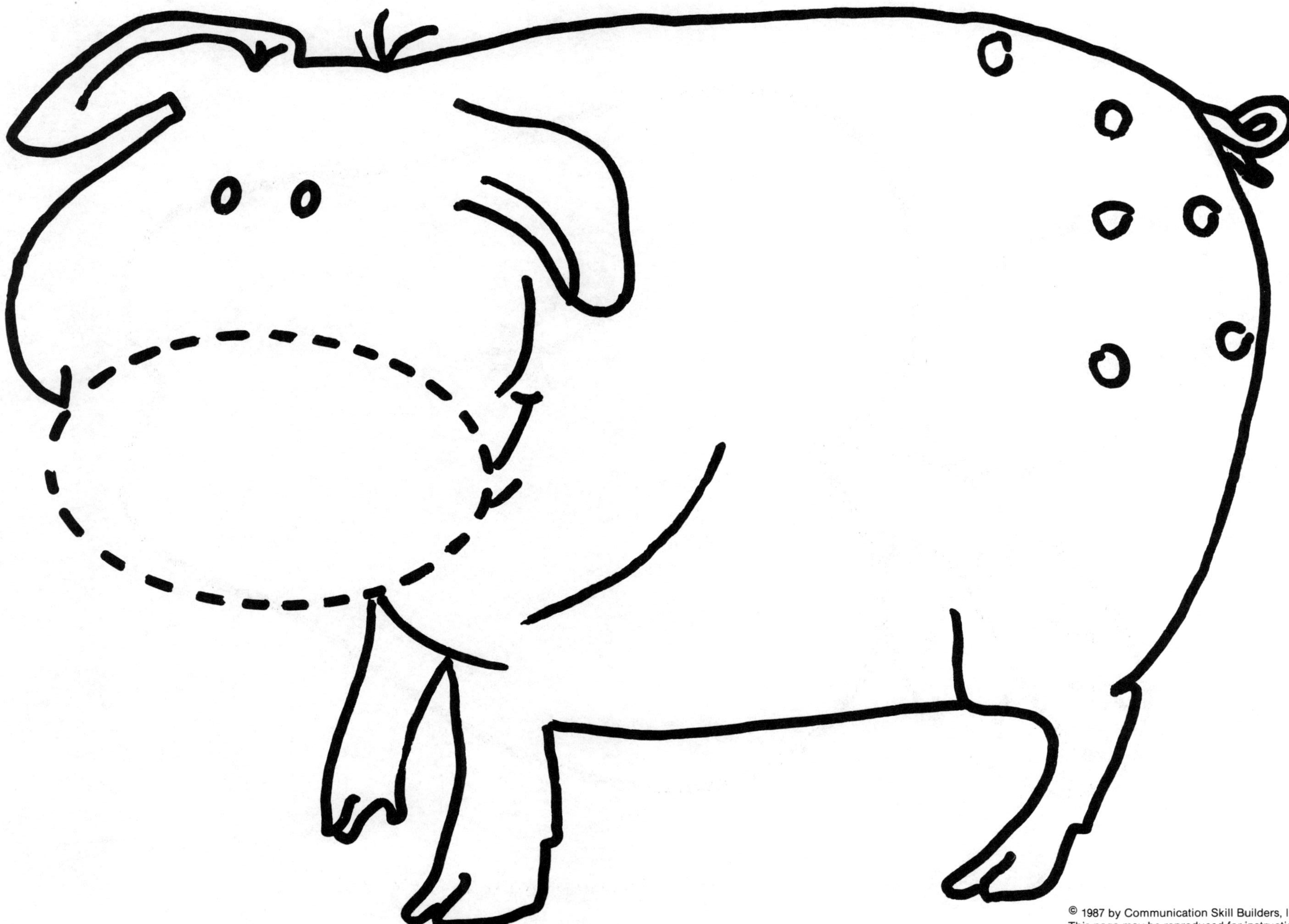

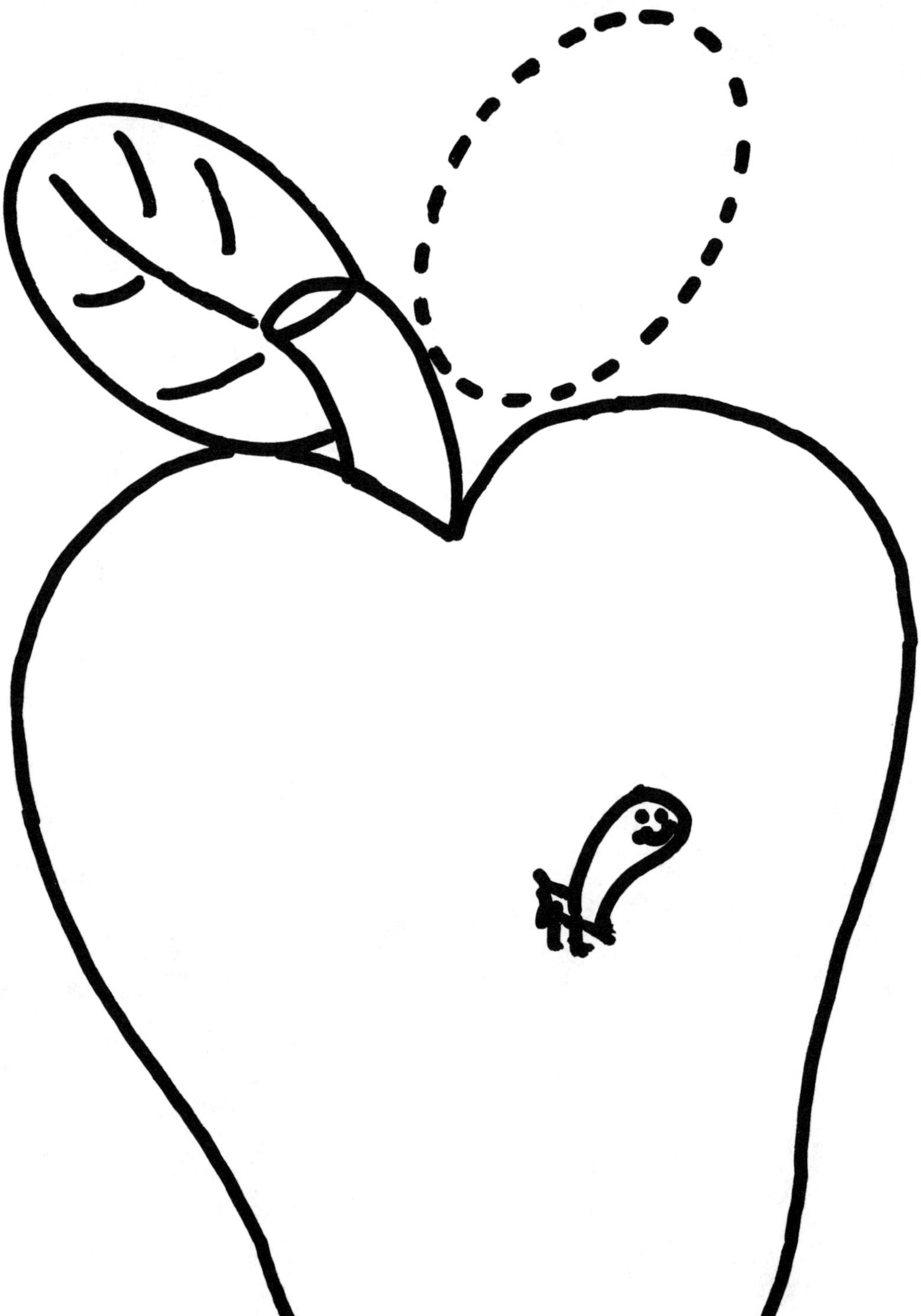

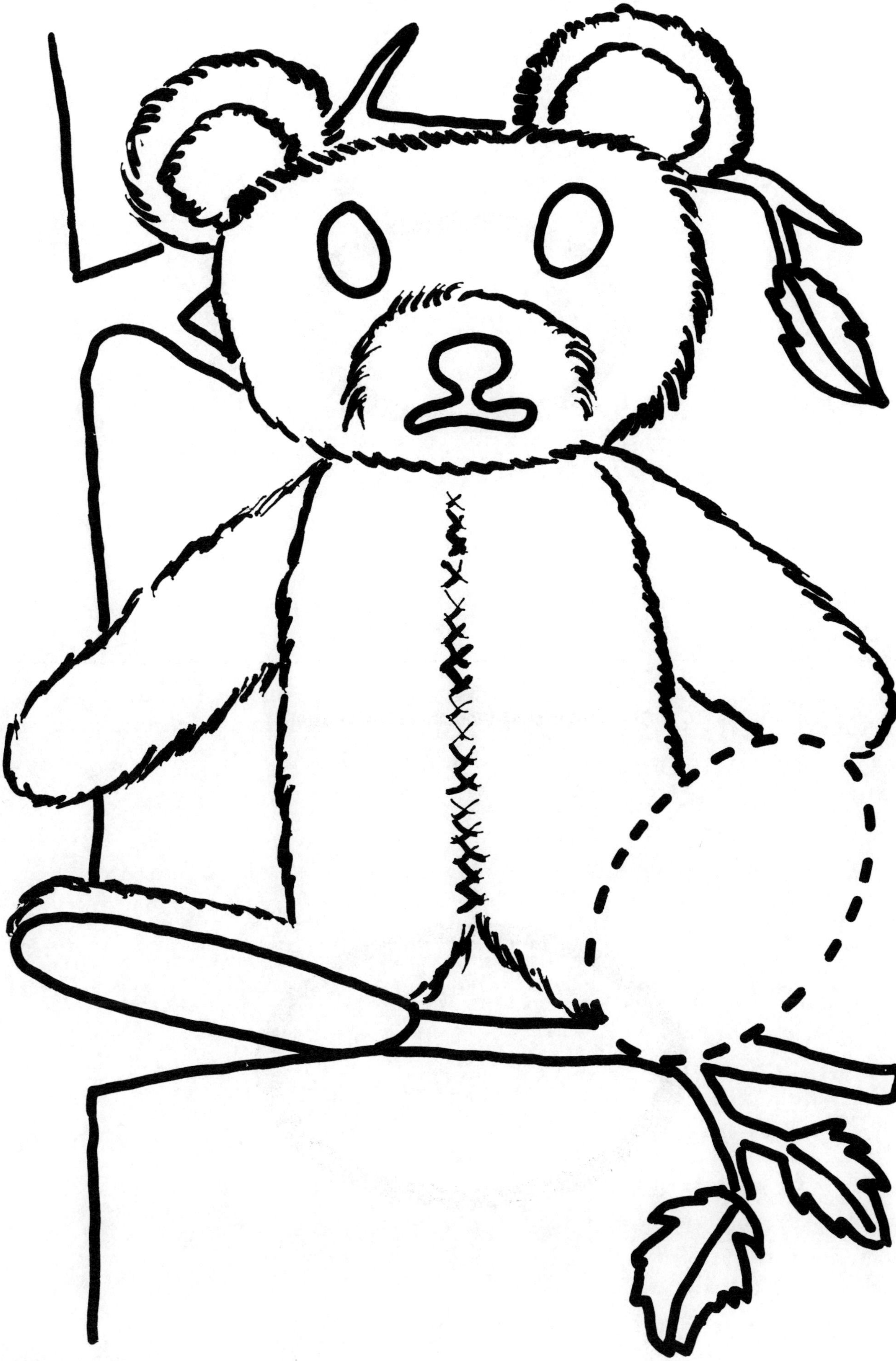

Skill 6
Step 2—Level #2 Pre/Posttest (flower petal)

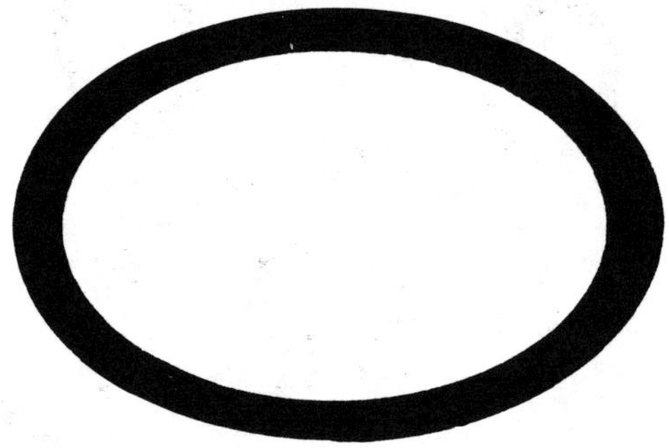

Skill 6
Step 2—Level #2 Worksheet (paint palette)

Skill 6
Step 2—Level #2 Worksheet (pig snout)

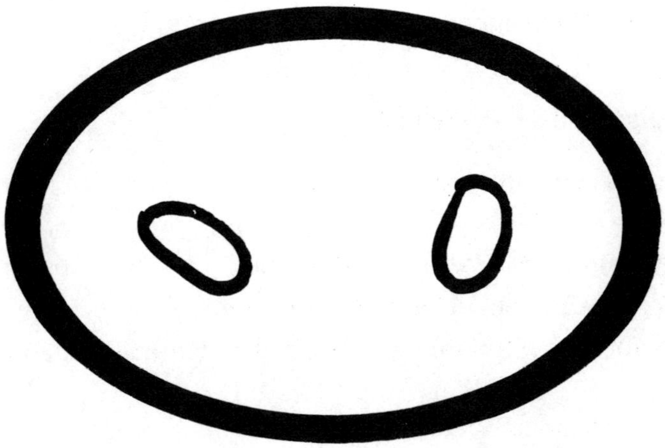

Skill 6
Step 2—Level #2 Worksheet (apple leaf)

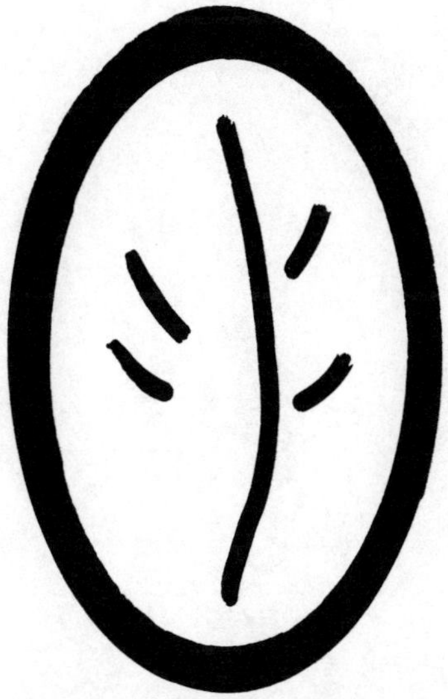

Skill 6
Step 2—Level #2 Worksheet (teddy bear's foot)

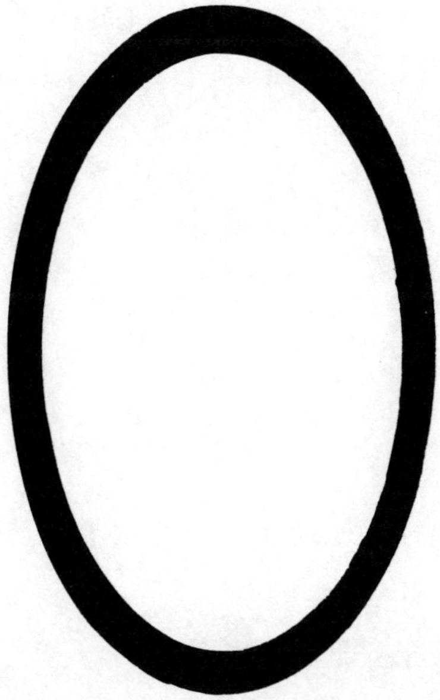

SKILL 6—STEP 3—CRESCENTS

Level #1—Crescents, 1/4" wide line
Pretest: Student takes Level #1 Pretest (girl in boat—4¾" crescent).

If criterion met: Student advances to Level #2.

If criterion not met:

1. Student cuts Level #1 worksheets:
   moon over tent—5¼"
   cow jumps over the moon—5"
   melon slices—4¾"
2. Student takes Level #1 Posttest (girl in boat).
   If criterion met: Student advances to Level #2.
   If criterion not met: Student repeats Level #1 worksheets and Posttest.

Level #2—Smaller Crescents, 1/4" wide line
Pretest: Student takes Level #2 Pretest (wizard's hat—2½" crescent).

If criterion met: Student advances to Step 4—Hearts.

If criterion not met:

1. Student cuts Level #2 worksheets:
   dancing crescent—4¾"
   clown's smile—2¾"
   swing—2¾"
   moon through the window—2¾"
2. Student takes Level #2 Posttest (wizard's hat).
   If criterion met: Student advances to Step 4—Hearts.
   If criterion not met: Student repeats Level #2 worksheets and Posttest.

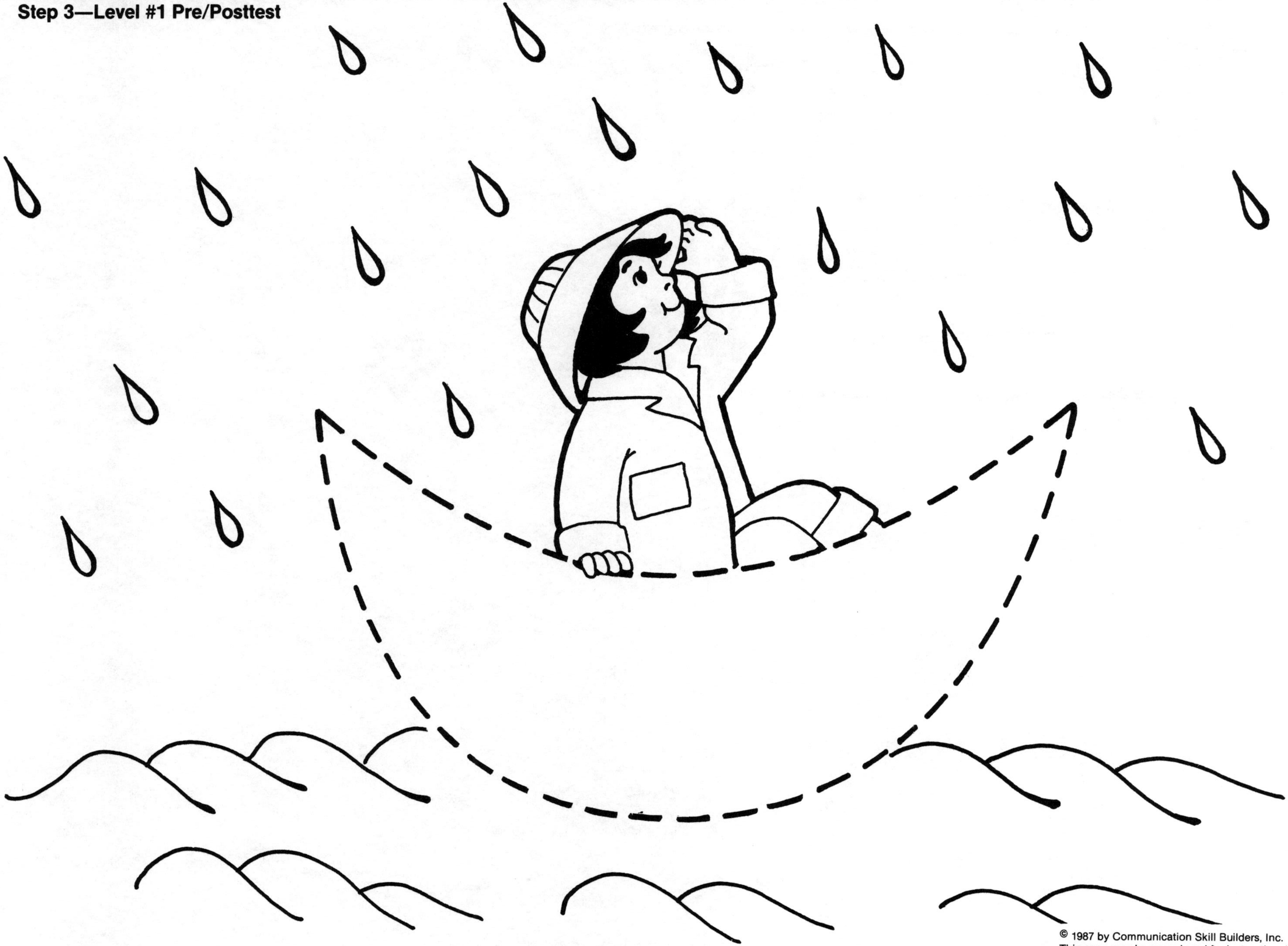

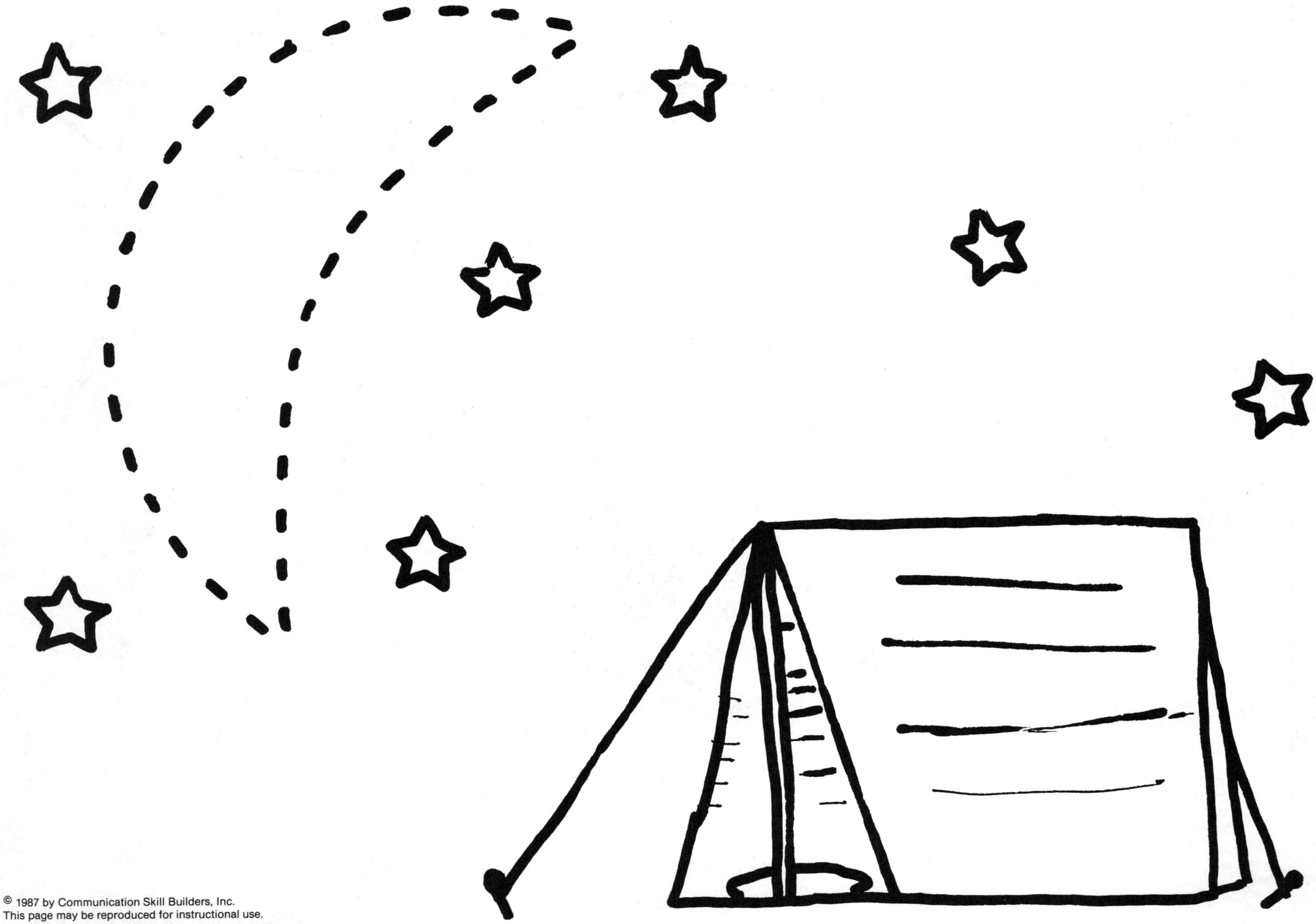

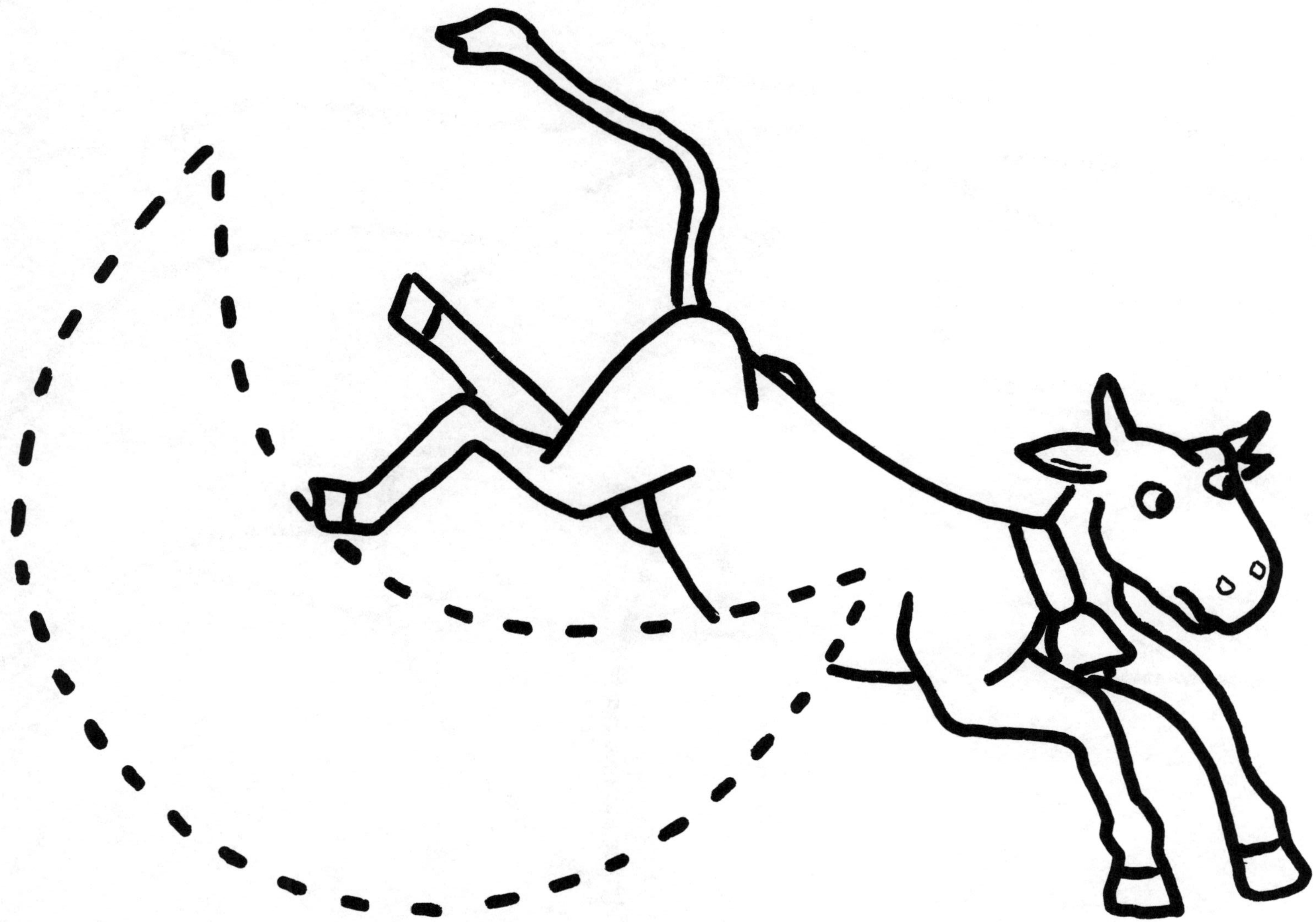

Step 3—Level #1 Worksheet

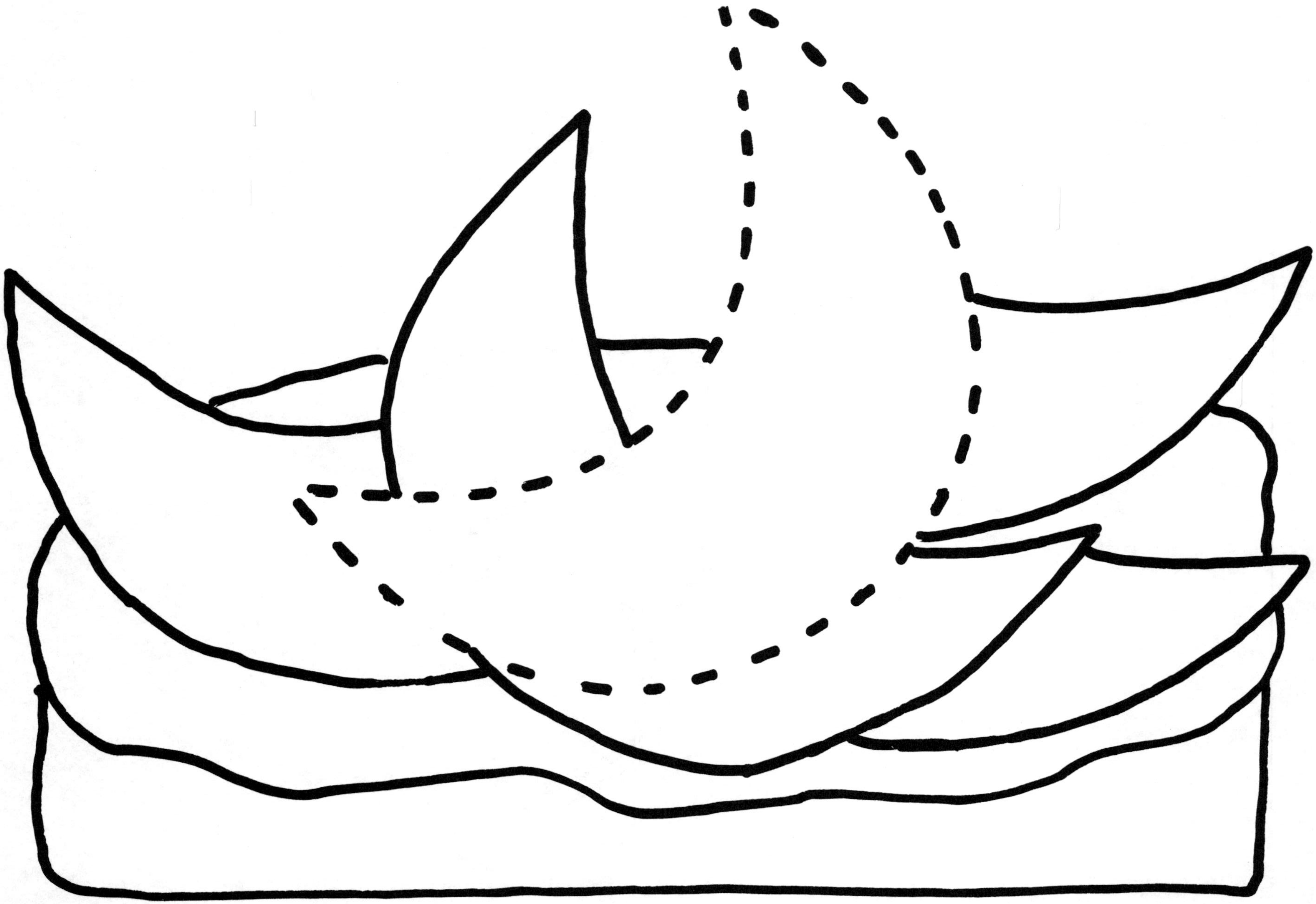

Skill 6
Step 3—Level #1 Pre/Posttest (girl in boat)

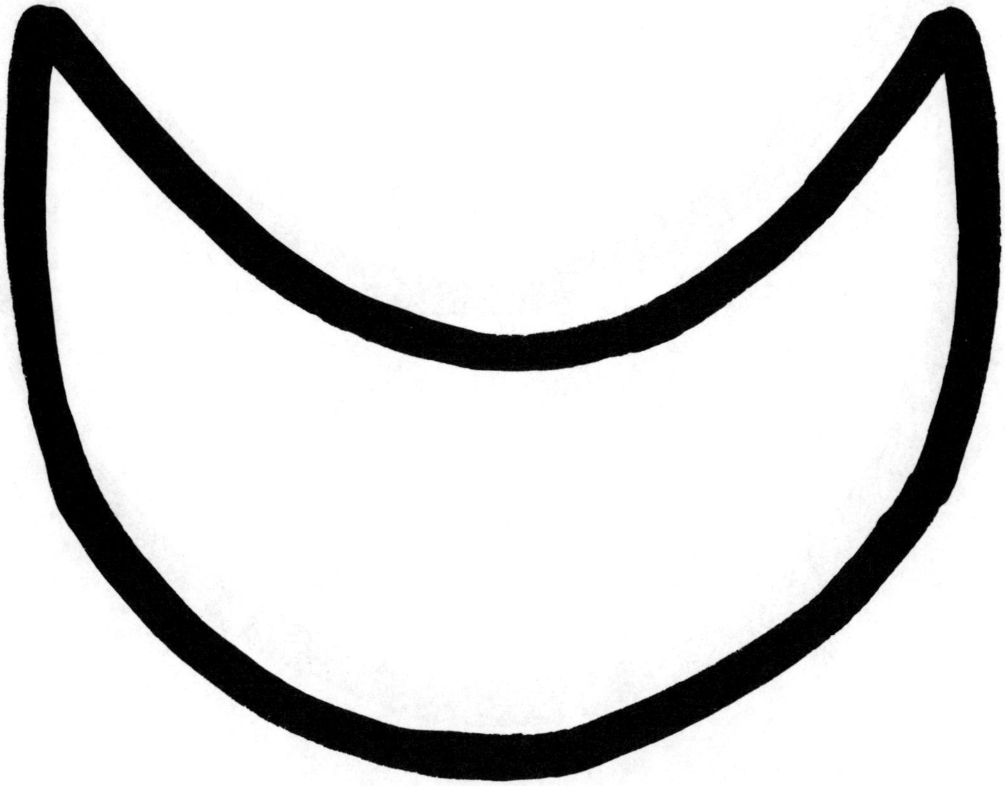

Skill 6
Step 3—Level #1 Worksheet (moon over tent)

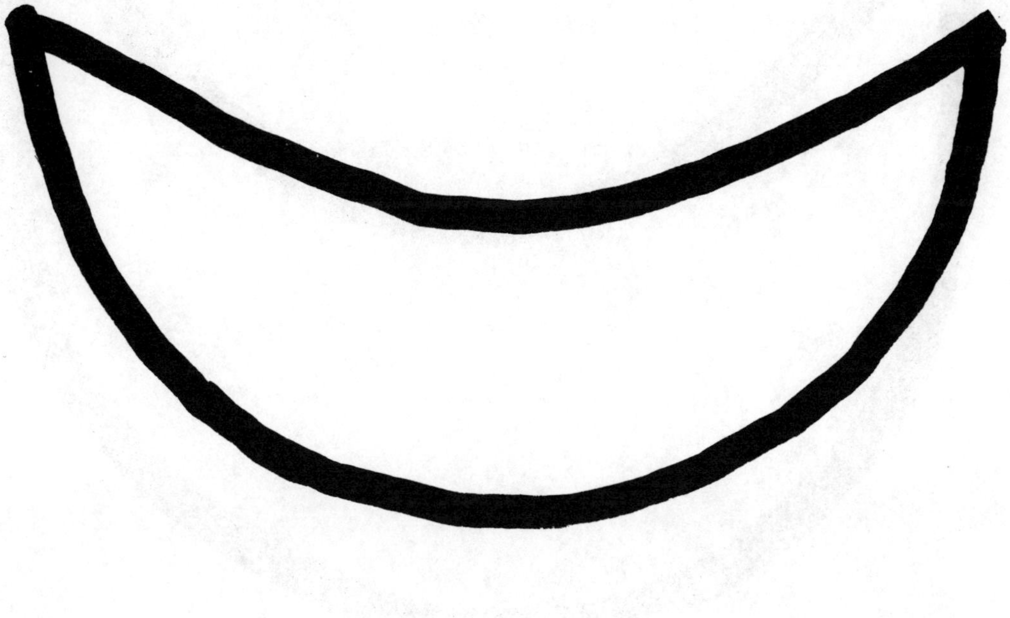

Skill 6
Step 3—Level #1 Worksheet (cow jumps over the moon)

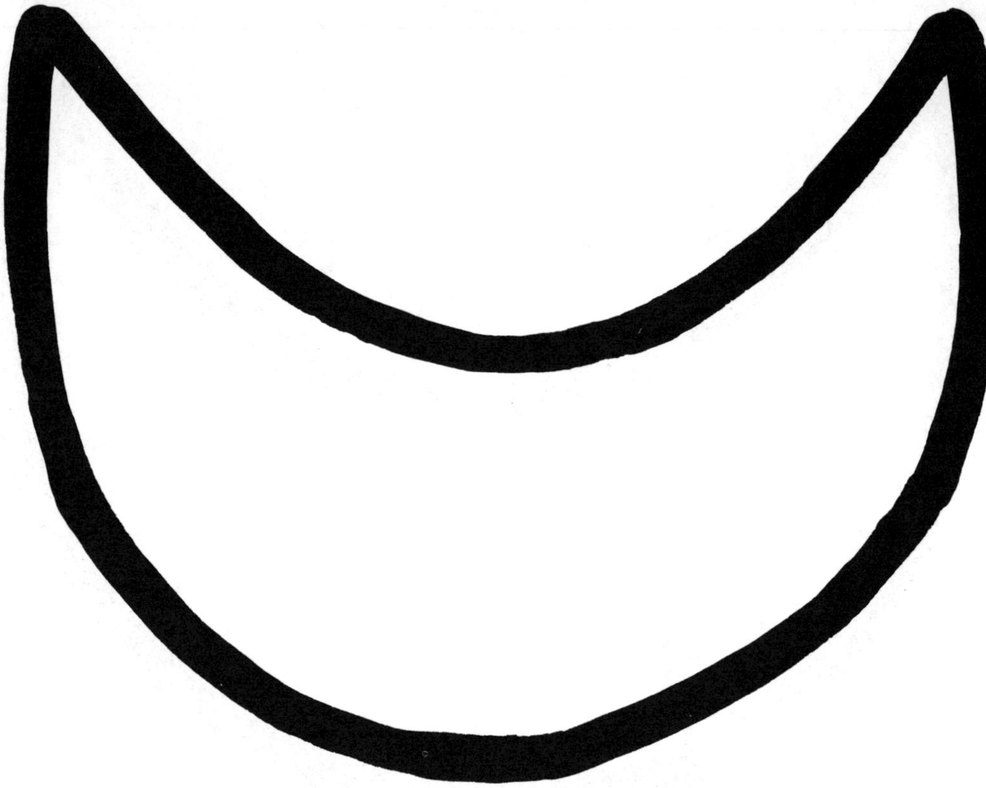

Skill 6
Step 3—Level #1 Worksheet (melon slices)

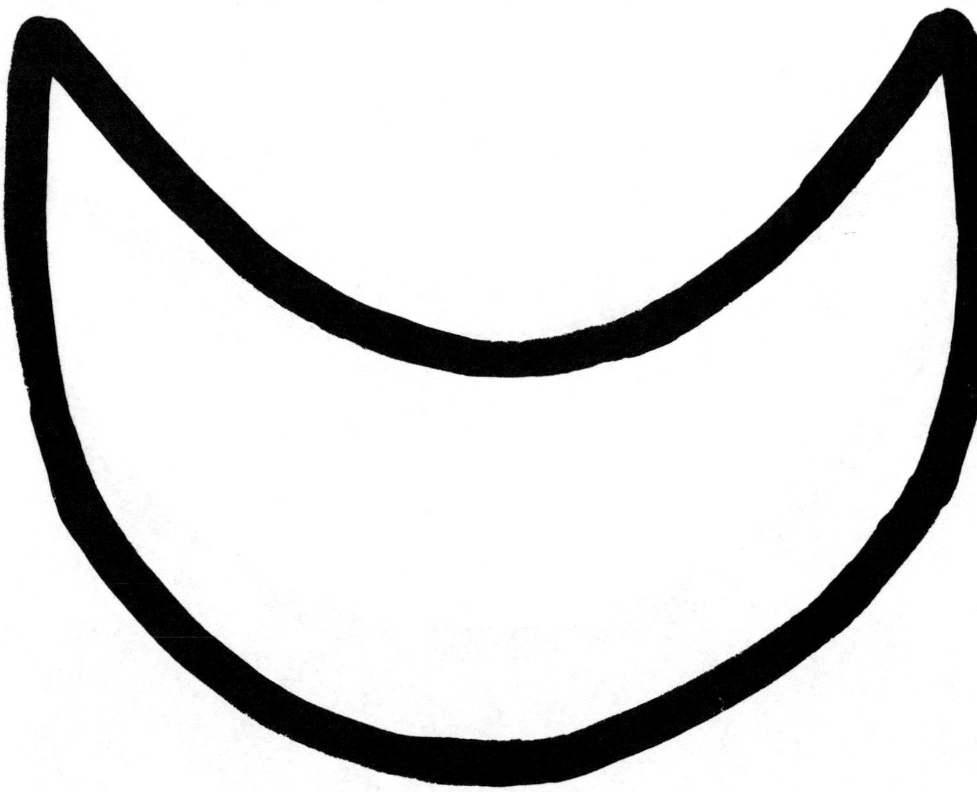

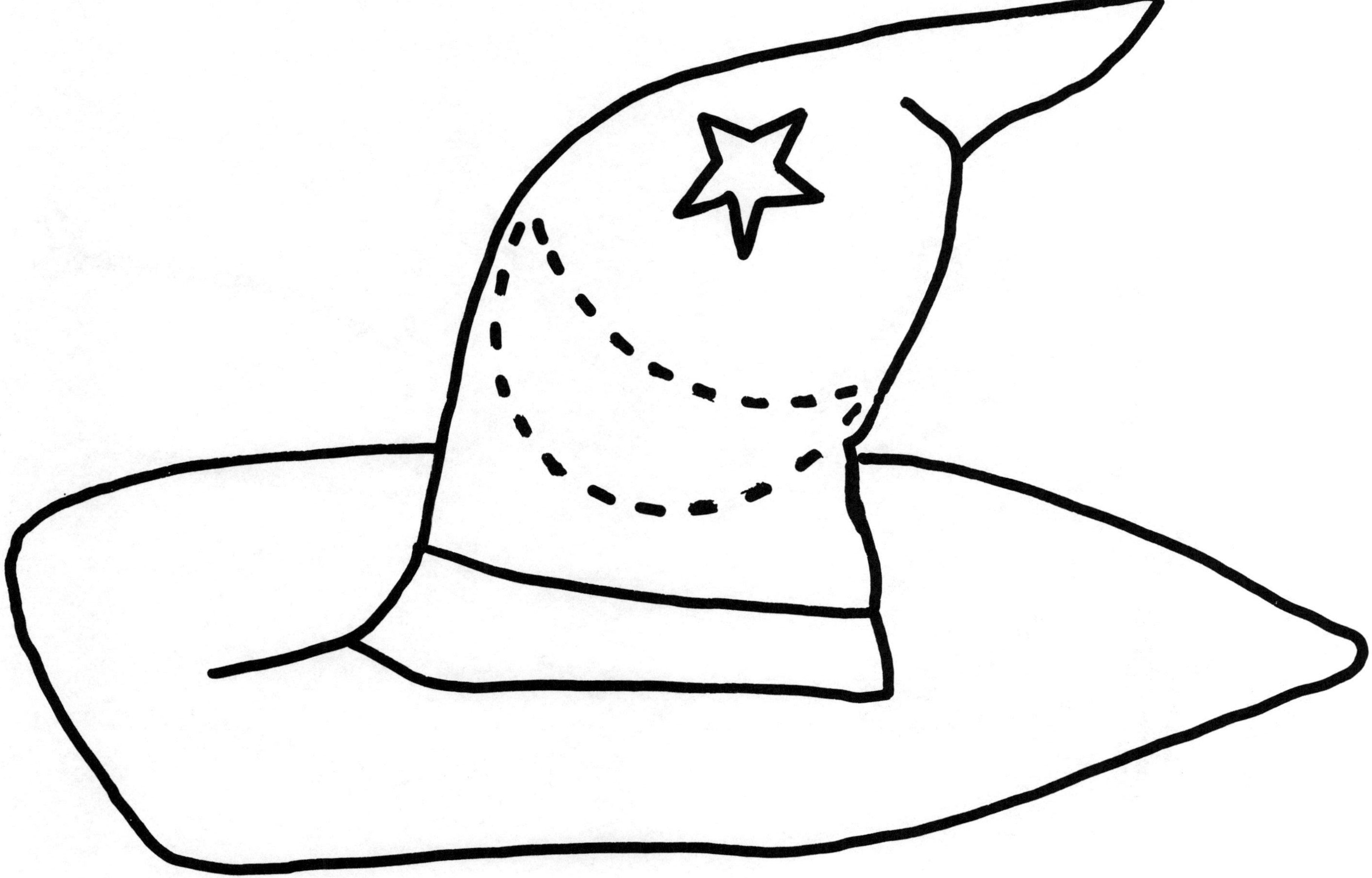

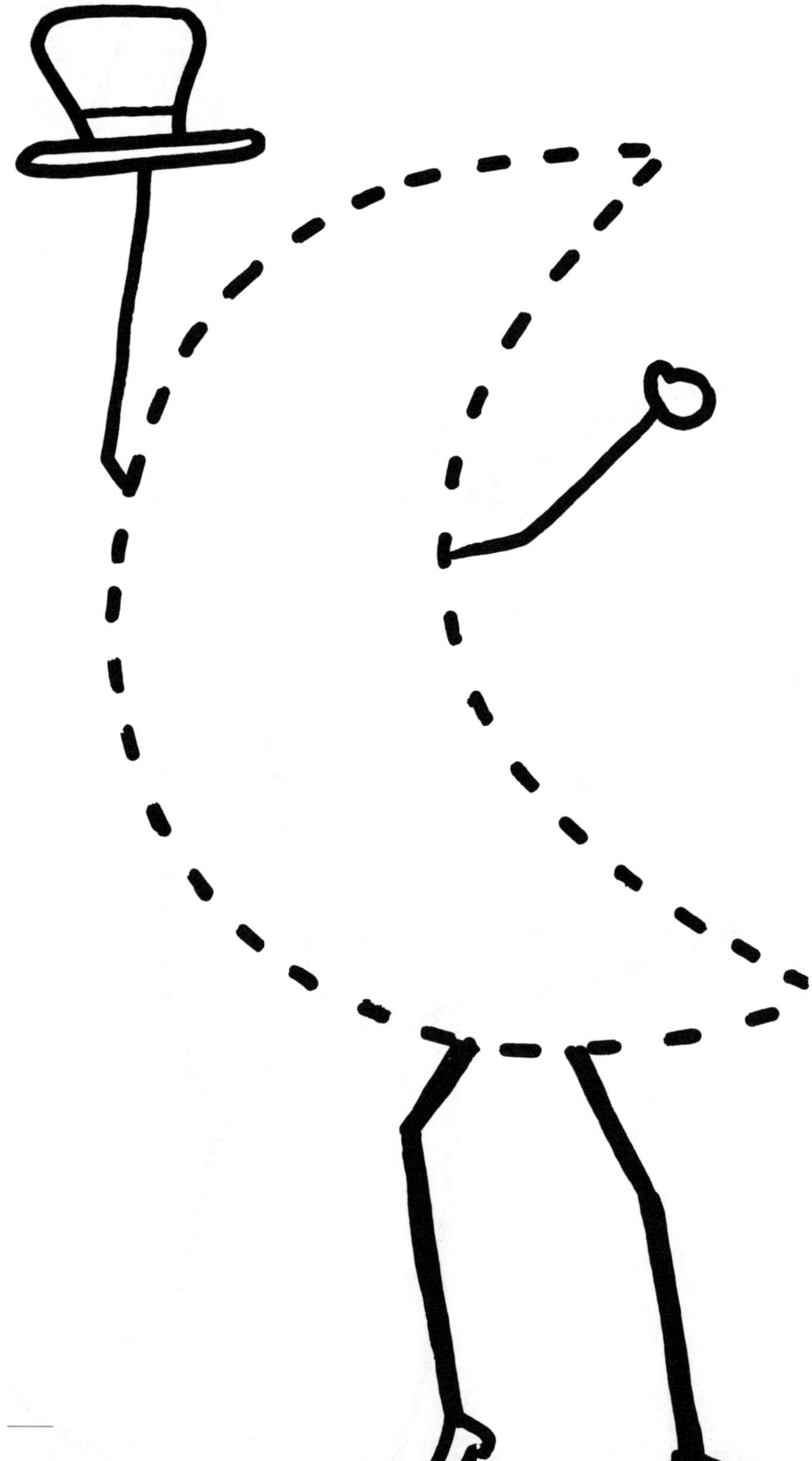

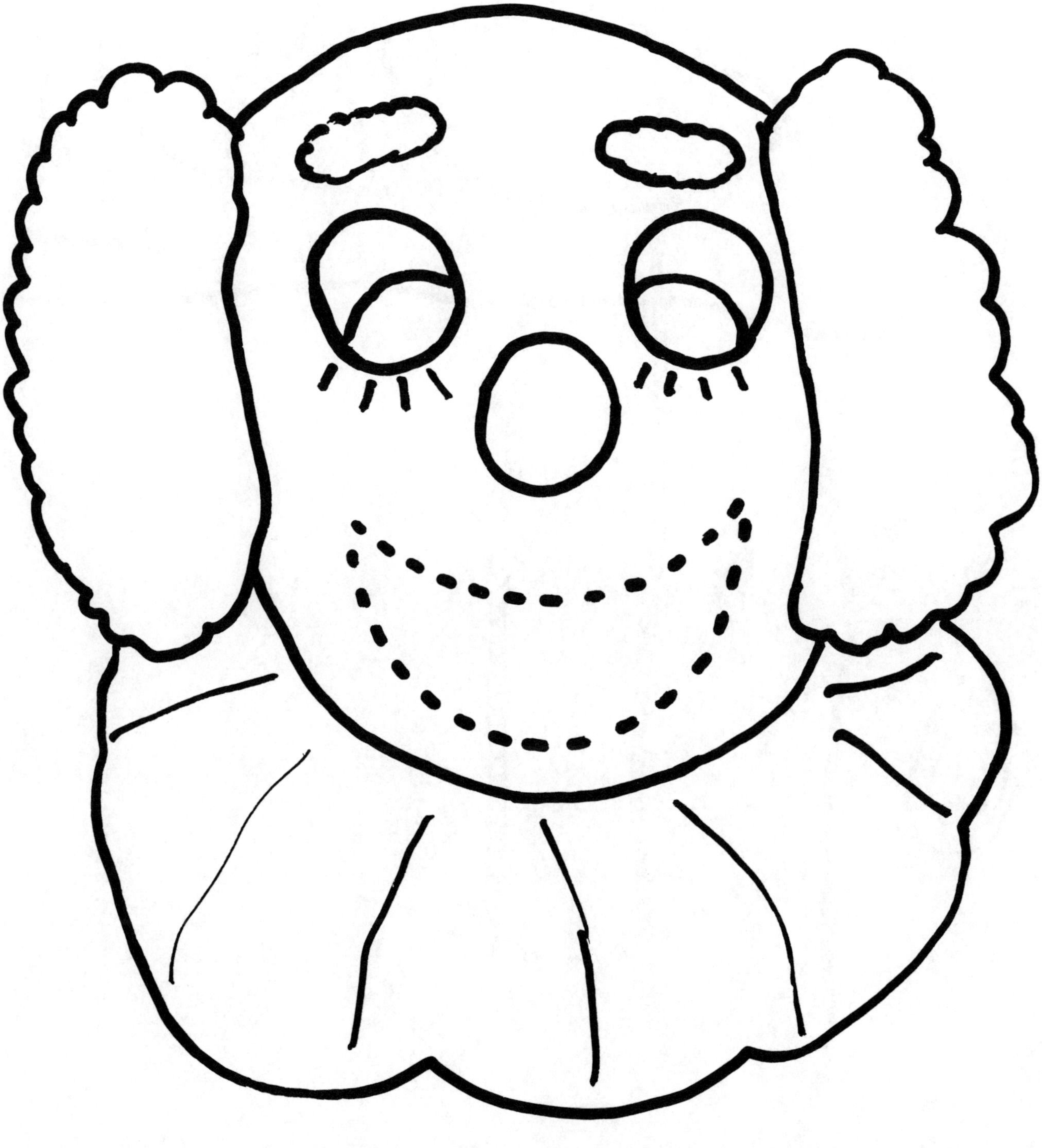

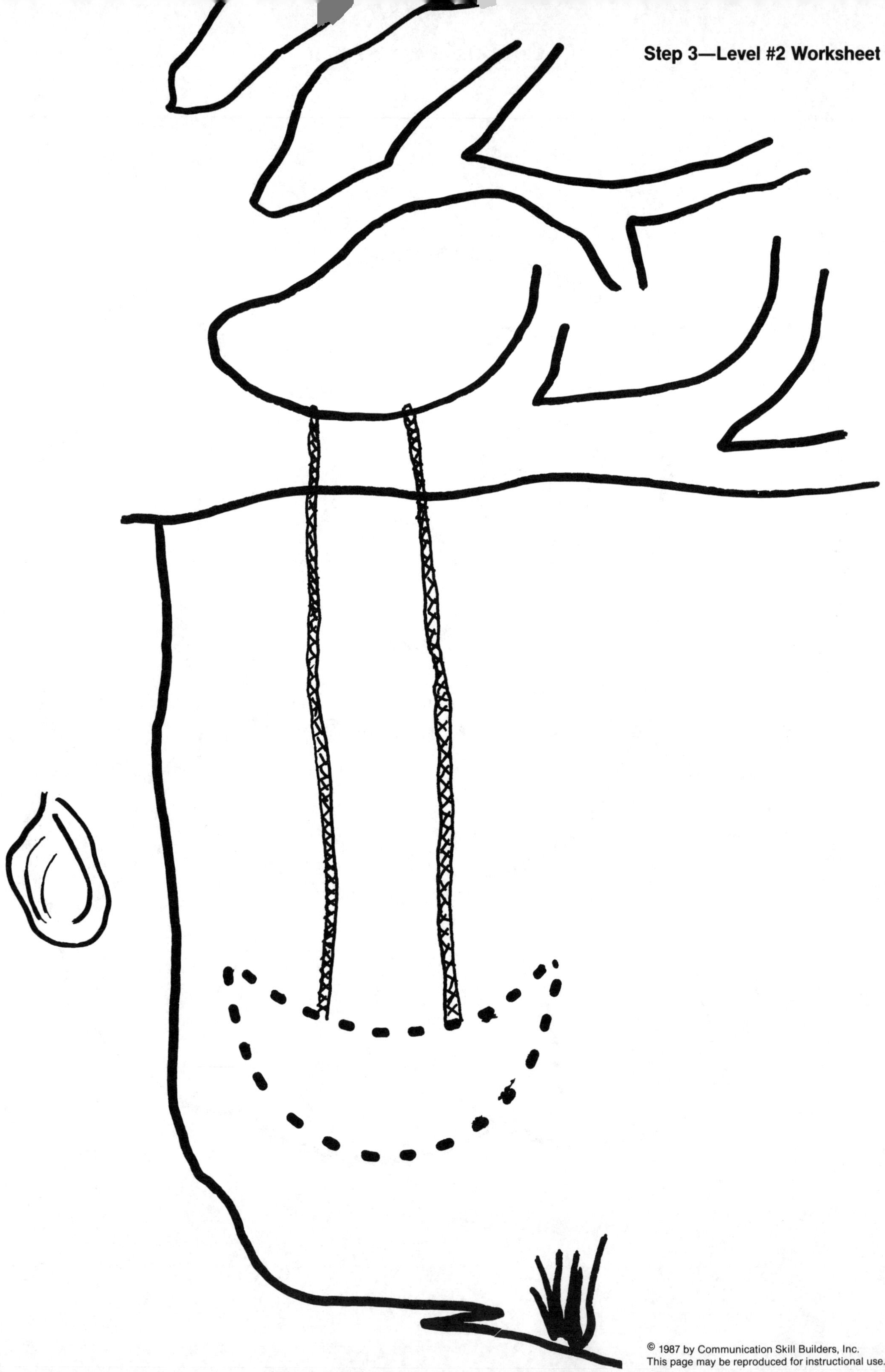

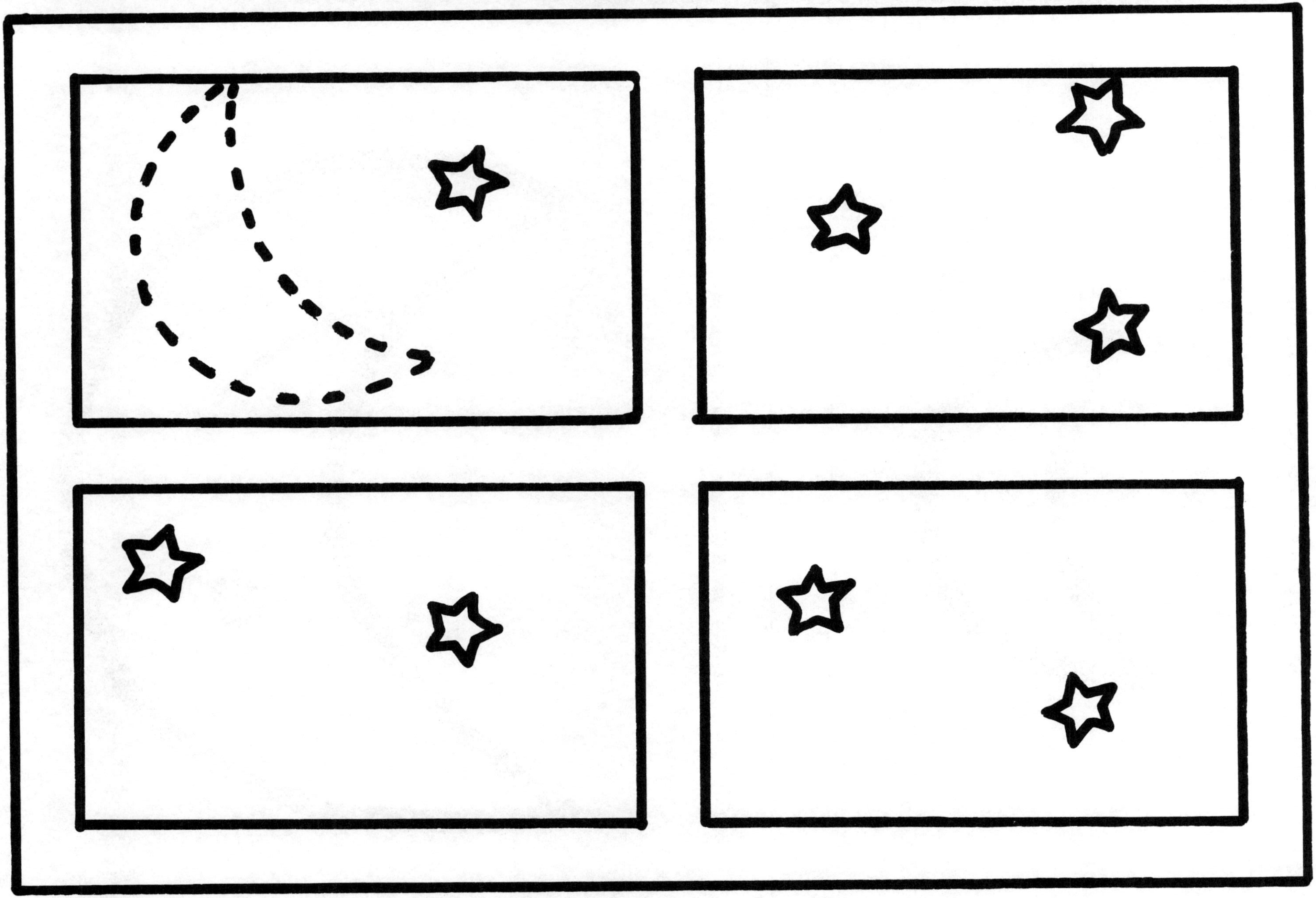

Step 3—Level #2 Worksheet

Skill 6
Step 3—Level #2 Pre/Posttest (wizard's hat)

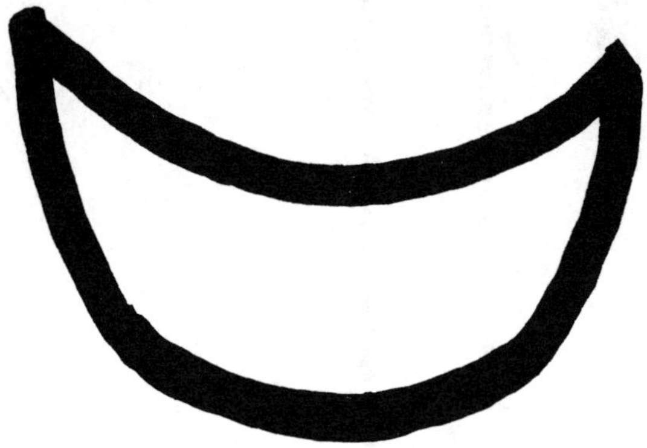

Skill 6
Step 3—Level #2 Worksheet (dancing crescent)

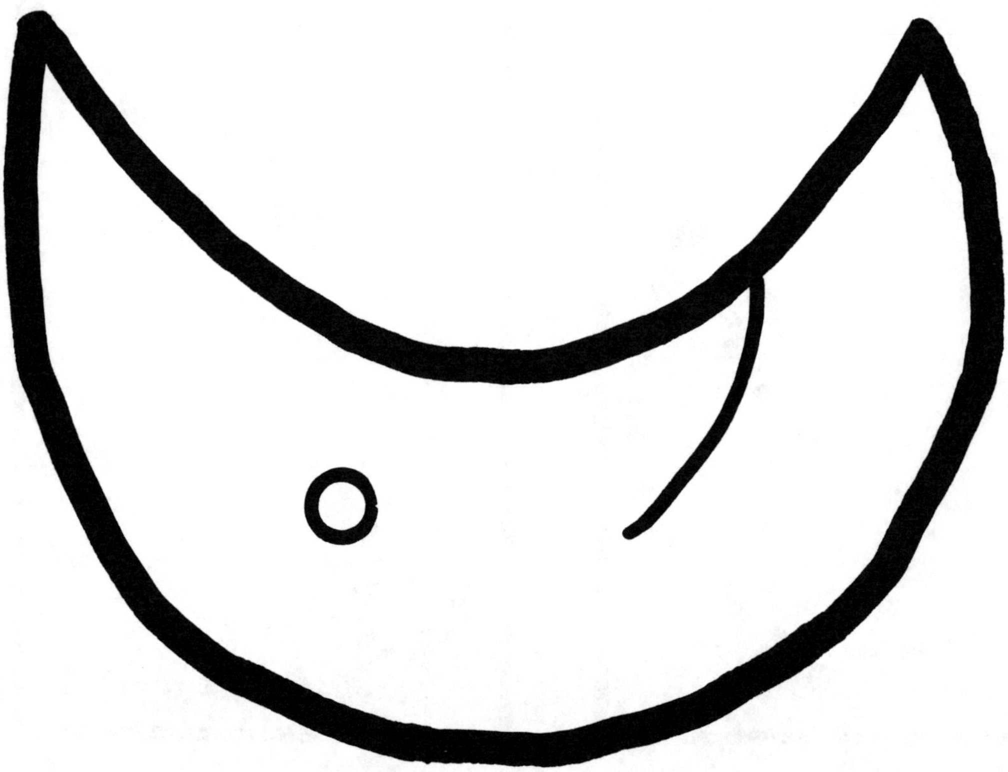

Skill 6
Step 3—Level #2 Worksheet (clown's smile)

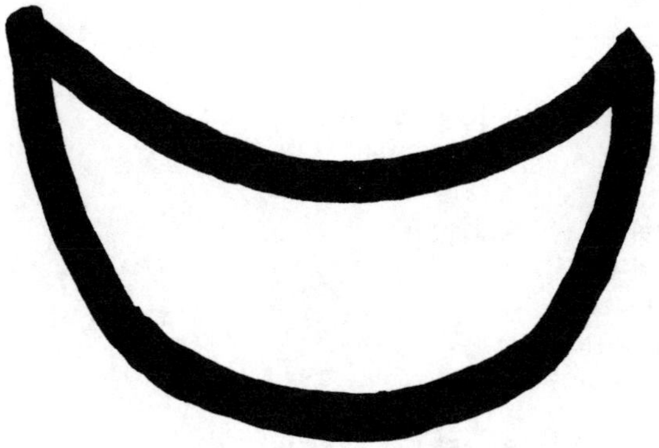

Skill 6
Step 3—Level #2 Worksheet (swing)

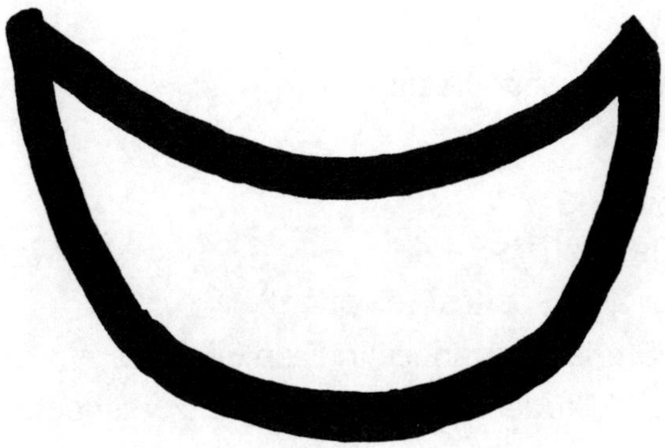

Skill 6
Step 3—Level #2 Worksheet (moon through the window)

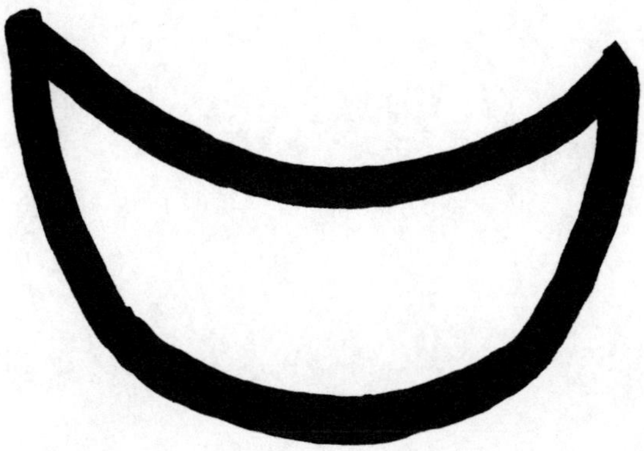

SKILL 6—STEP 4—HEARTS

Level #1—Hearts, ¼" wide line
Pretest: Student takes Level #1 Pretest (lovebirds—4½" heart).

If criterion met: Student advances to Level #2.

If criterion not met:

1. Student cuts Level #1 worksheets:
   - valentine card—4¾"
   - balloon heart—4¾"
   - girl holding heart—4¾"
   - three hearts—4½"
2. Student takes Level #1 Posttest (lovebirds).

   If criterion met: Student advances to Level #2.

   If criterion not met: Student repeats Level #1 worksheets and Posttest.

Level #2—Smaller Hearts, ¼" wide line
Pretest: Student takes Level #2 Pretest (elephant—3" heart).

If criterion met: Student advances to Step 5—Stars.

If criterion not met:

1. Student cuts Level #2 worksheets:
   - girl heart—4"
   - boy heart—4"
   - four-leaf clover—3"
   - kitten holding heart—3"
2. Student takes Level #2 Posttest (elephant).

   If criterion met: Student advances to Step 5—Stars.

   If criterion not met: Student repeats Level #2 worksheets and Posttest.

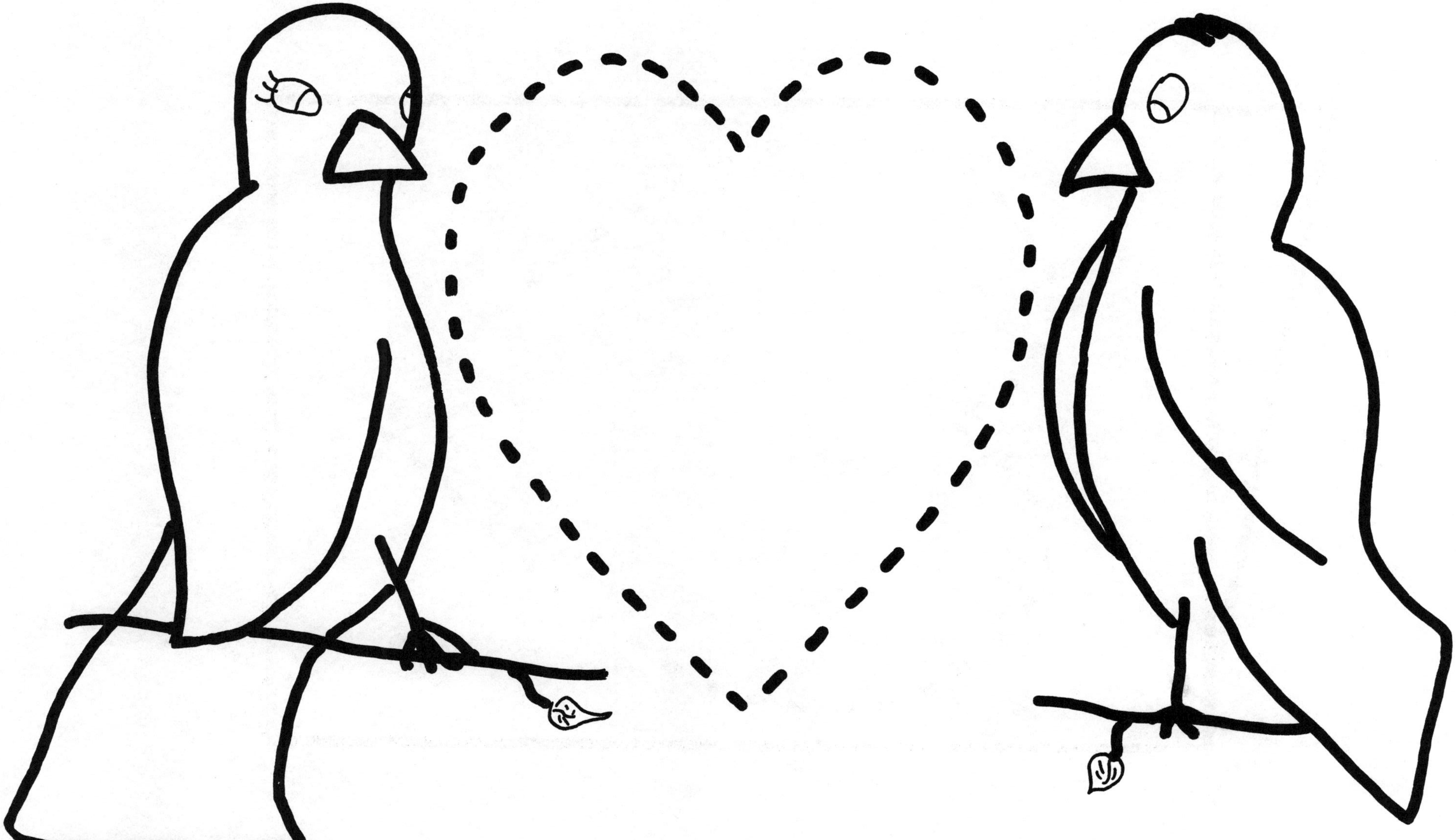

Step 4—Level #1 Worksheet

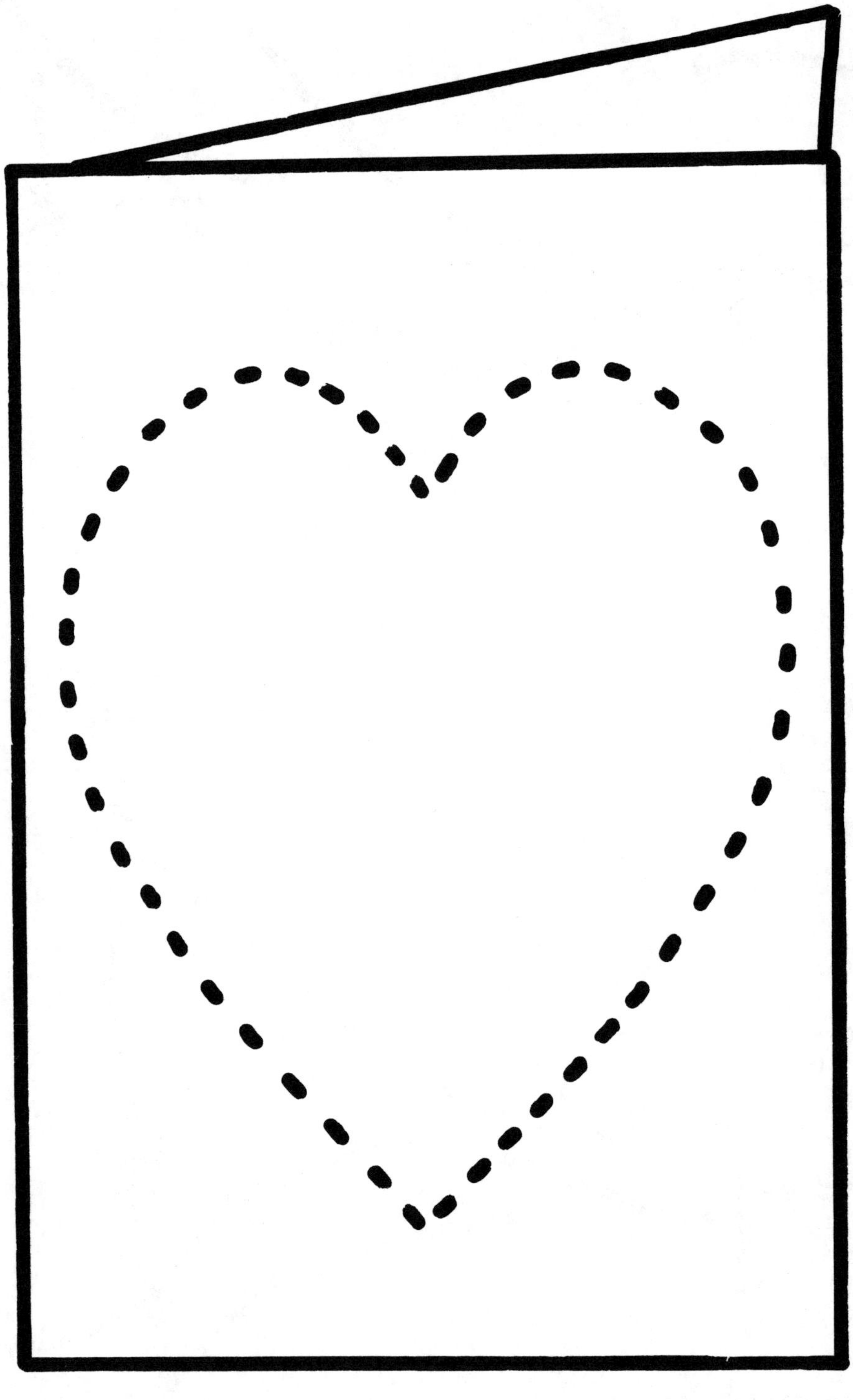

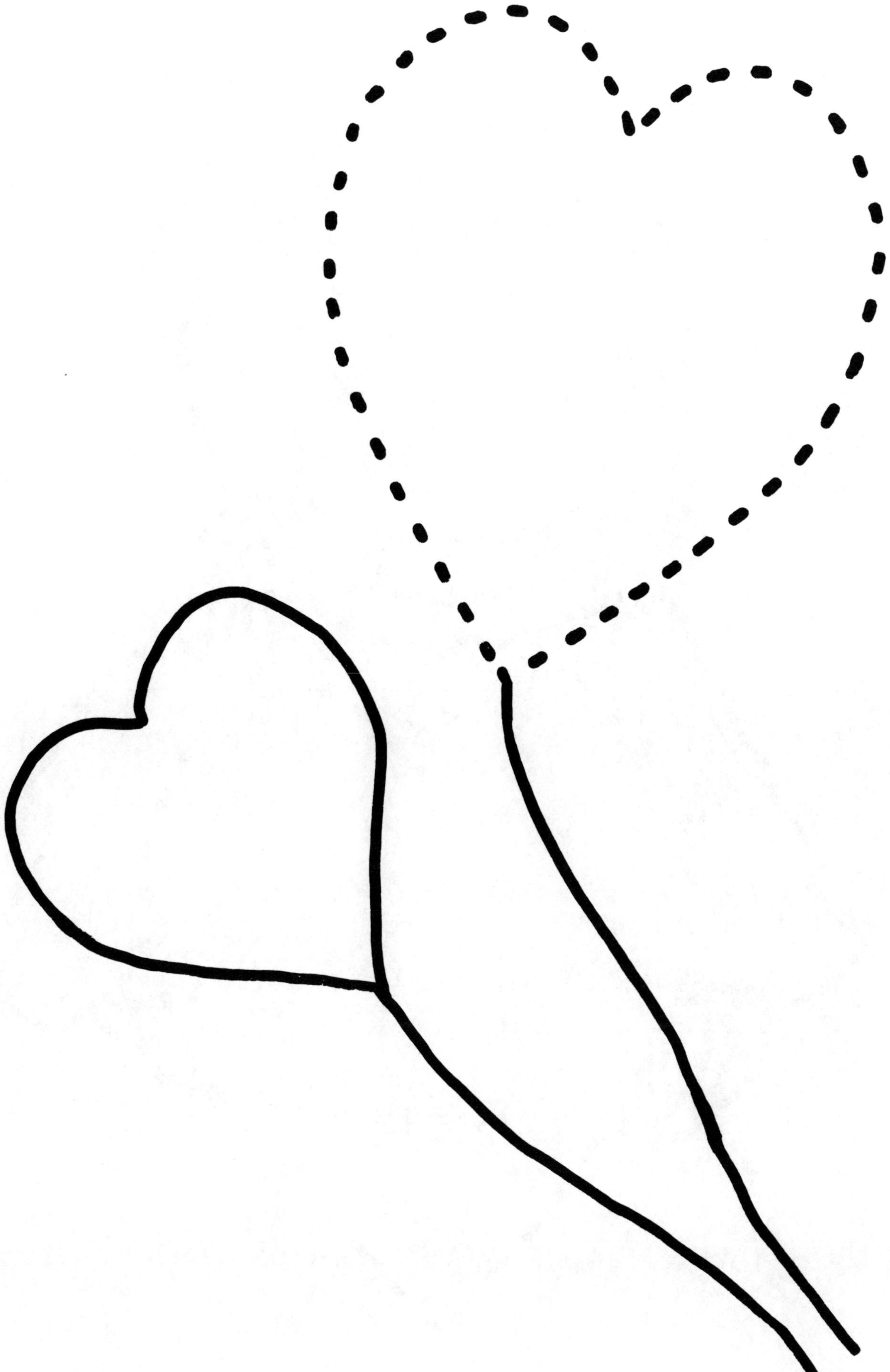

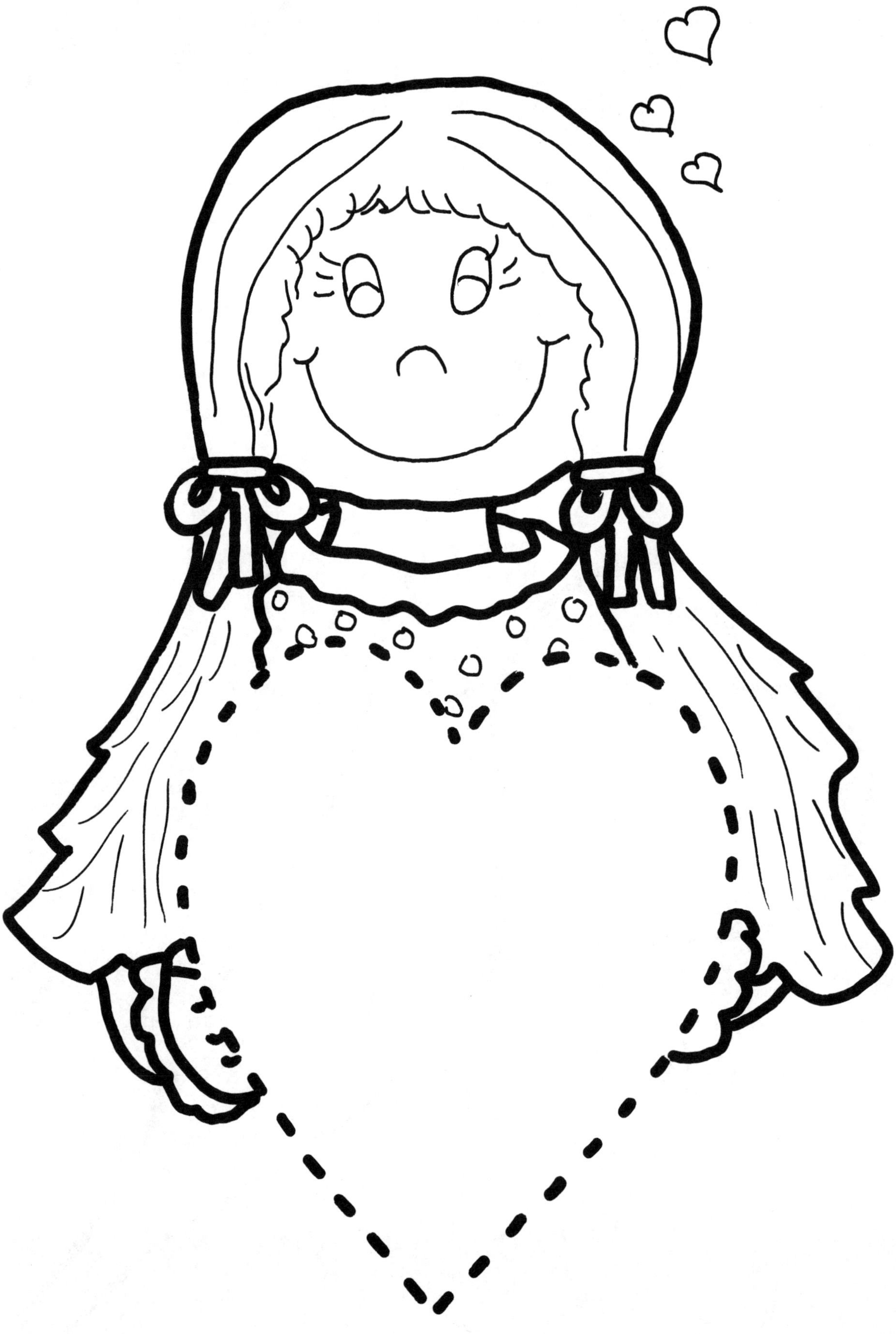

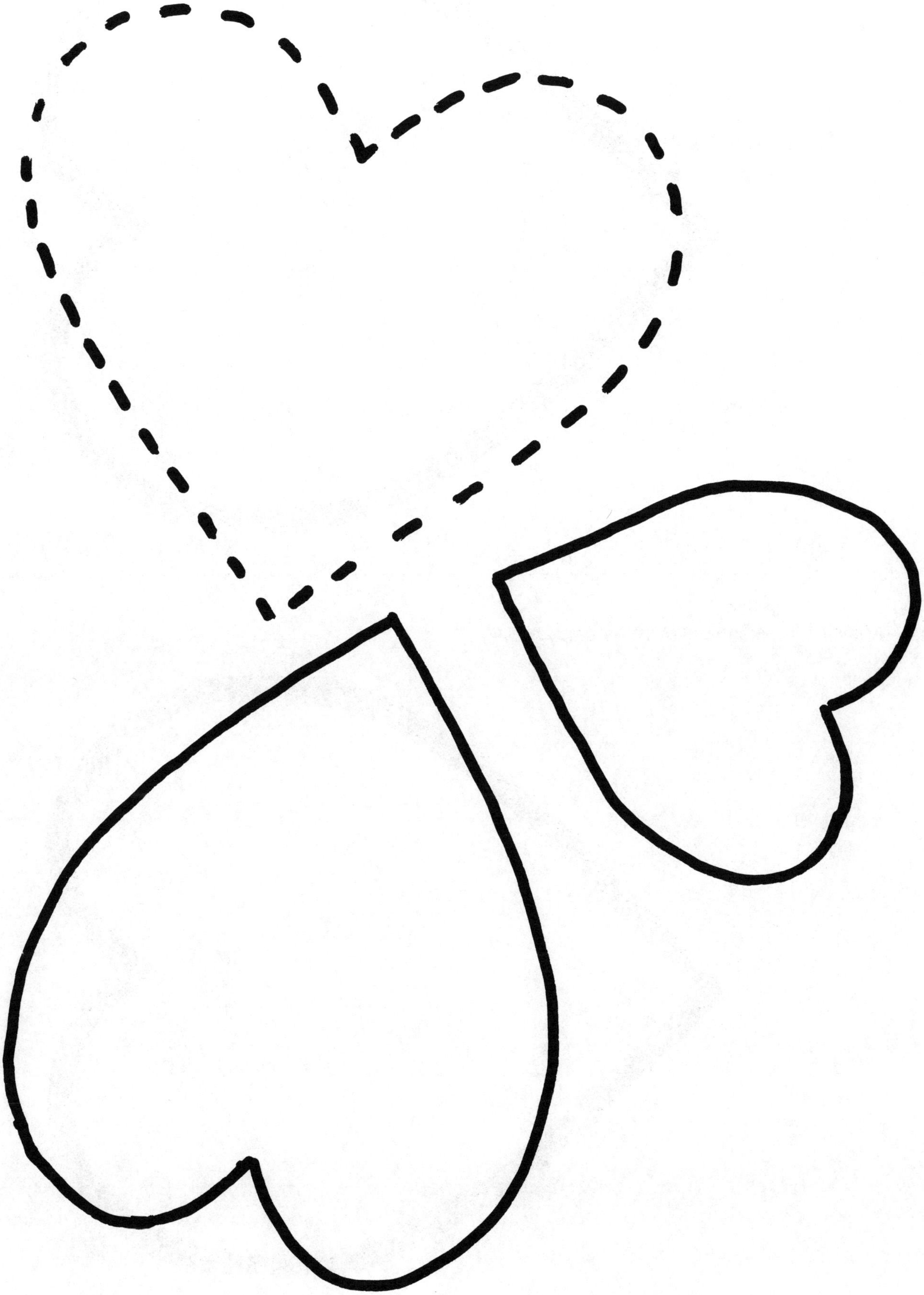

Skill 6
Step 4—Level #1 Pre/Posttest (lovebirds)

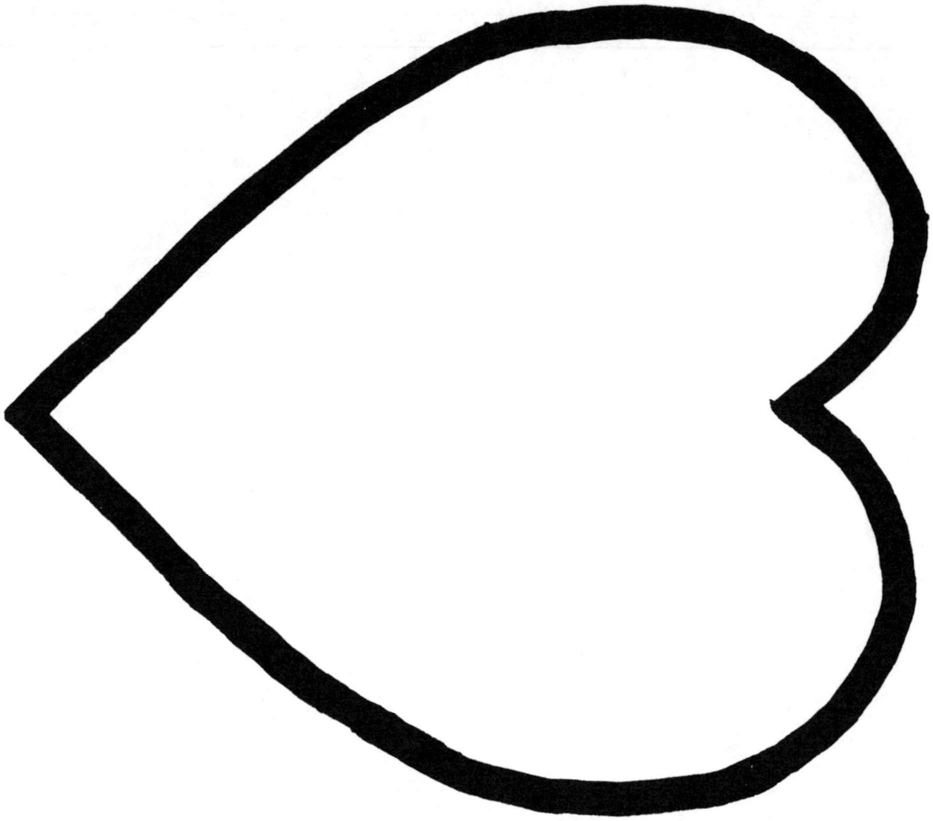

Skill 6
Step 4—Level #1 Worksheet (valentine card)

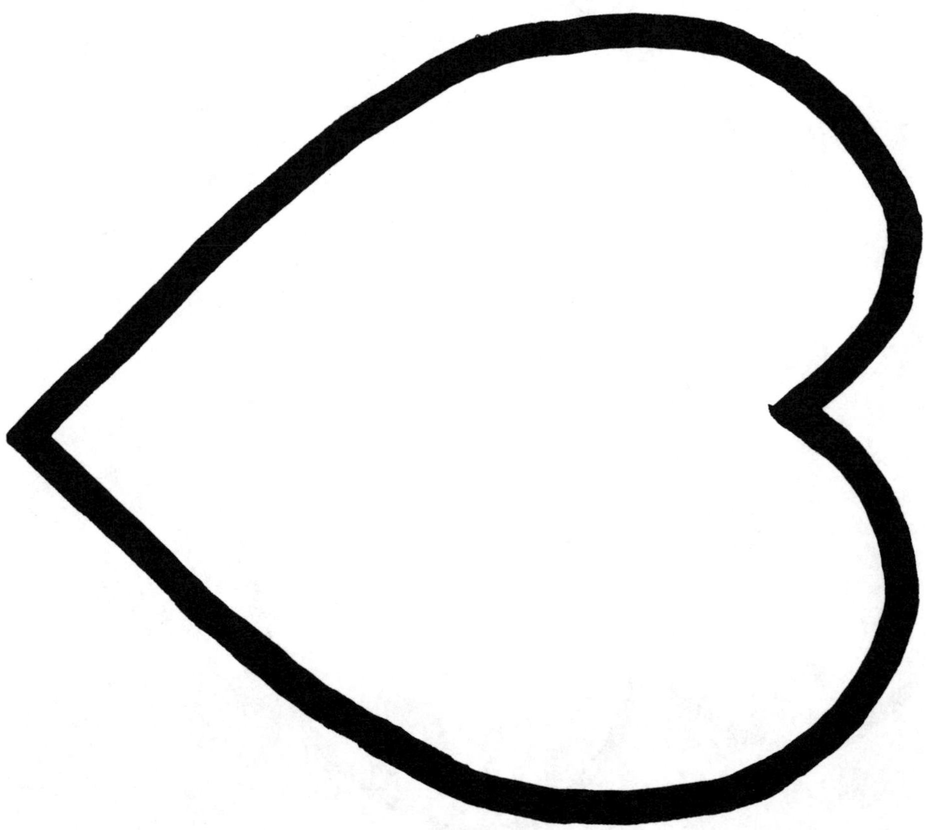

Skill 6
Step 4—Level #1 Worksheet (balloon heart)

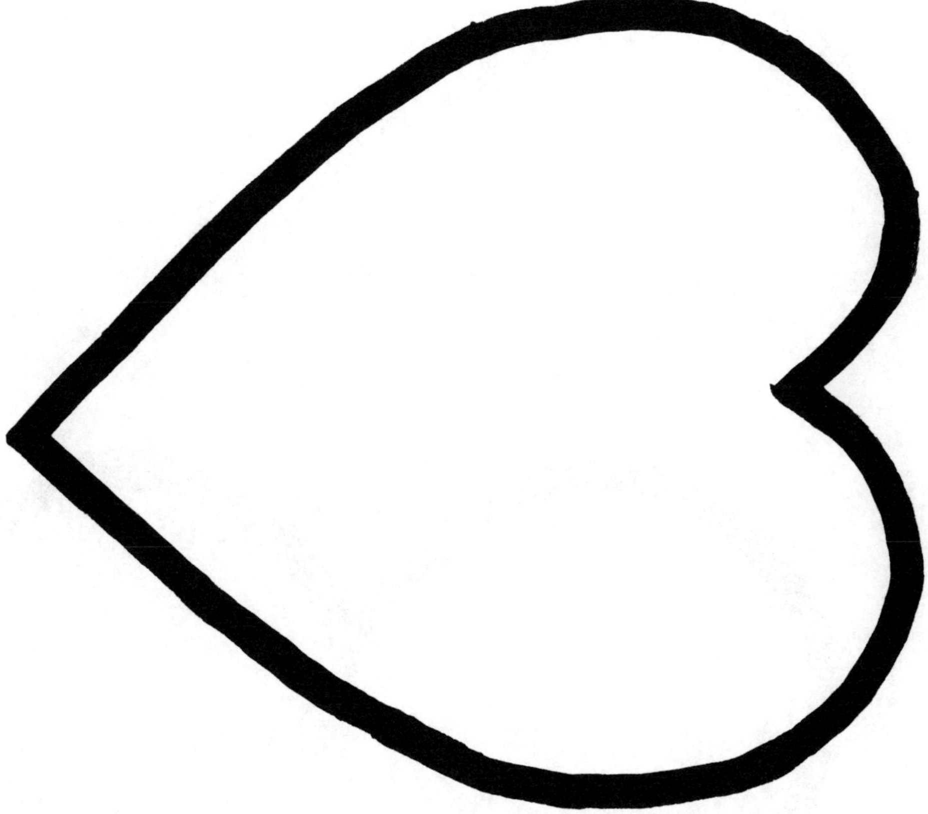

Skill 6
Step 4—Level #1 Worksheet (girl holding heart)

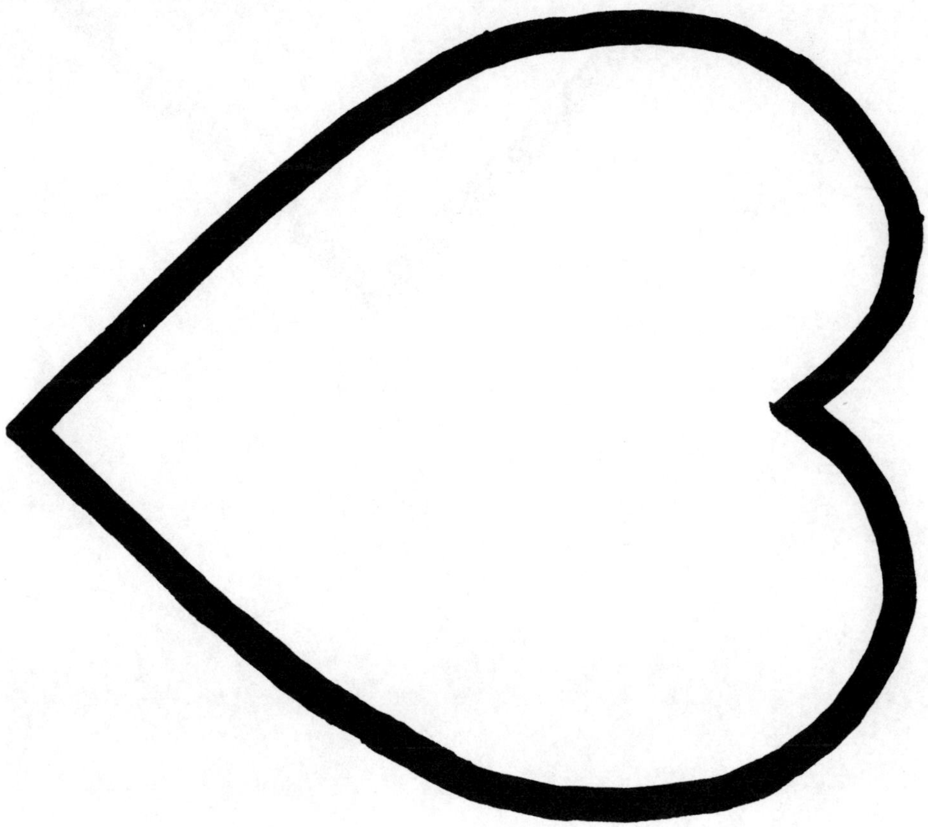

Skill 6
Step 4—Level #1 Worksheet (three hearts)

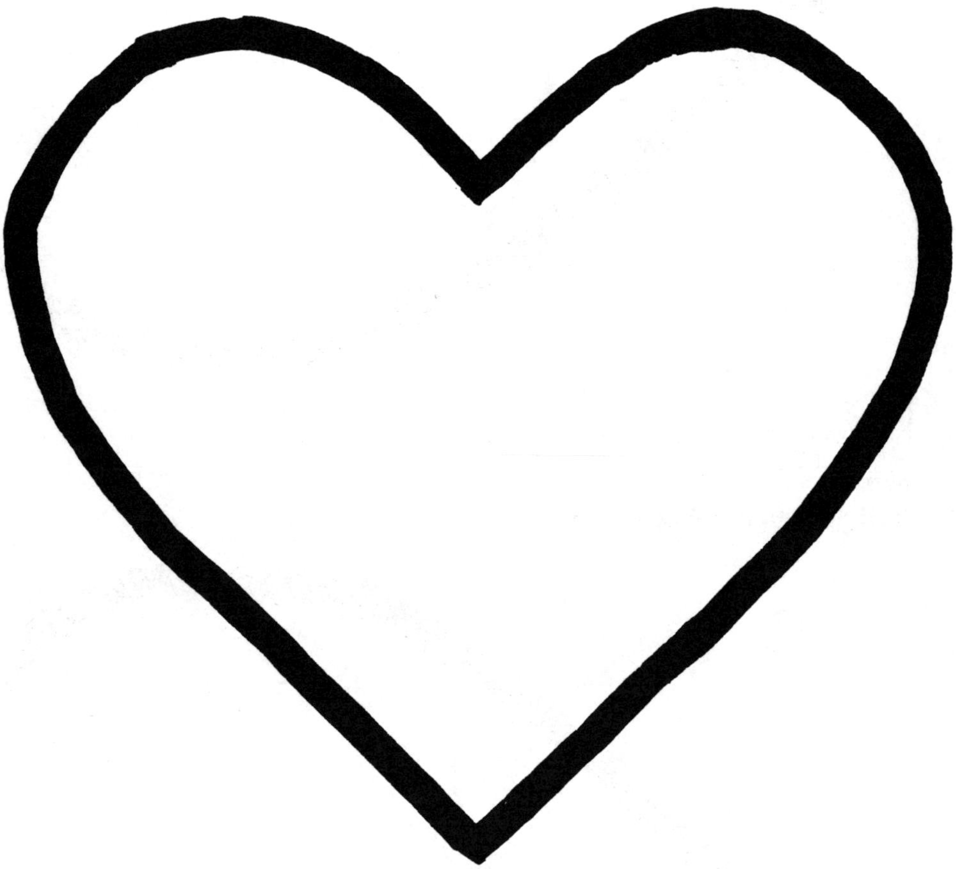

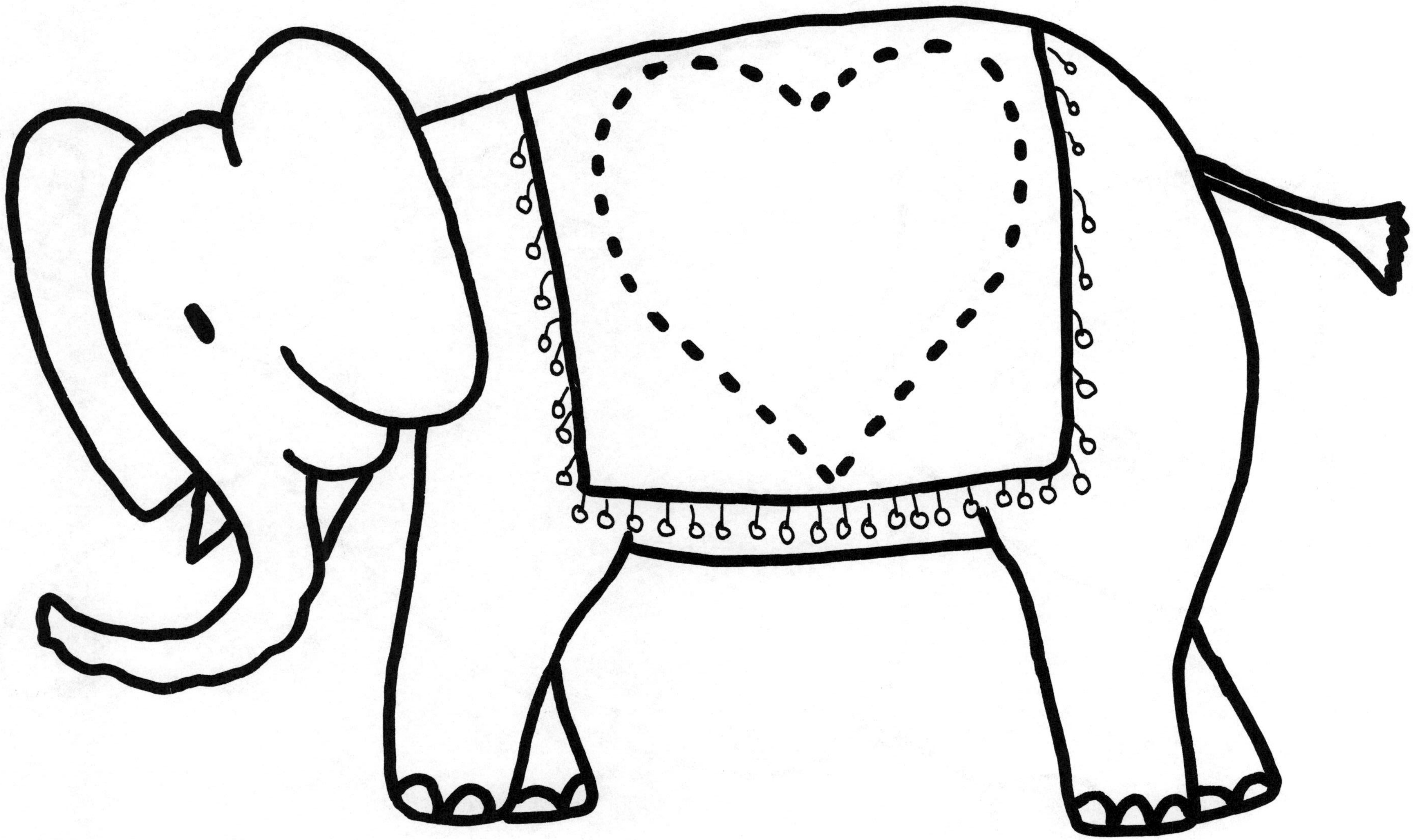

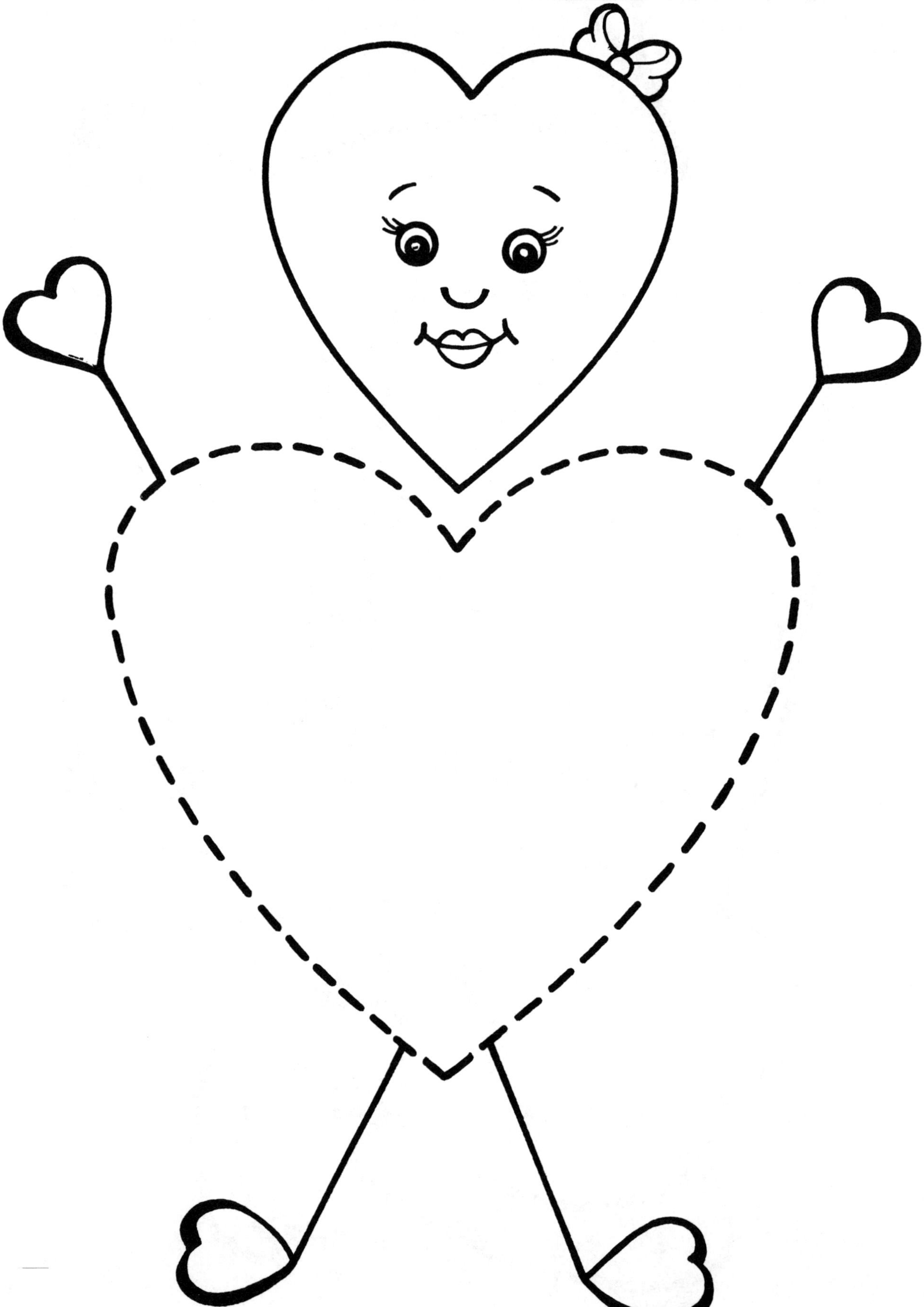

Step 4—Level #2 Worksheet

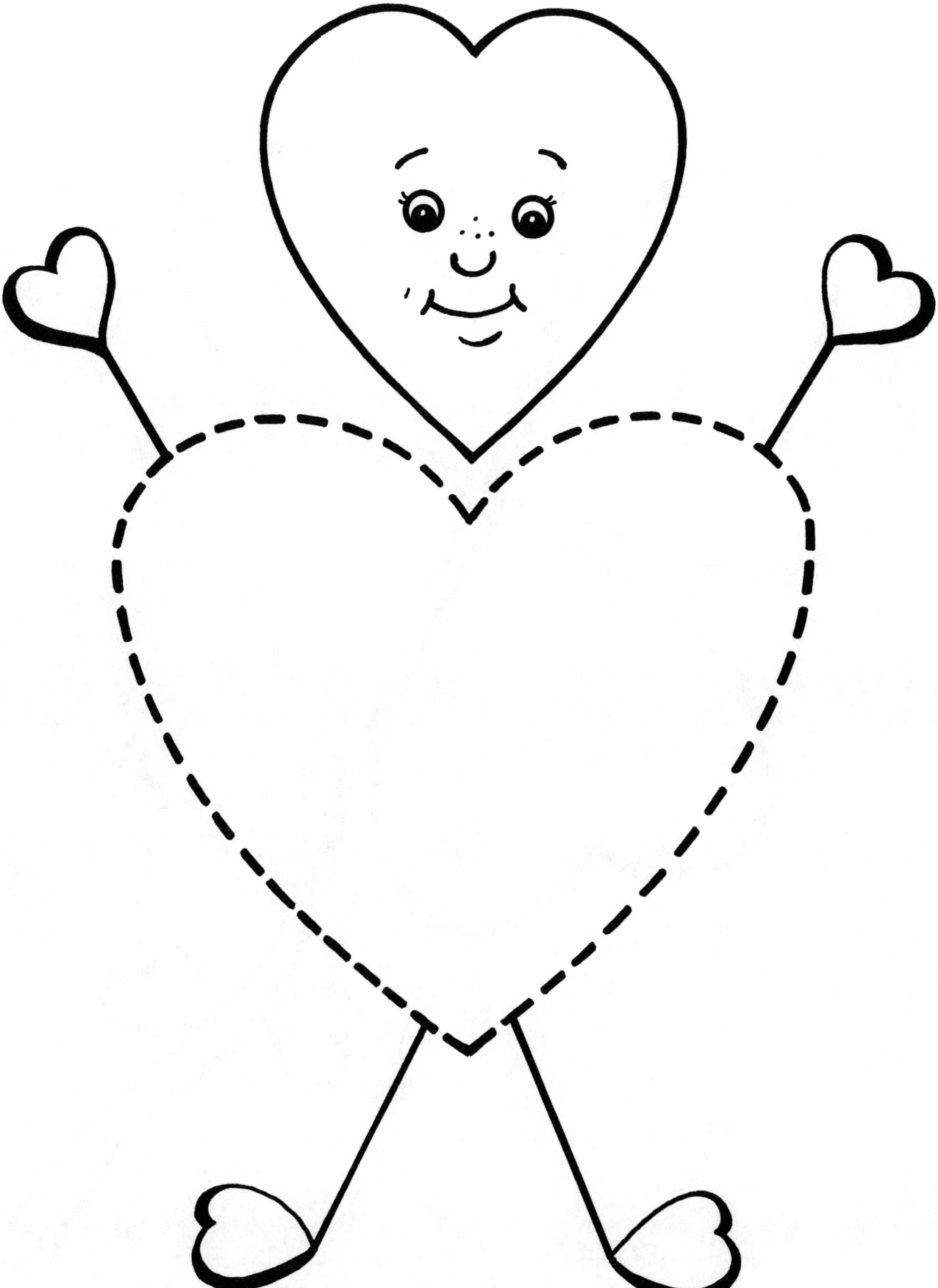

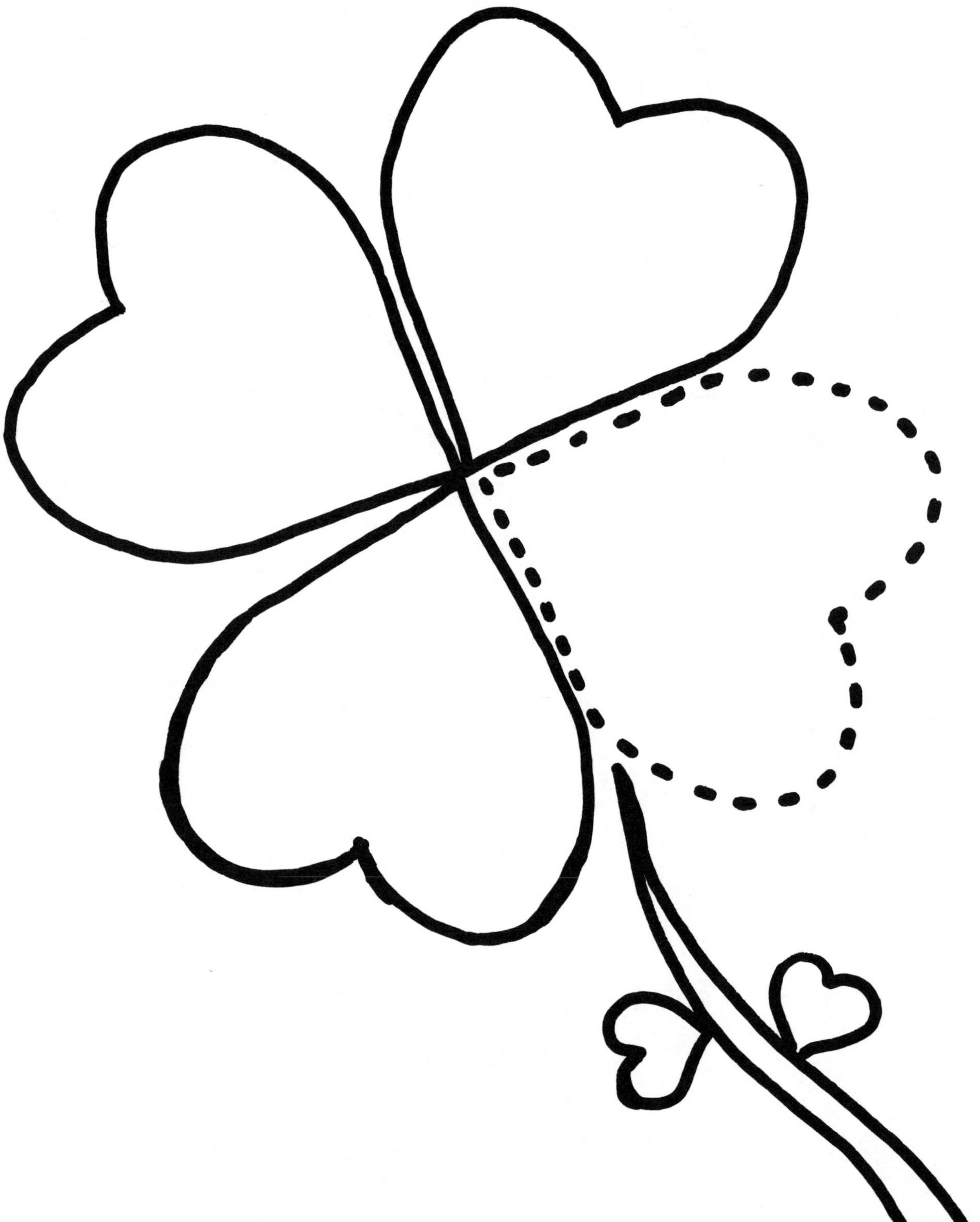

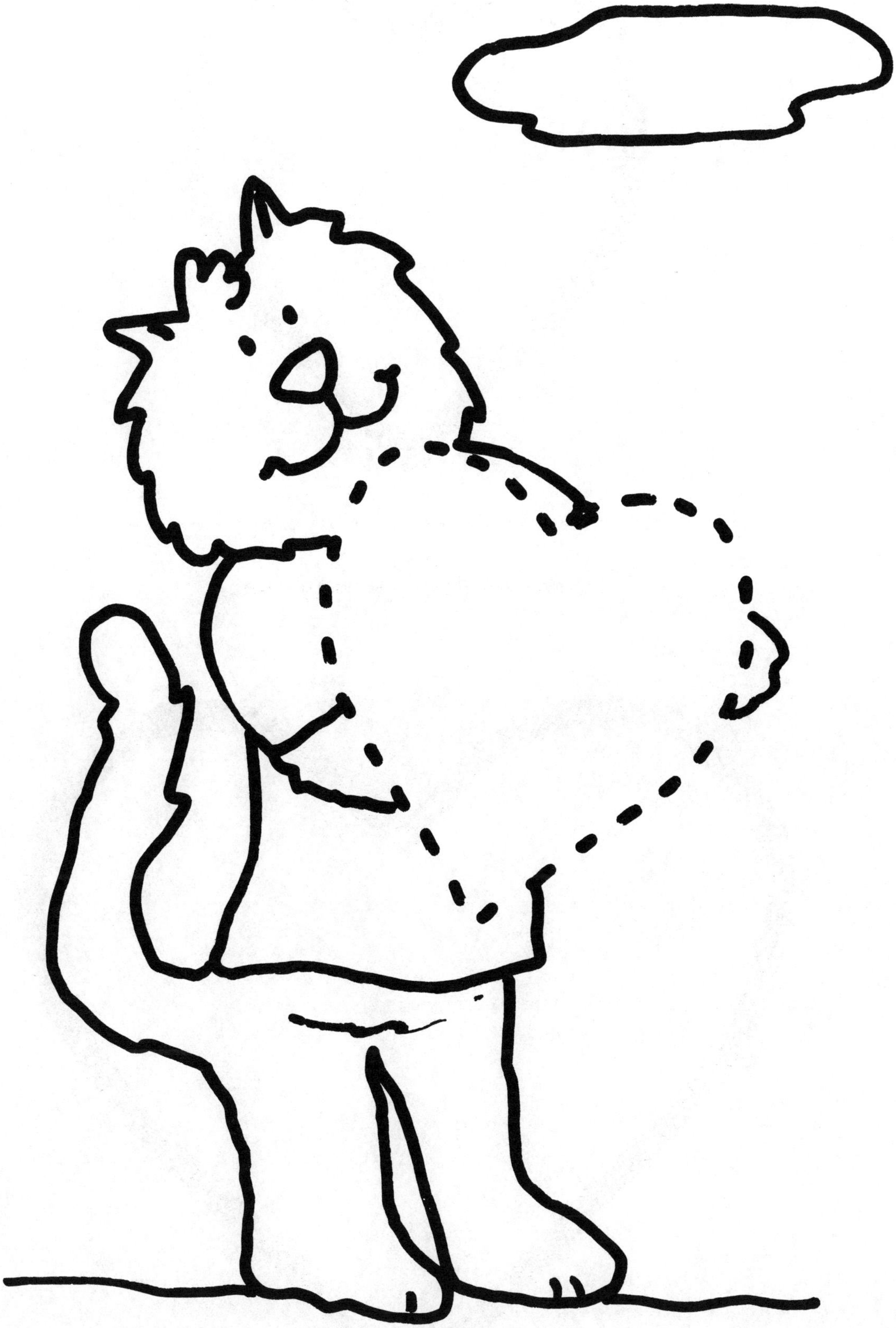

Skill 6
Step 4—Level #2 Pre/Posttest (elephant)

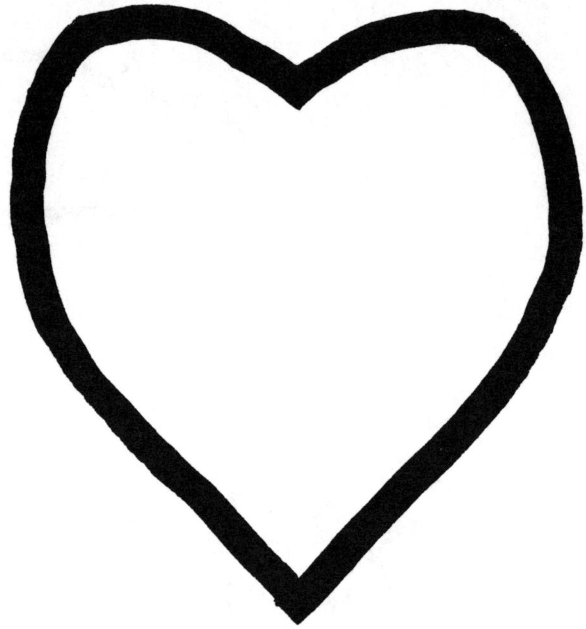

Skill 6
Step 4—Level #2 Worksheet (girl heart)

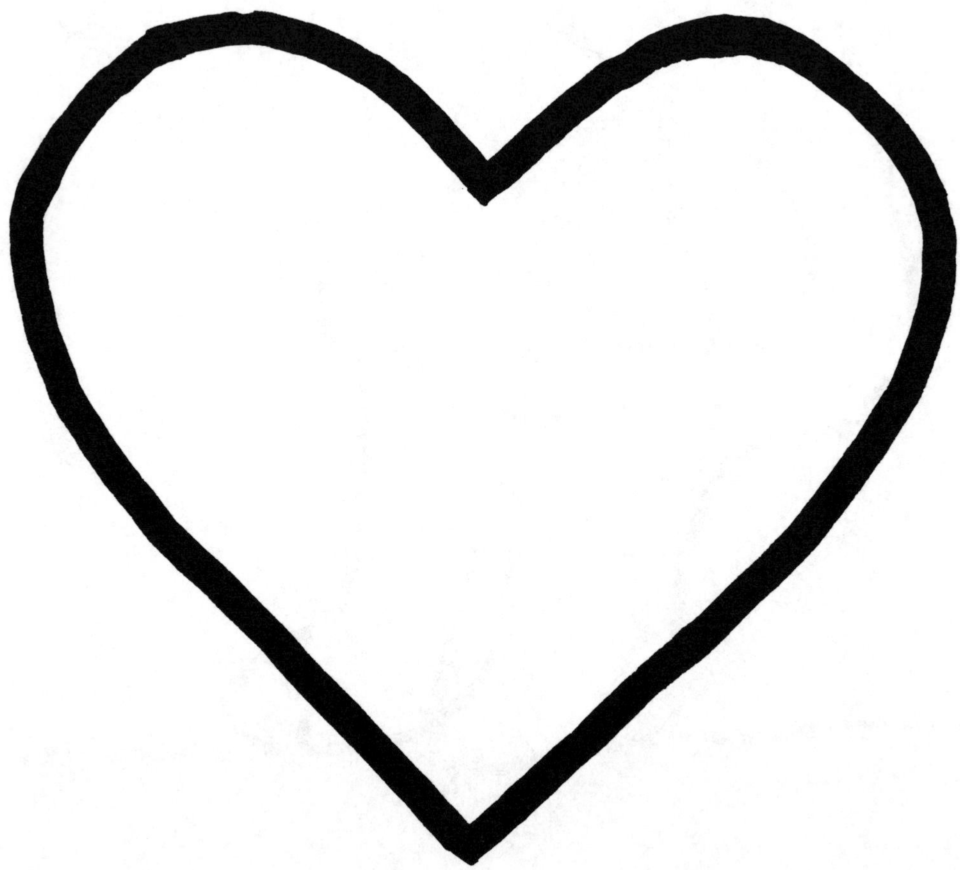

Skill 6
Step 4—Level #2 Worksheet (boy heart)

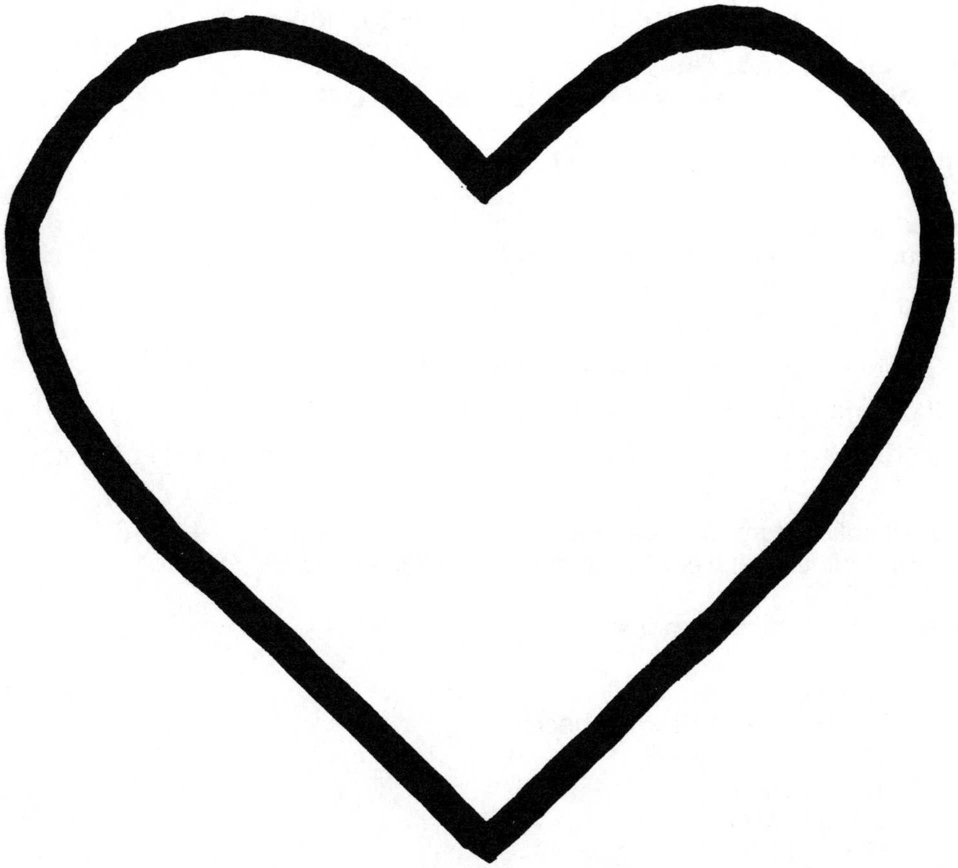

Skill 6
Step 4—Level #2 Worksheet (four-leaf clover)

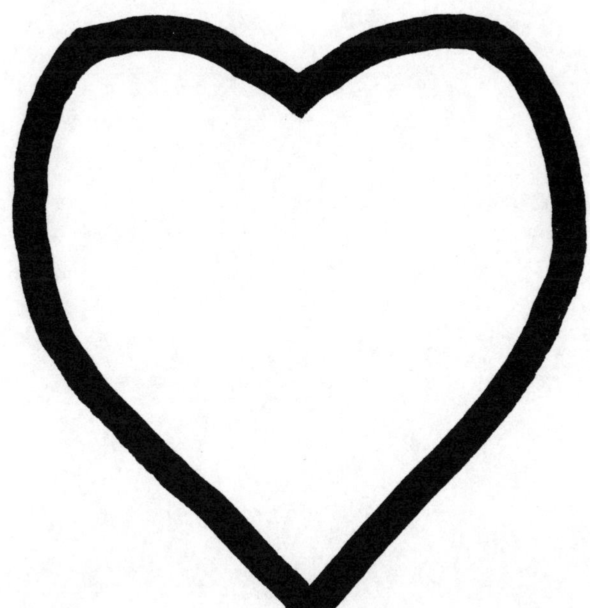

Skill 6
Step 4—Level #2 Worksheet (kitten holding heart)

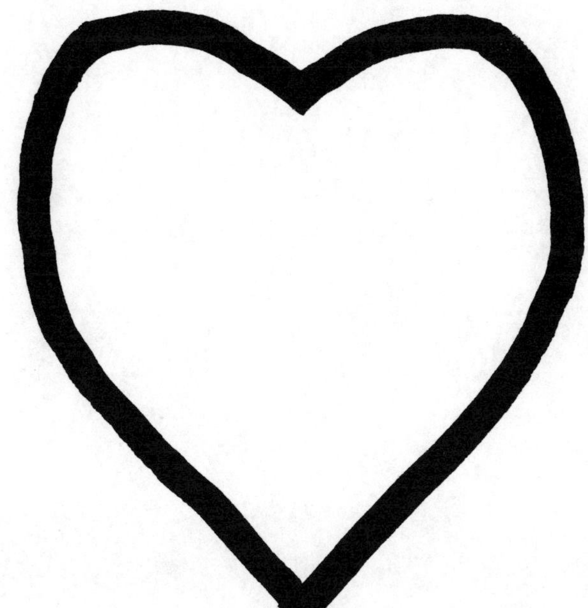

SKILL 6—STEP 5—STARS

Level #1—Stars, 1/4″ wide line
Pretest: Student takes Level #1 Pretest (star on door—4¾″ star).

If criterion met: Student advances to Level #2.

If criterion not met:
1. Student cuts Level #1 worksheets:
   cloud and star—4¾″
   magic wand—4¾″
2. Student takes Level #1 Posttest (star on door).
   If criterion met: Student advances to Level #2.
   If criterion not met: Student repeats Level #1 worksheets and Posttest.

Level #2—Smaller Stars, 1/4″ wide line
Pretest: Student takes Level #2 Pretest (star on flag—3″ star).

If criterion met: Student advances to Skill 7.

If criterion not met:
1. Student cuts Level #2 worksheets:
   football helmet—3″
   star on box—3″
   star on easel—3″
   star on ball—3″
   star on baby's bib—3″
   star on clown—3″
2. Student takes Level #2 Posttest (star on flag).
   If criterion met: Student advances to Skill 7.
   If criterion not met: Student repeats Level #2 worksheets and Posttest.

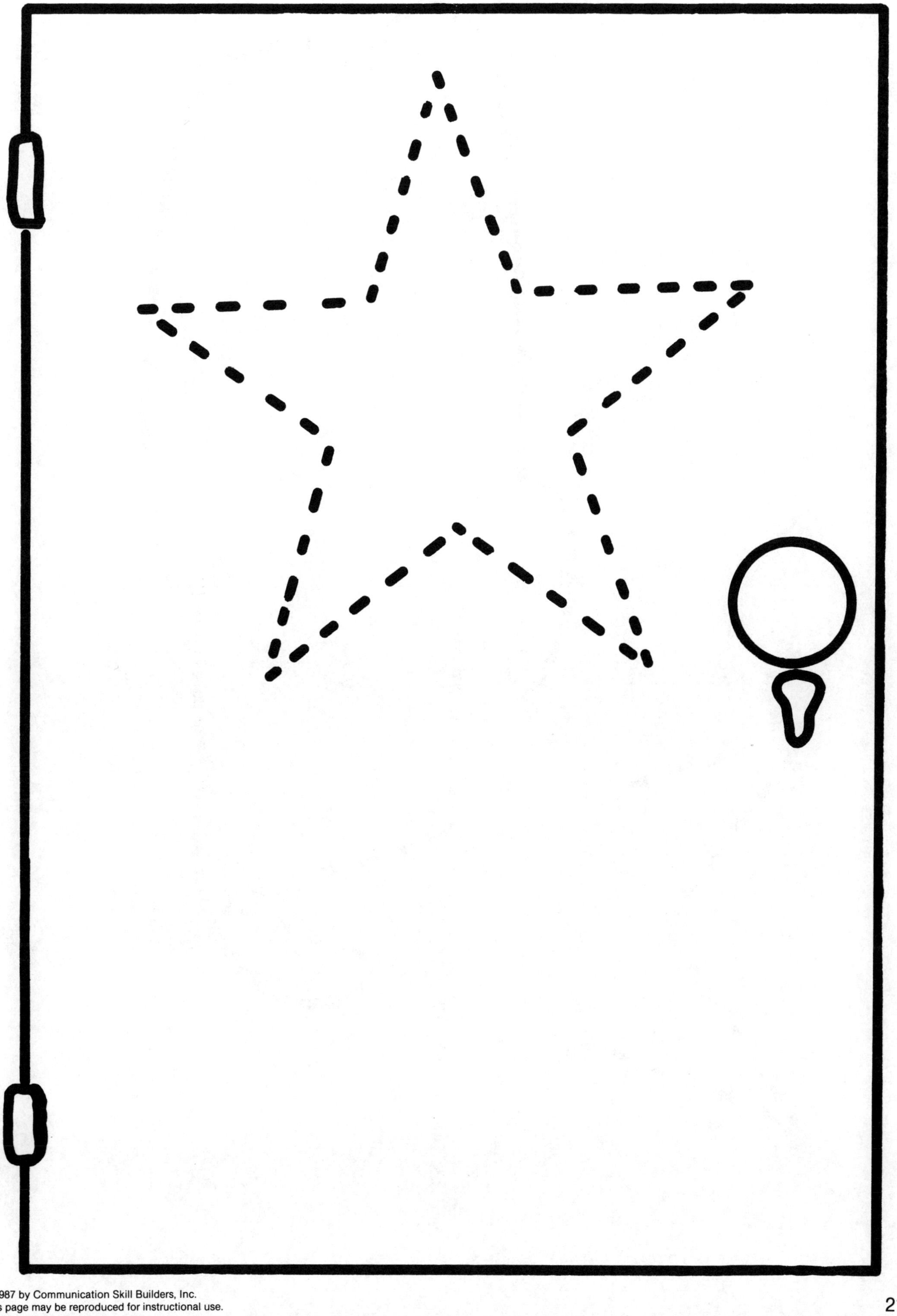

Step 5—Level #1 Worksheet

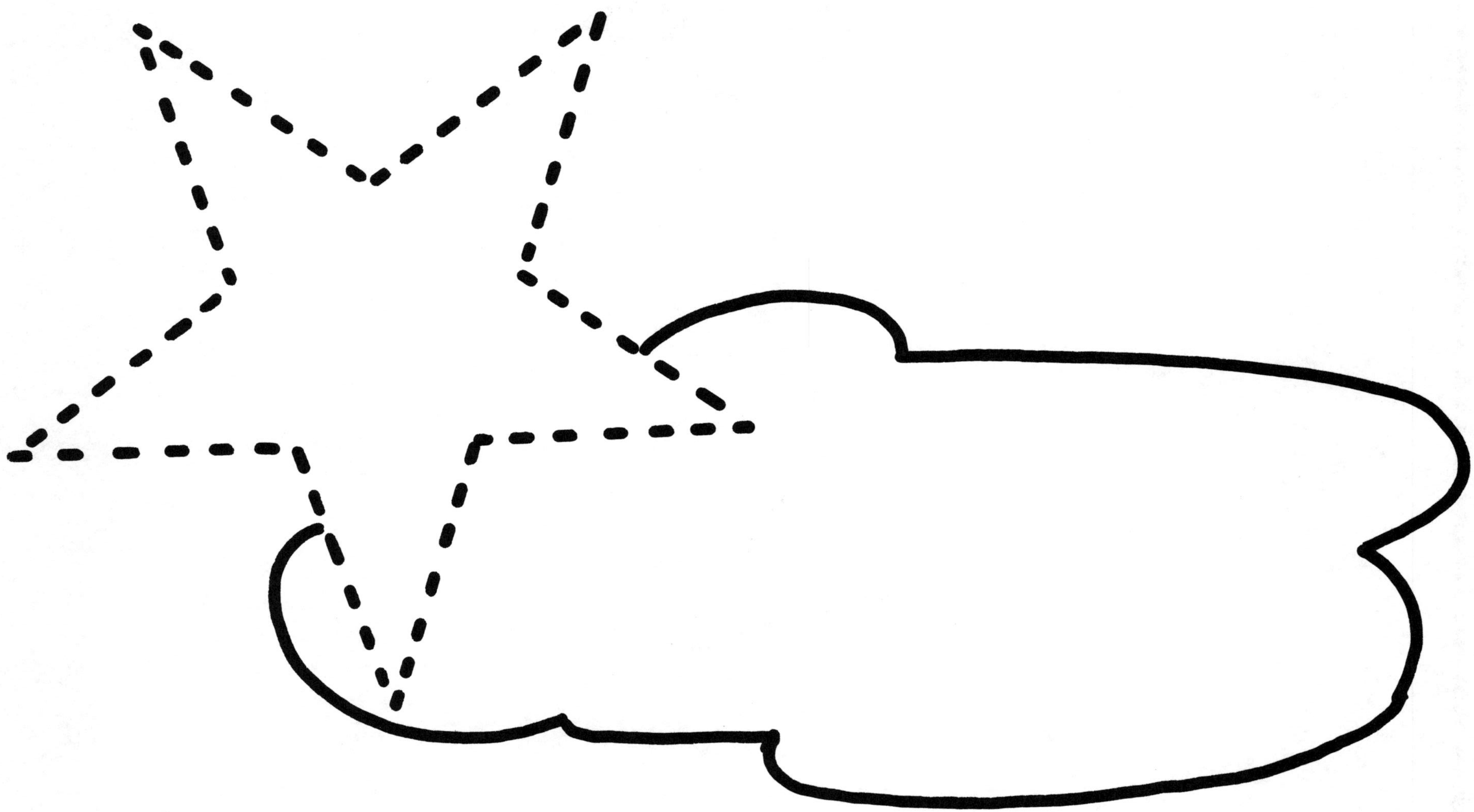

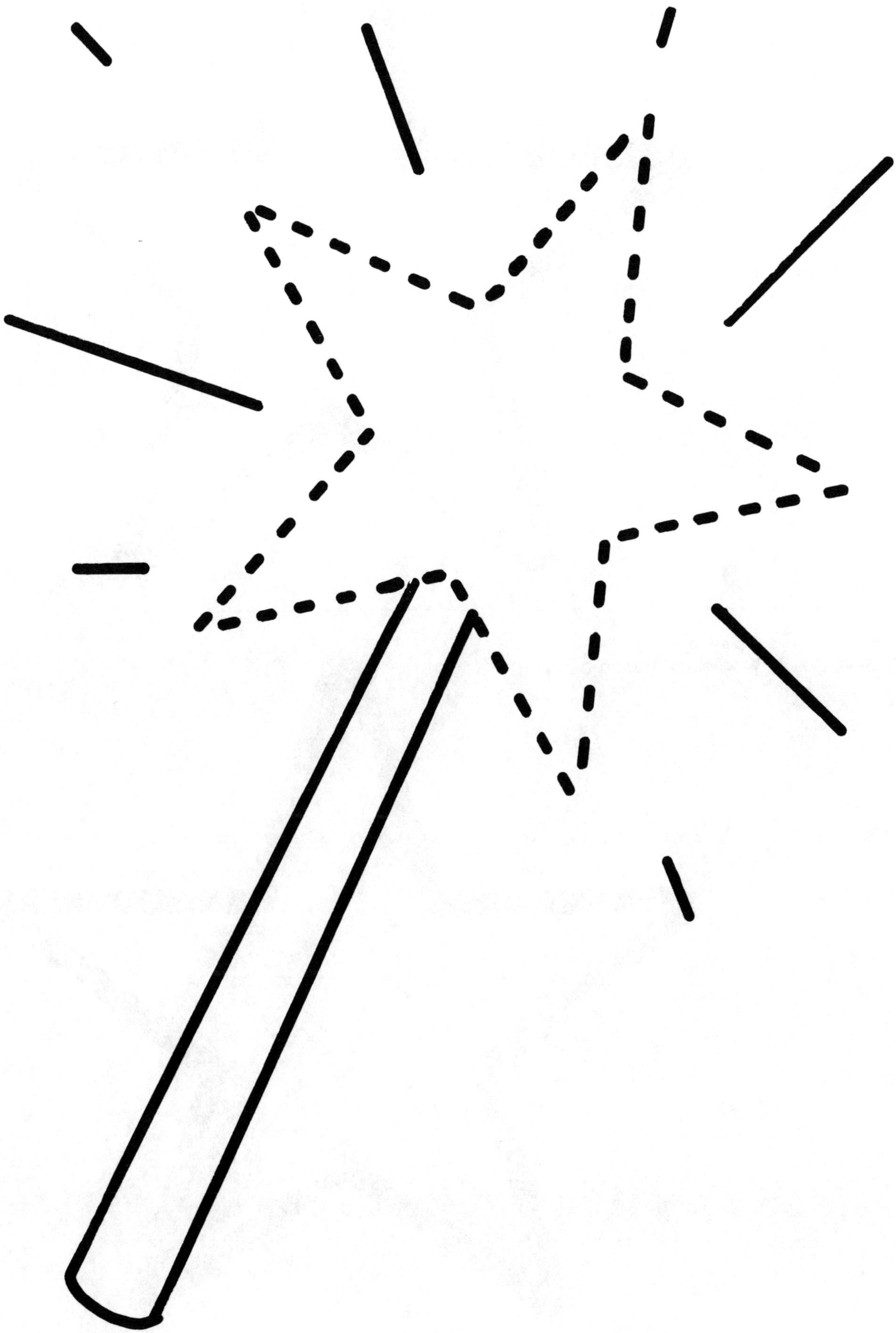

Skill 6
Step 5—Level #1 Pre/Posttest (star on door)

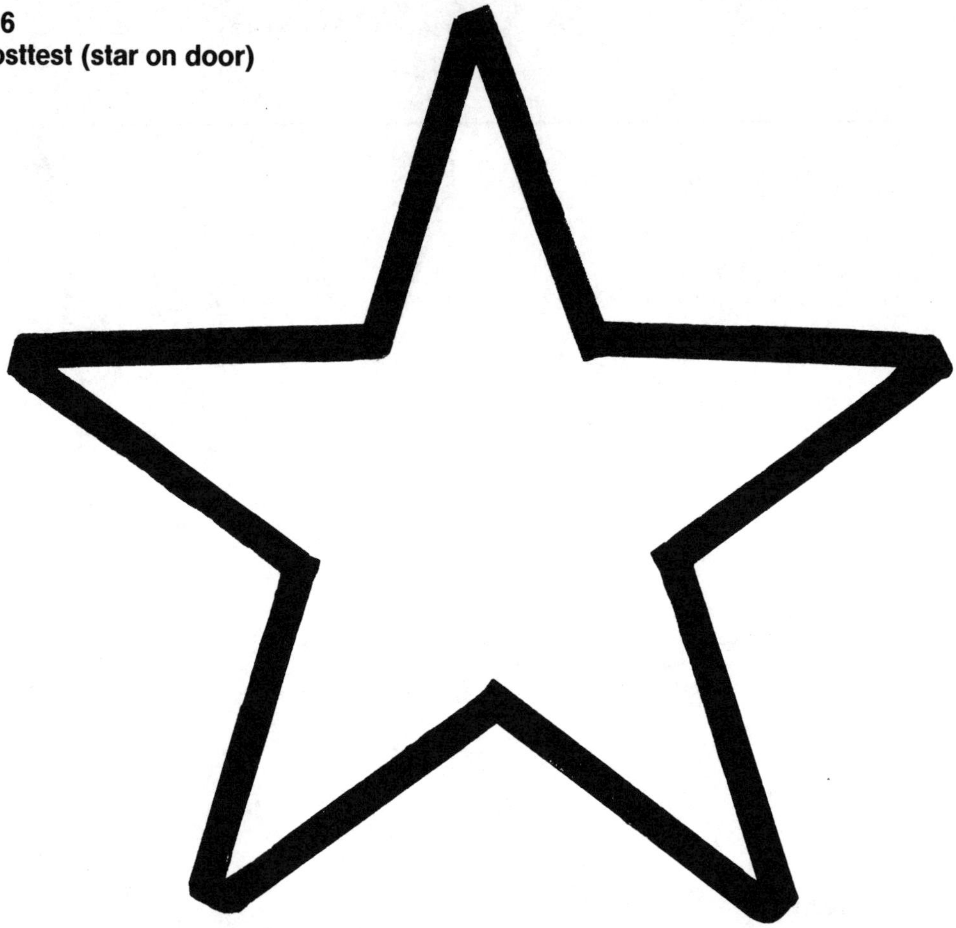

Skill 6
Step 5—Level #1 Worksheet (cloud and star)

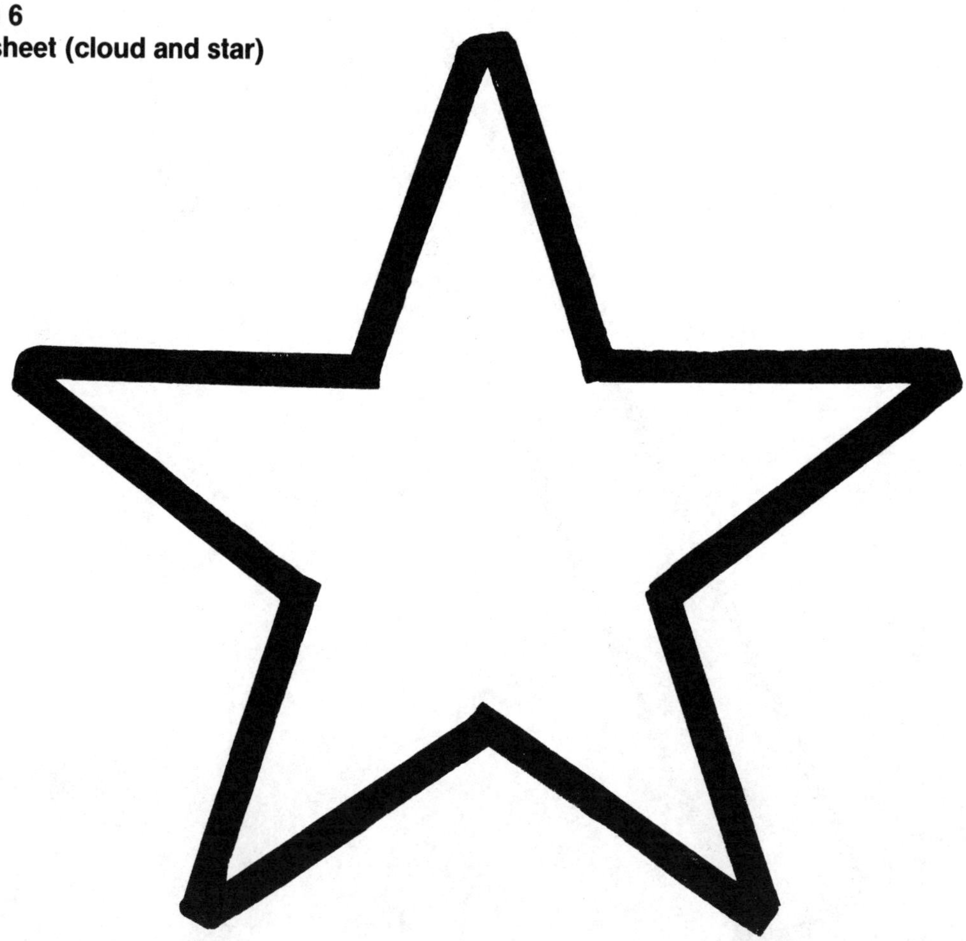

Skill 6
Step 5—Level #1 Worksheet (magic wand)

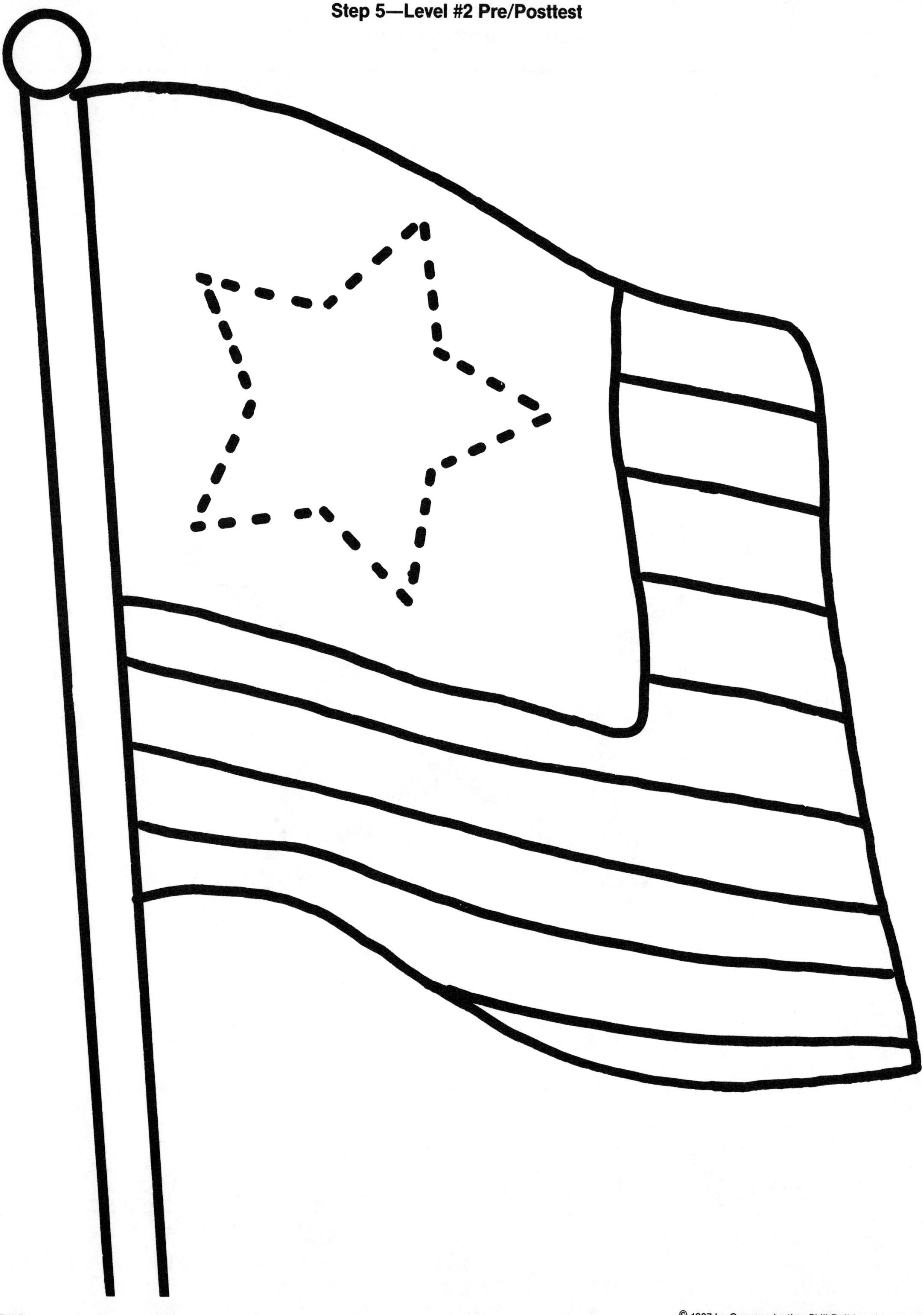

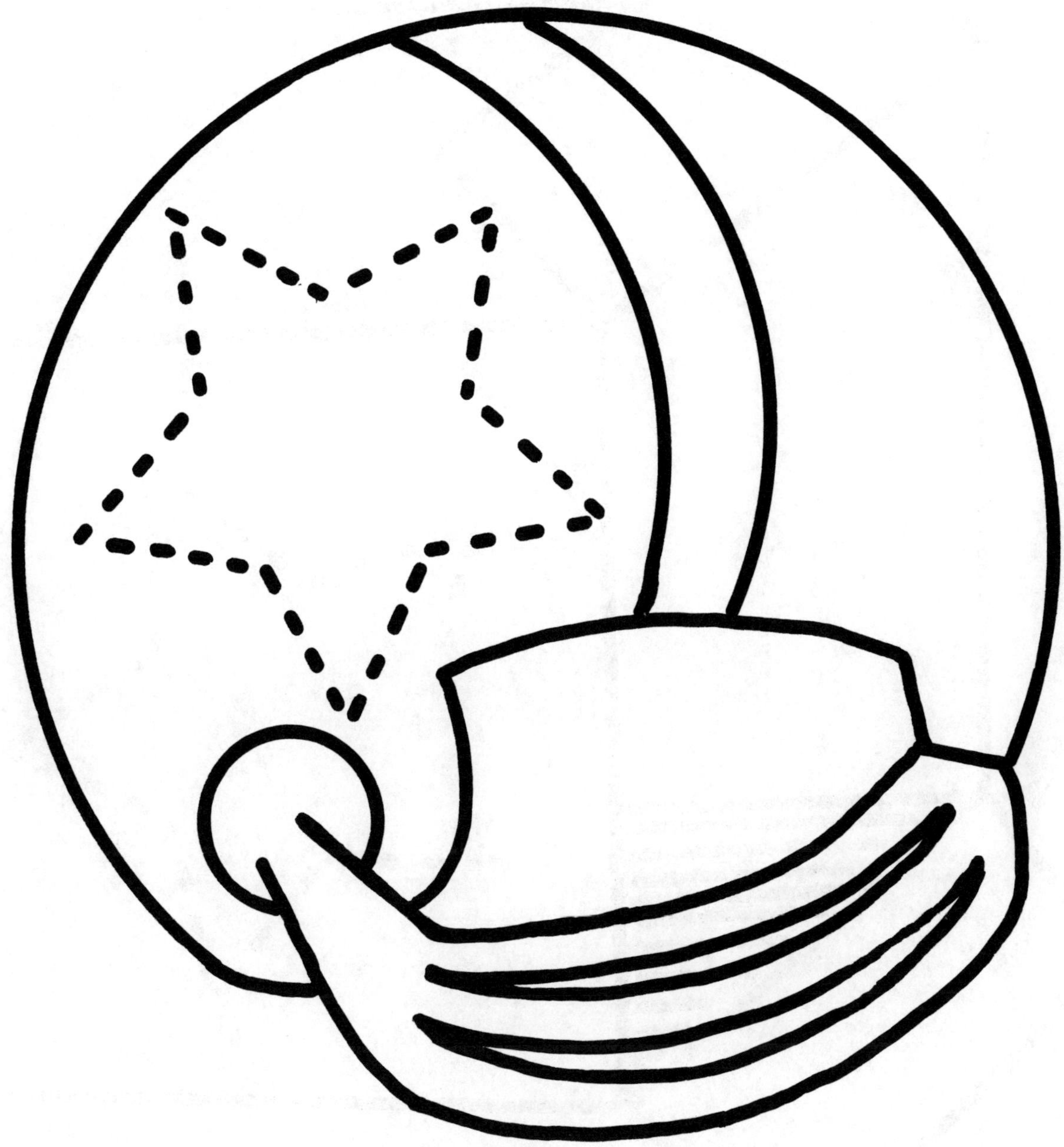

Step 5—Level #2 Worksheet

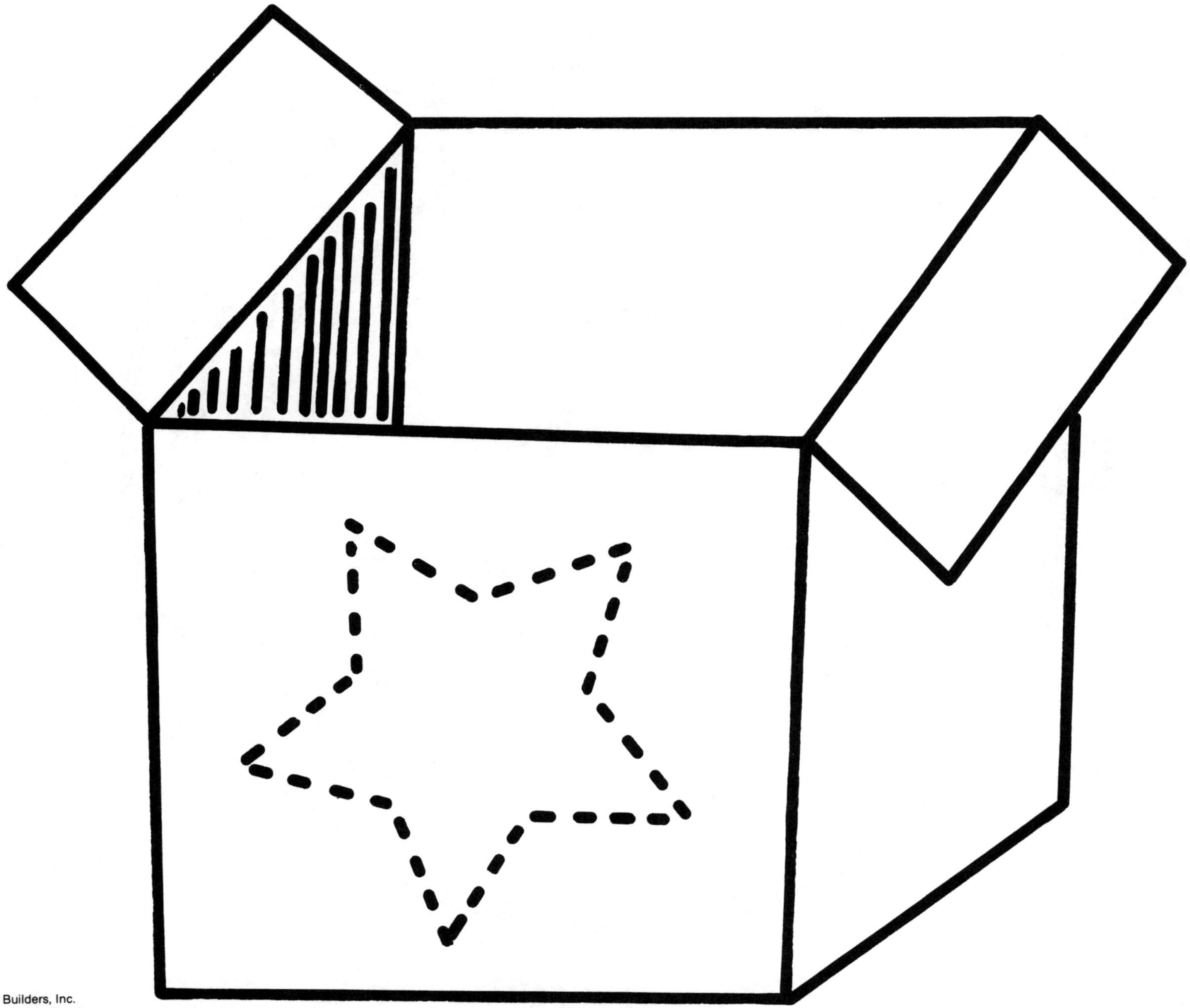

Step 5—Level #2 Worksheet

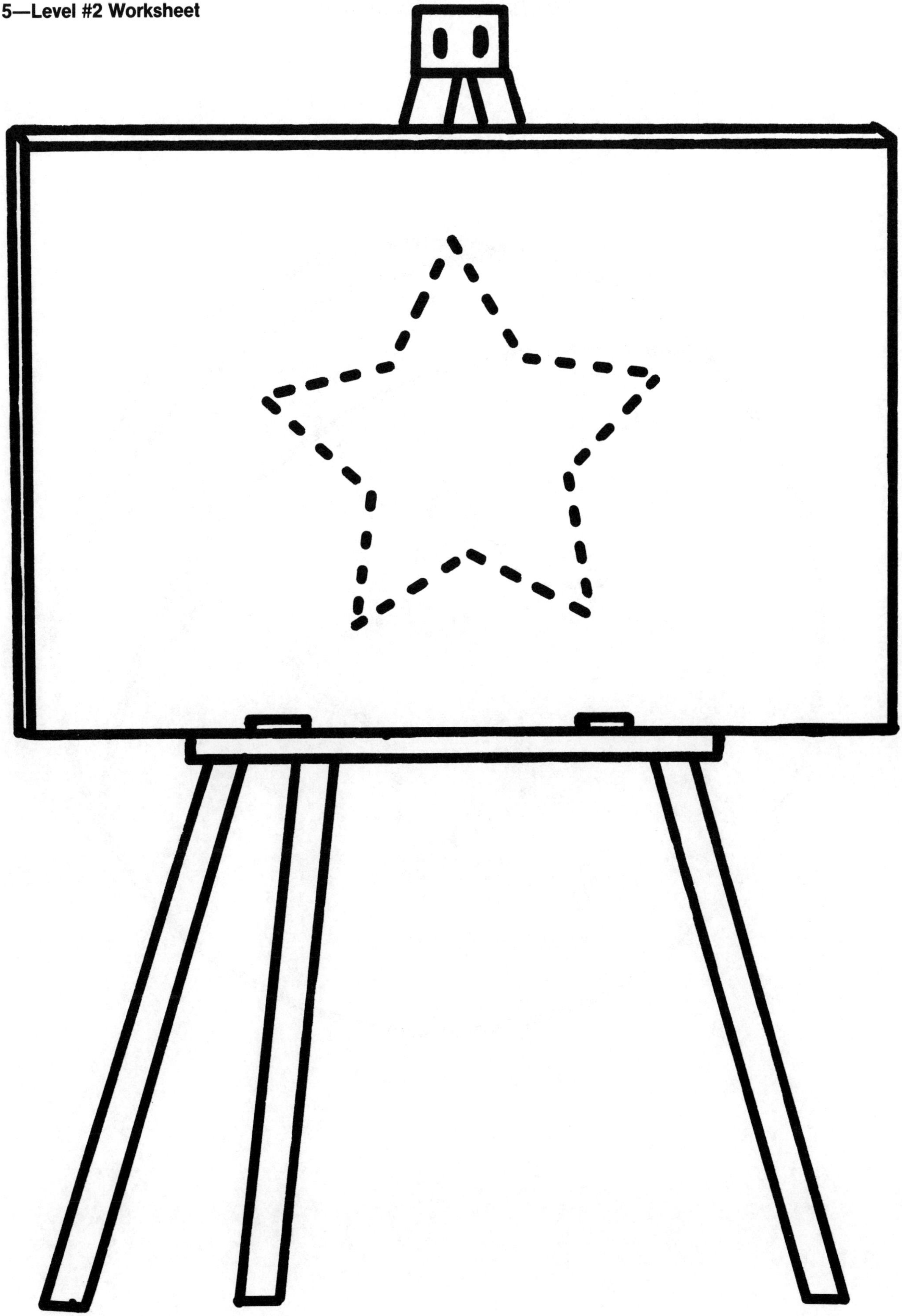

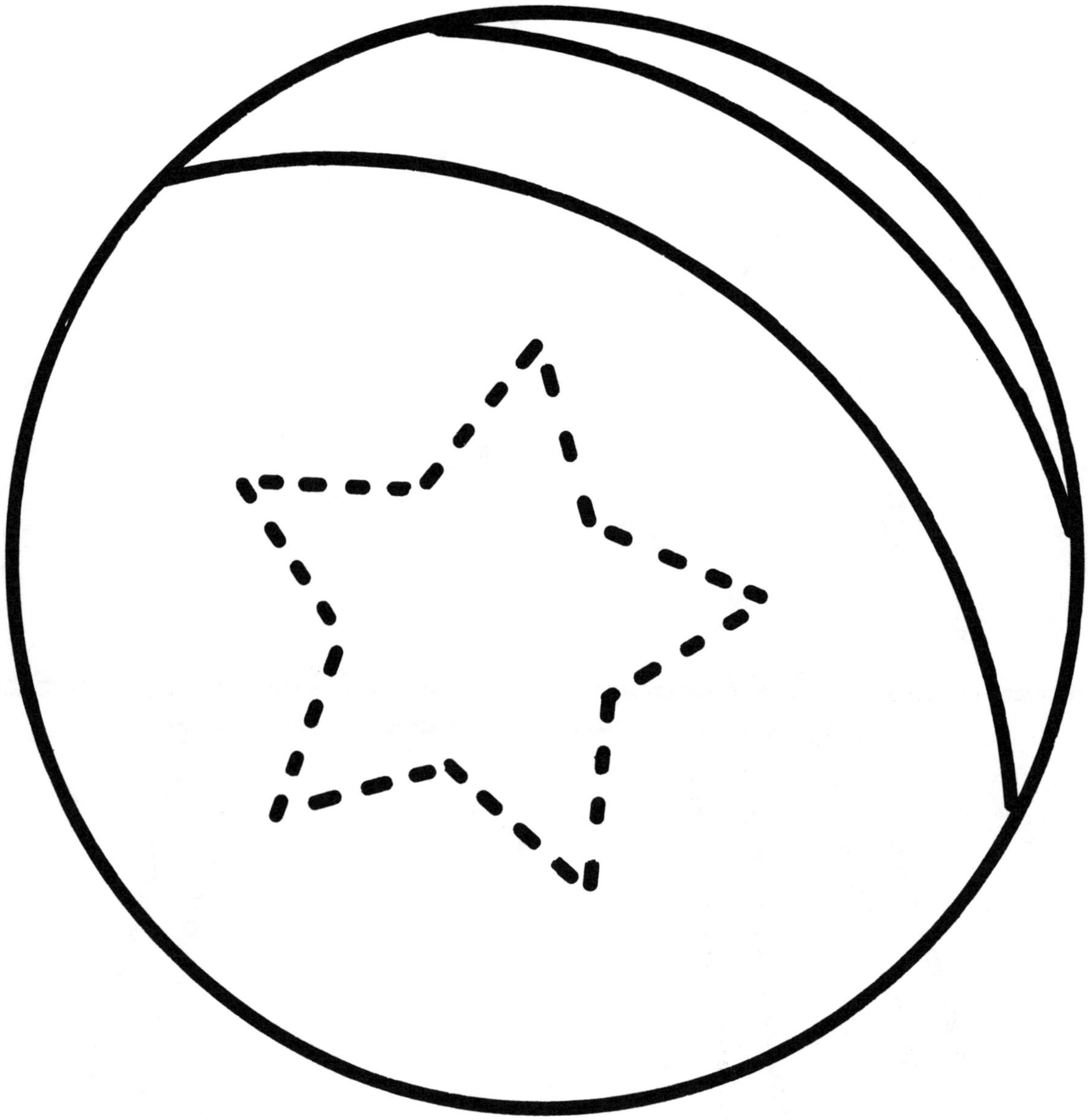

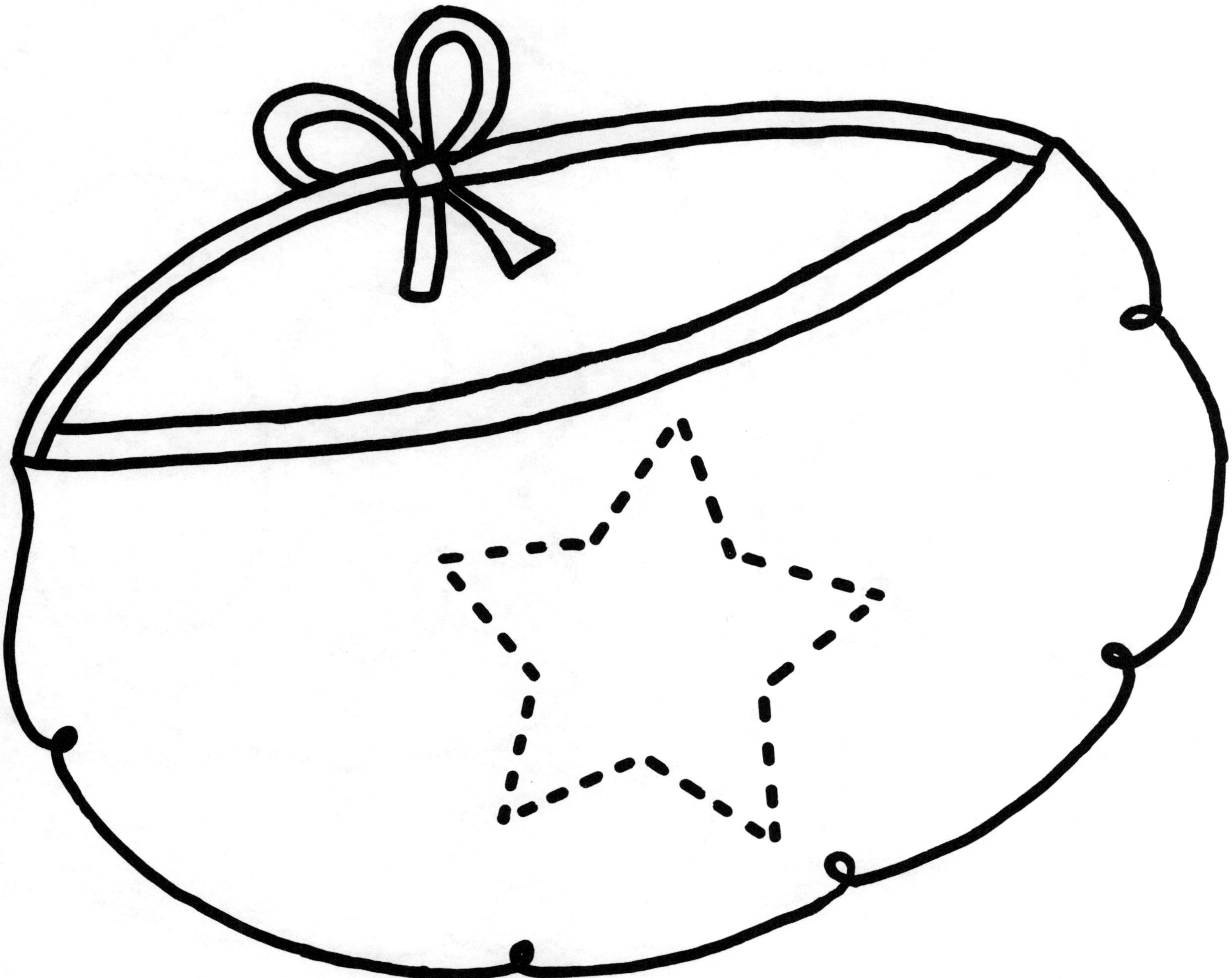

Skill 6
Step 5—Level #2 Pre/Posttest (star on flag)

Skill 6
Step 5—Level #2 Worksheet (football helmet)

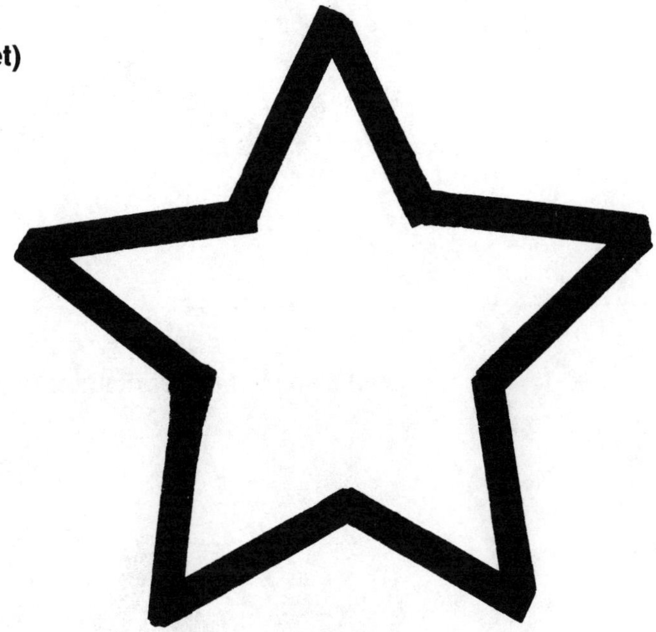

Skill 6
Step 5—Level #2 Worksheet (star on box)

Skill 6
Step 5—Level #2 Worksheet (star on easel)

Skill 6
Step 5—Level #2 Worksheet (star on ball)

Skill 6
Step 5—Level #2 Worksheet (star on baby's bib)

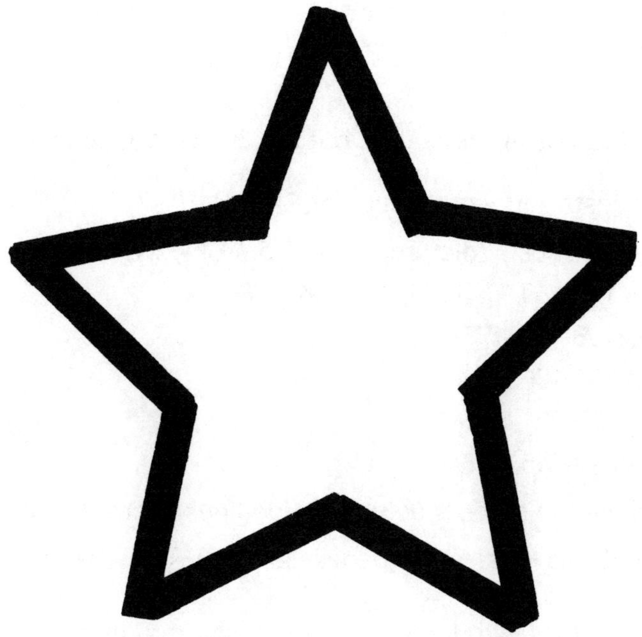

Skill 6
Step 5—Level #2 Worksheet (star on clown)

Skill 7—Cutting Circles and Complex Shapes—⅛″ Line

Objective: Student cuts out circles and complex shapes of varying sizes with a line ⅛″ wide, and pastes them on the corresponding fixed outlines, with 80% accuracy.

Procedure
All Skill 6 Steps and Levels are repeated, but the line is reduced to ⅛″ wide.

To prepare Pre/Posttests and worksheets for Skill 7:

1. Reproduce the worksheets (pictures only) from Skill 6 at each Step and Level:
   - Step 1: pages 145-150, 154-158, 161-164
   - Step 2: pages 168-172, 175-179
   - Step 3: pages 183-186, 189-193
   - Step 4: pages 197-201, 205-209
   - Step 5: pages 213-215, 218-224
2. DO NOT reproduce the cutouts (with ¼″ wide lines) from Skill 6.
3. Reproduce the cutouts that follow (pages 229-253). These shapes have ⅛″ wide lines needed for Skill 7.

   Use these Skill 7 shapes with the worksheets (pictures) from Skill 6.

Skill 7
Step 1—Level #1 Pre/Posttest (shape person)

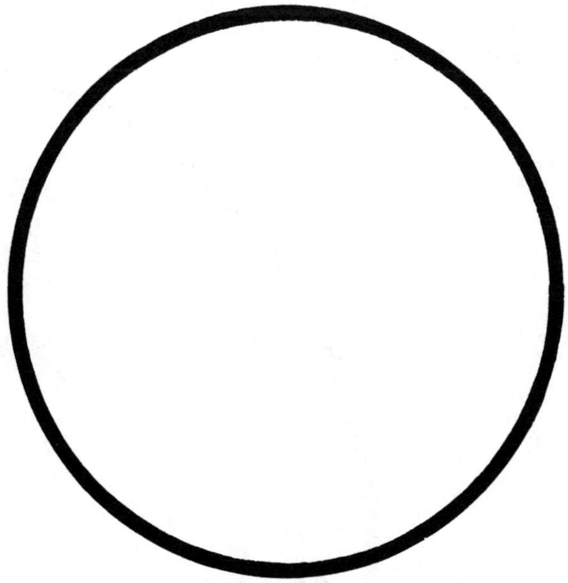

Skill 7
Step 1—Level #1 Worksheet (snail)

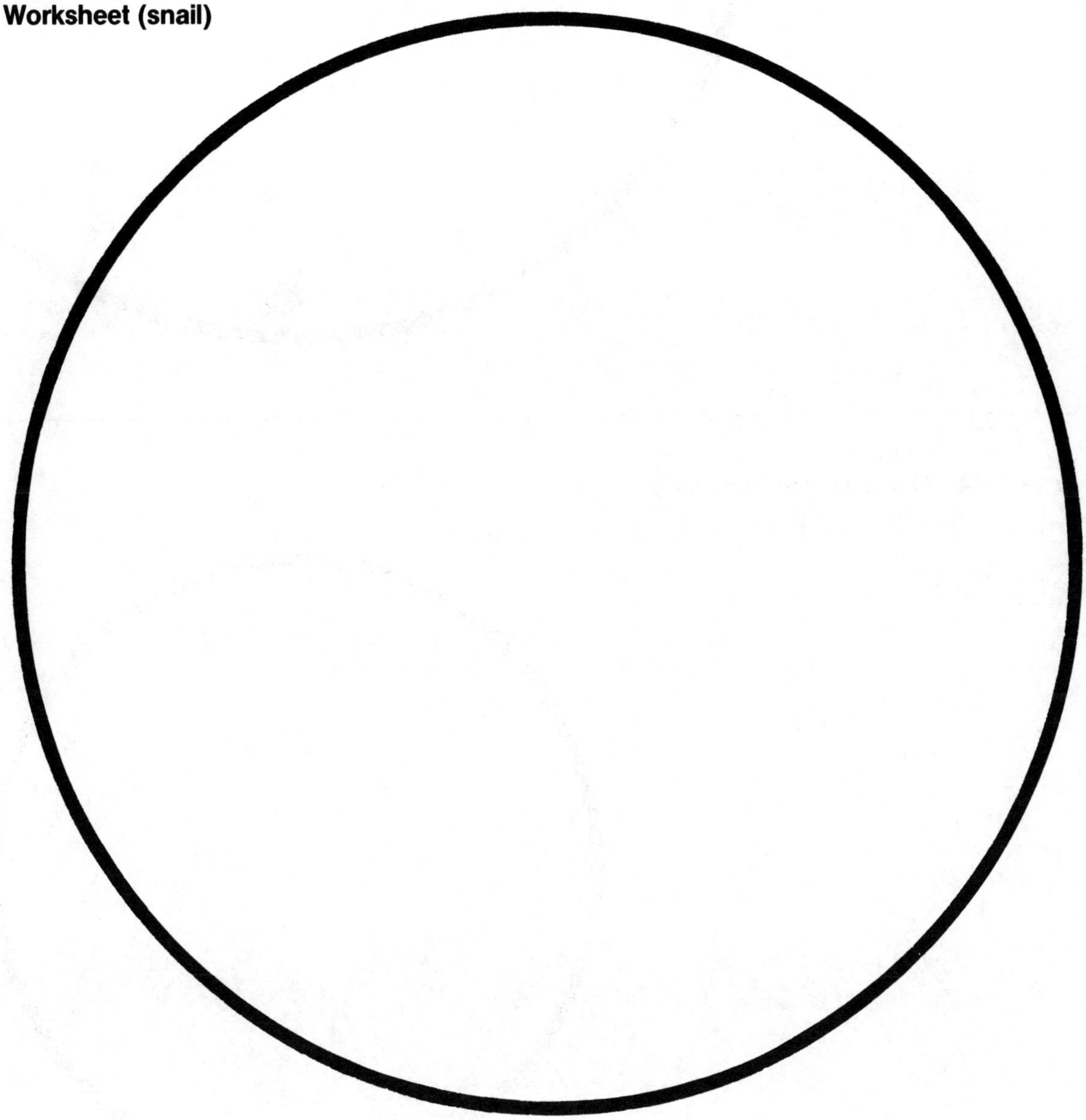

Skill 7
Step 1—Level #1 Worksheet (clock)

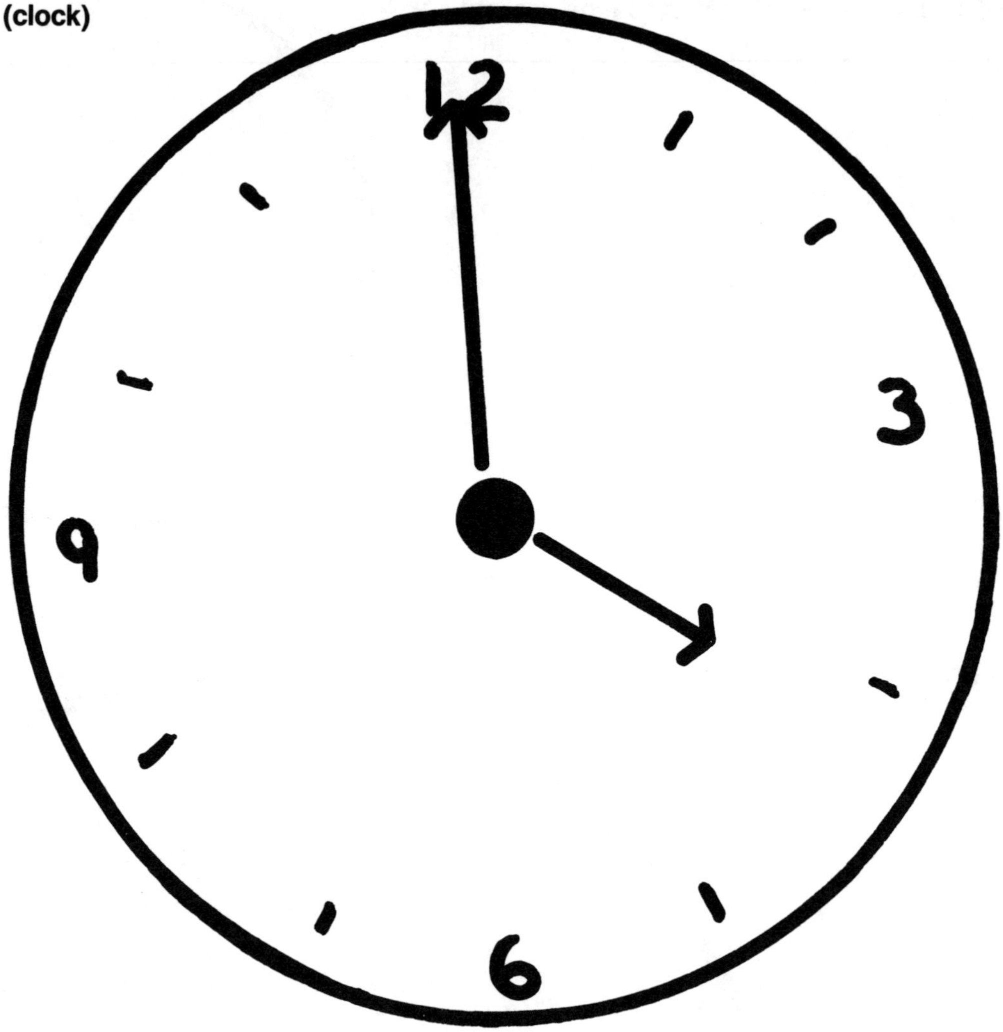

Skill 7
Step 1—Level #1 Worksheet (baseball)

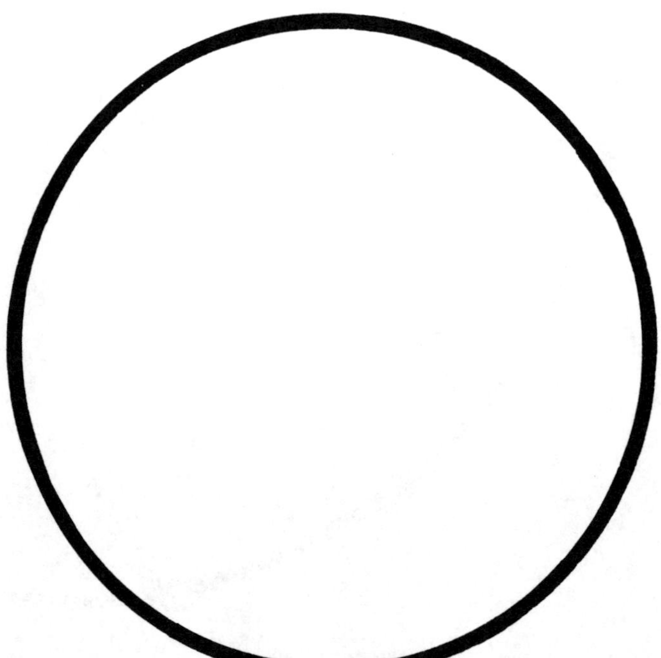

Skill 7
Step 1—Level #1 Worksheet (tricycle)

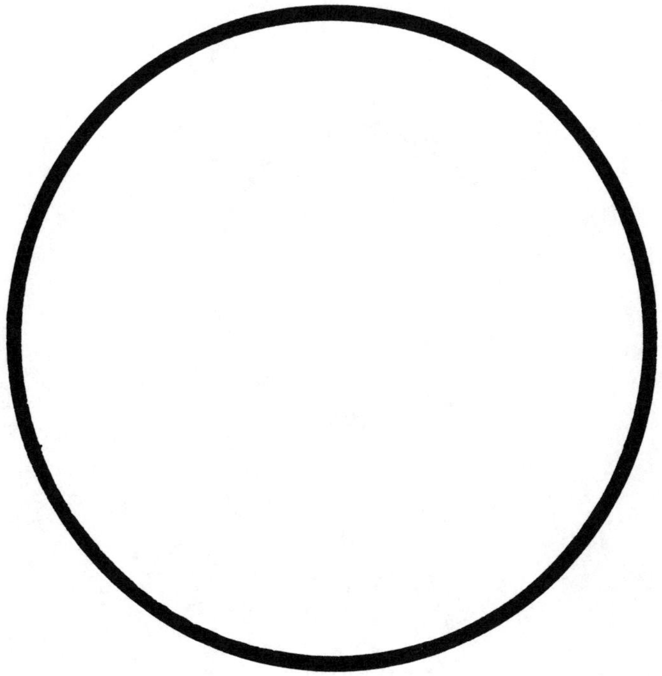

Skill 7
Step 1—Level #1 Worksheet (sun)

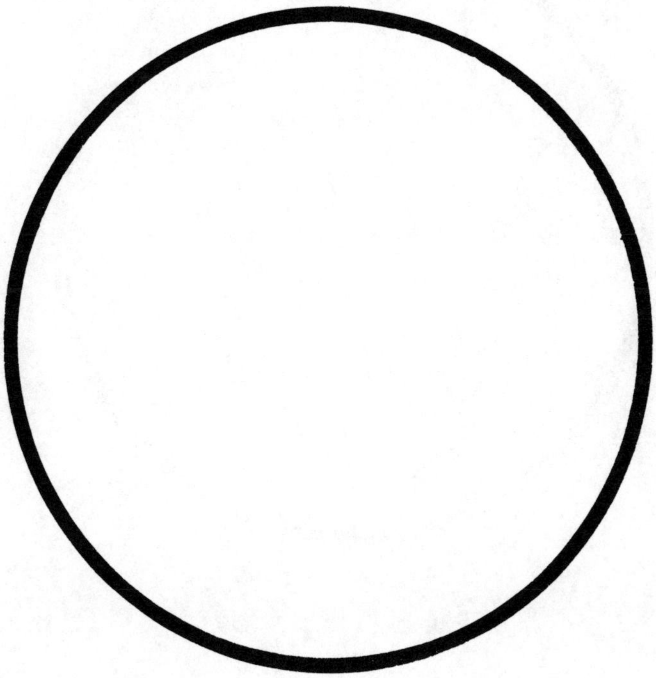

Skill 7
Step 1—Level #2 Pre/Posttest (fish with air bubble)

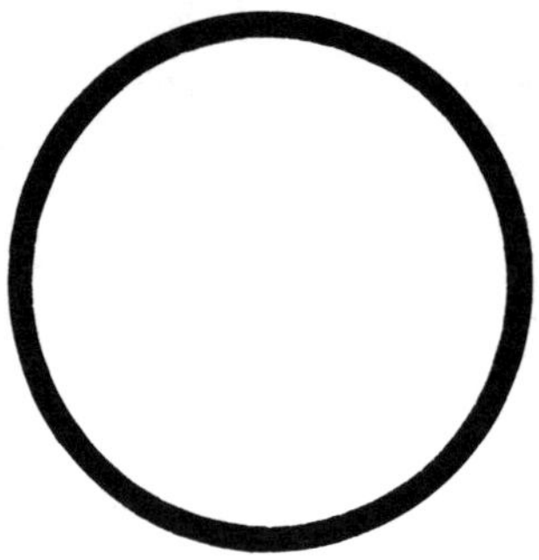

Skill 7
Step 1—Level #2 Worksheet (balloon)

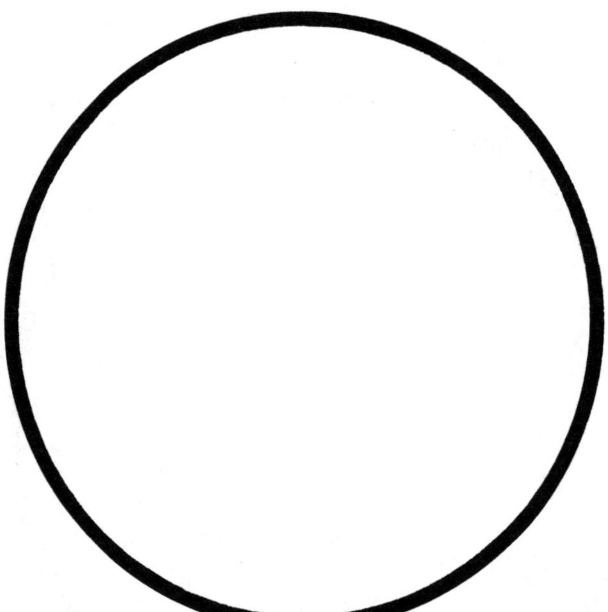

Skill 7
Step 1—Level #2 Worksheet (soap bubble)

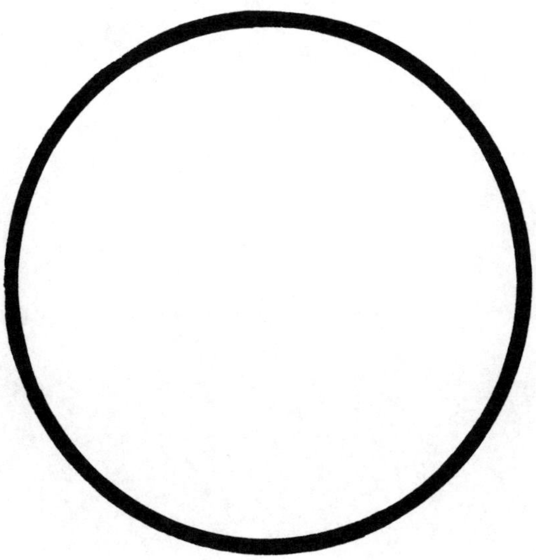

Skill 7
Step 1—Level #2 Worksheet (traffic signal)

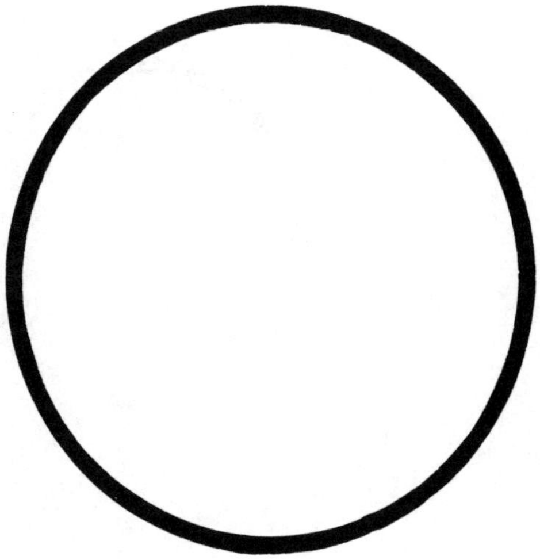

Skill 7
Step 1—Level #2 Worksheet (flower)

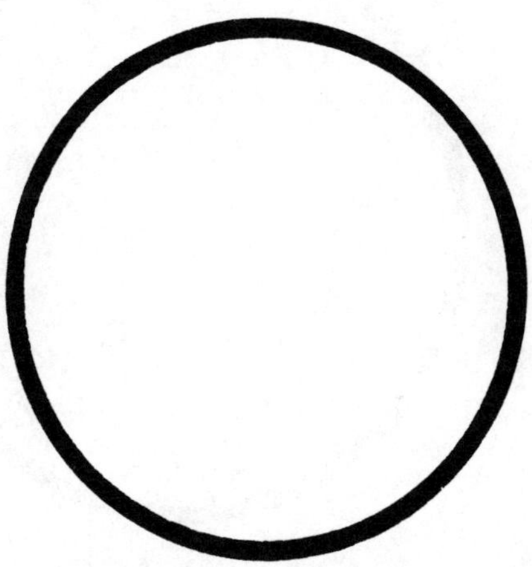

Skill 7
Step 1—Level #3 Pre/Posttest (sunglasses)

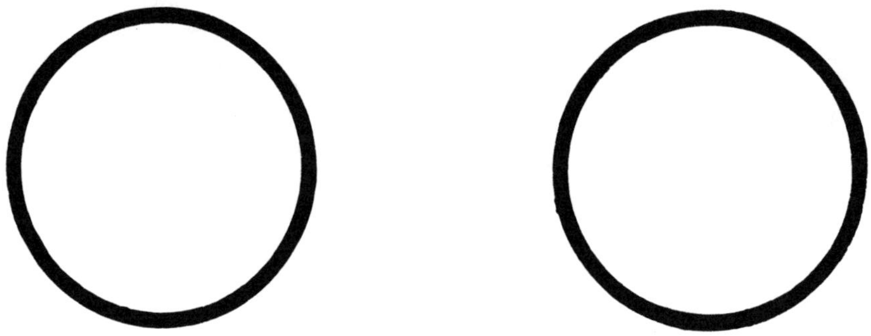

Skill 7
Step 1—Level #3 Worksheet (golf cart)

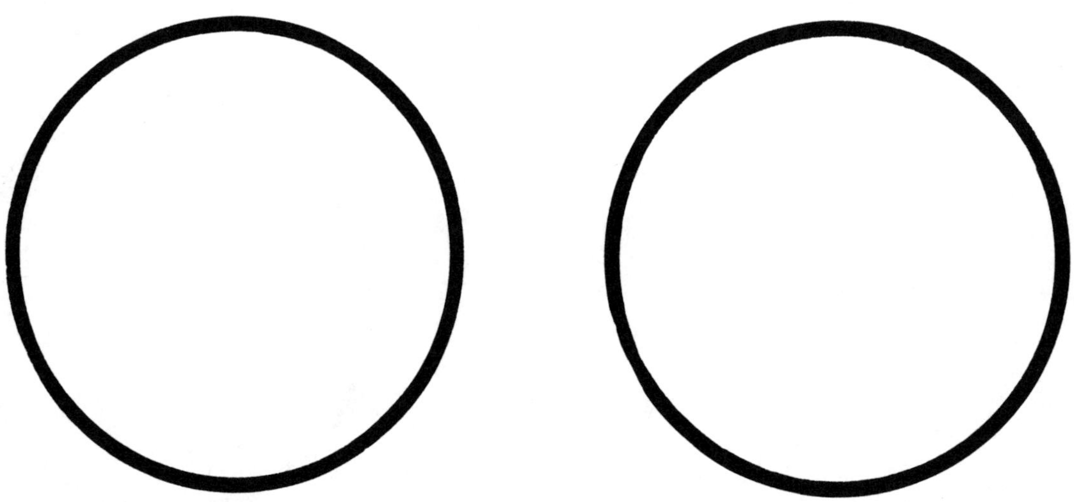

Skill 7
Step 1—Level #3 Worksheet (car)

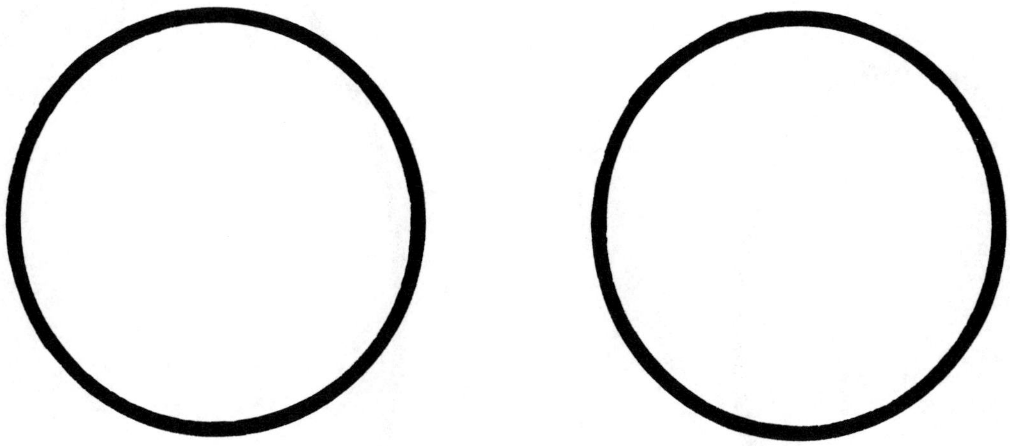

Skill 7
Step 1—Level #3 Worksheet (baby carriage)

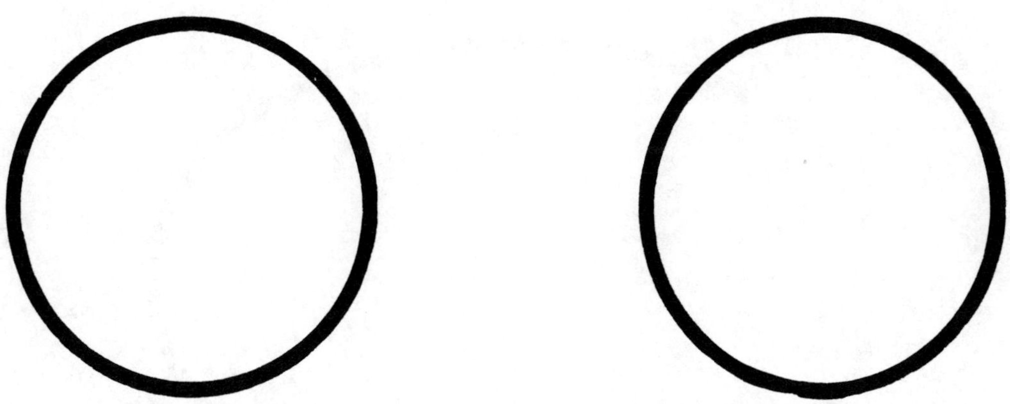

Skill 7
Step 2—Level #1 Pre/Posttest (cattail plant)

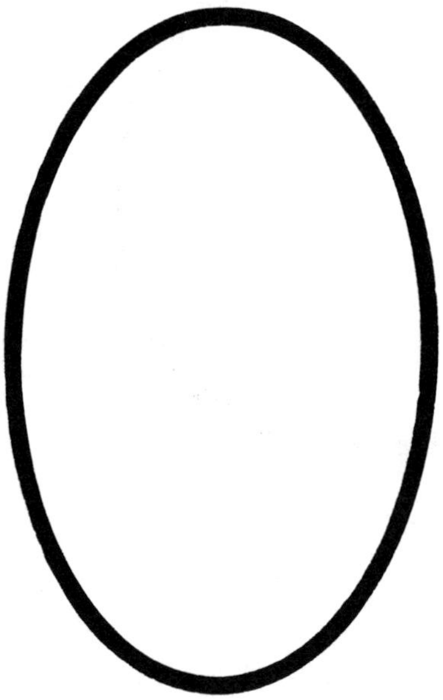

Skill 7
Step 2—Level #1 Worksheet (clown with balloon)

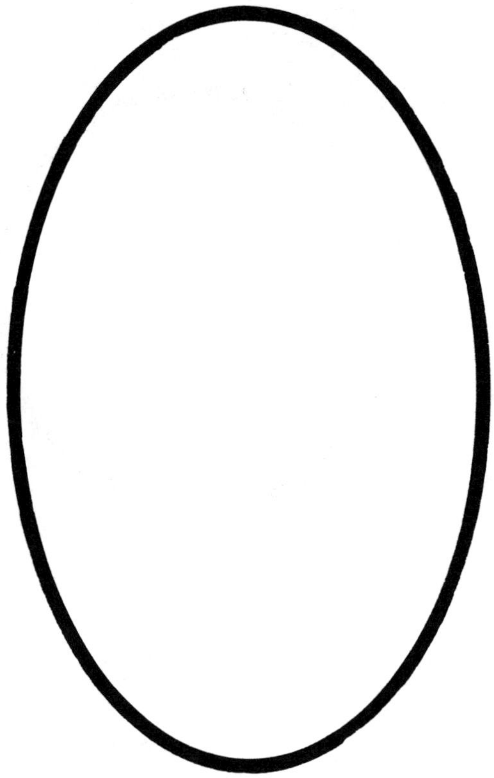

Skill 7
Step 2—Level #1 Worksheet (egg)

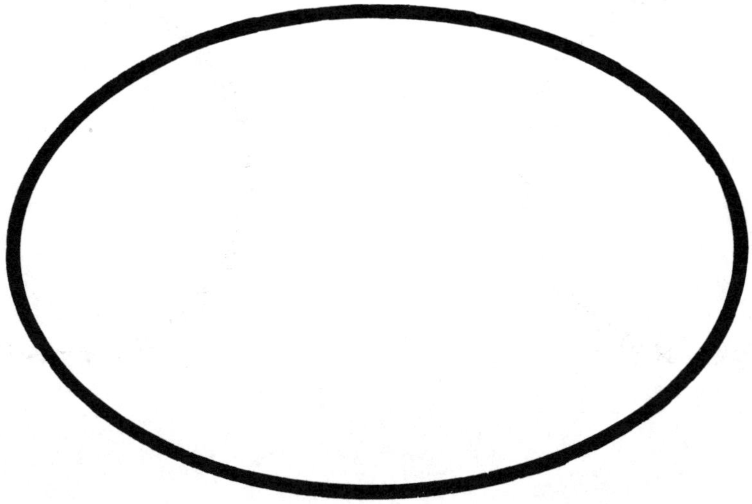

Skill 7
Step 2—Level #1 Worksheet (mirror)

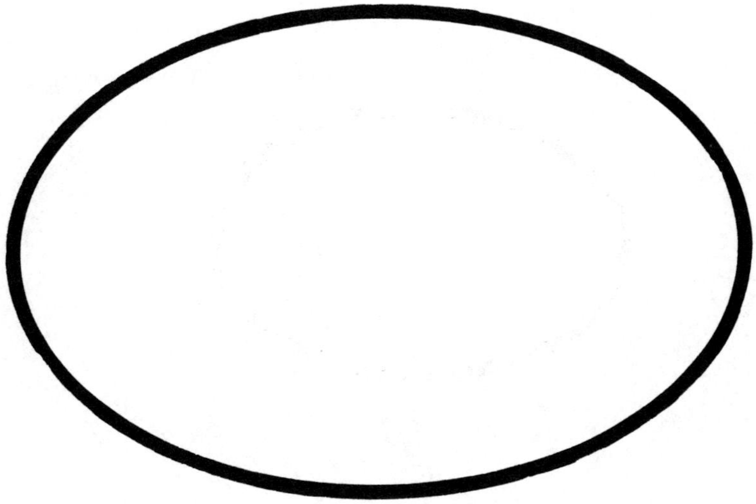

Skill 7
Step 2—Level #1 Worksheet (garbage can cover)

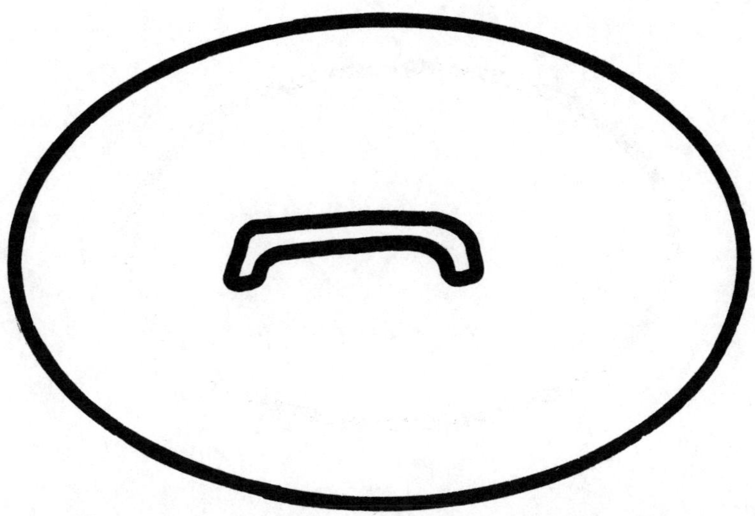

Skill 7
Step 2—Level #2 Pre/Posttest (flower petal)

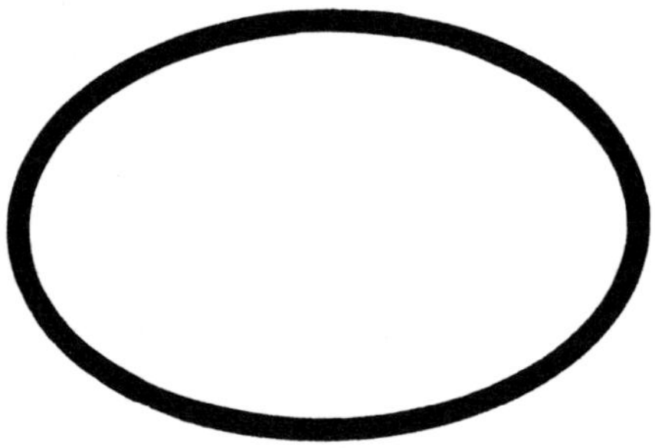

Skill 7
Step 2—Level #2 Worksheet (paint palette)

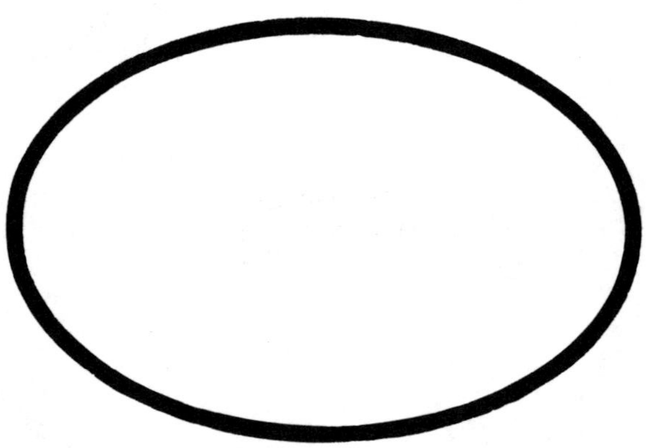

Skill 7
Step 2—Level #2 Worksheet (pig snout)

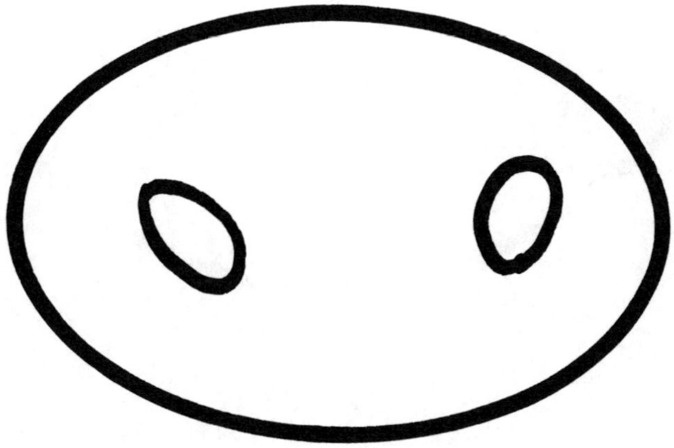

Skill 7
Step 2—Level #2 Worksheet (apple leaf)

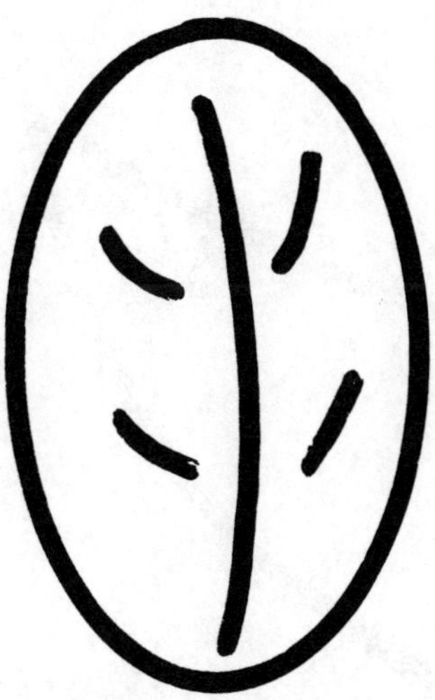

Skill 7
Step 2—Level #2 Worksheet (teddy bear's foot)

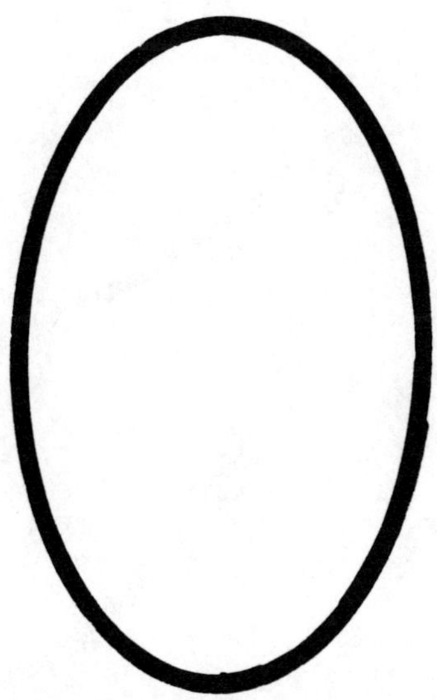

Skill 7
Step 3—Level #1 Pre/Posttest (girl in boat)

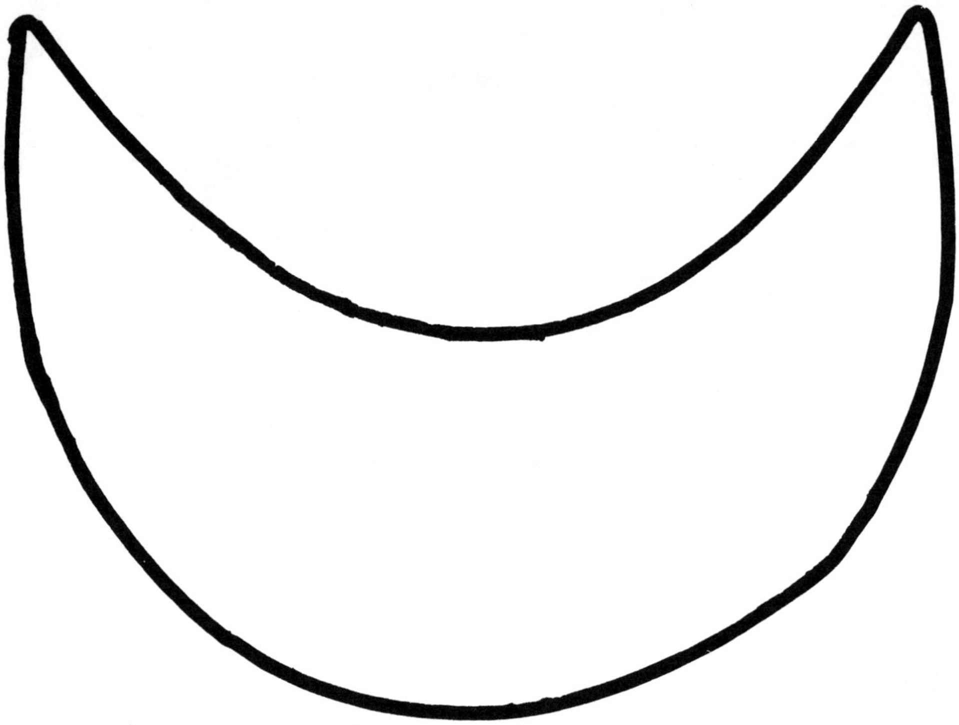

Skill 7
Step 3—Level #1 Worksheet (moon over tent)

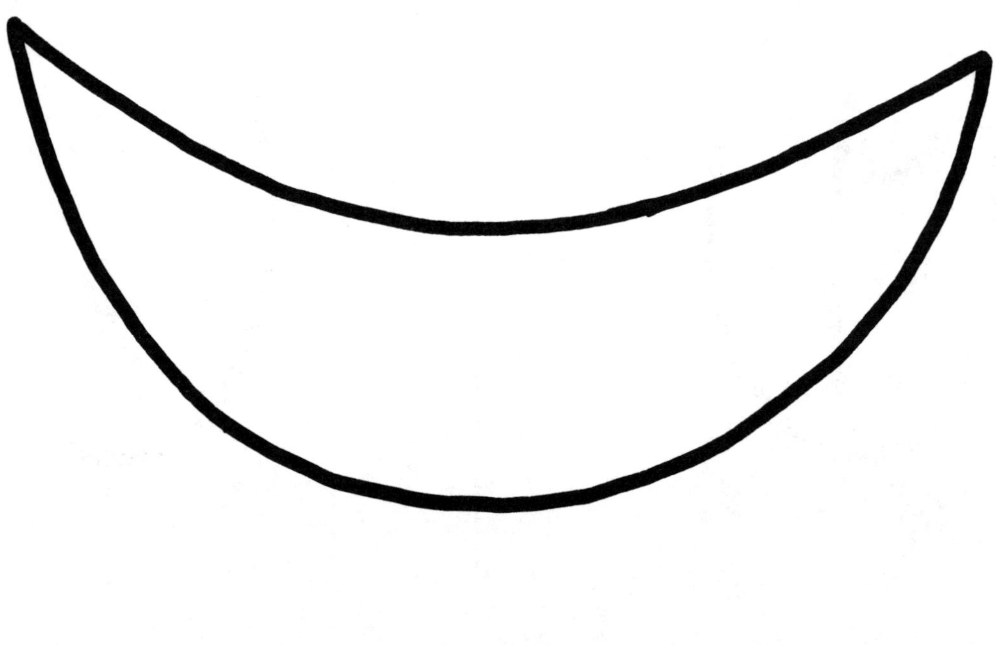

Skill 7
Step 3—Level #1 Worksheet (cow jumps over the moon)

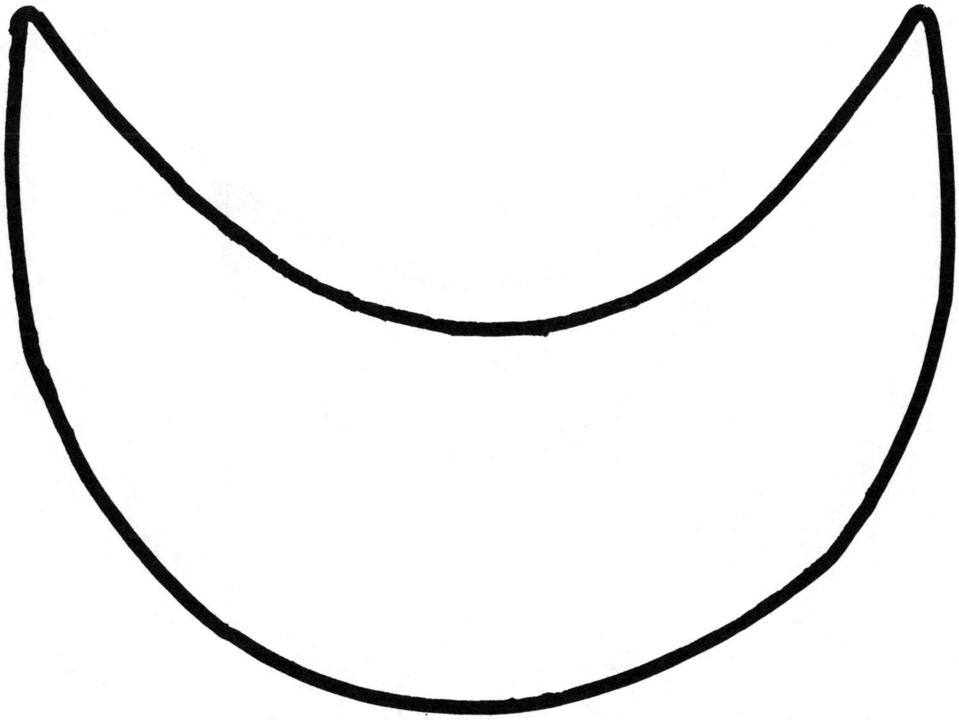

Skill 7
Step 3—Level #1 Worksheet (melon slices)

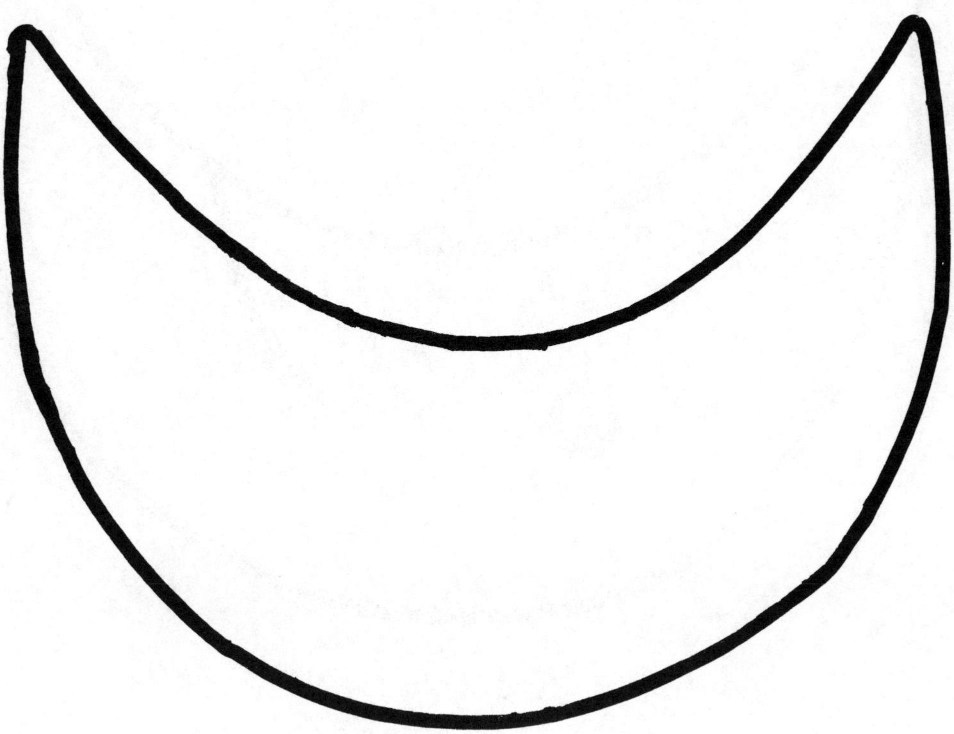

Skill 7
Step 3—Level #2 Pre/Posttest (wizard's hat)

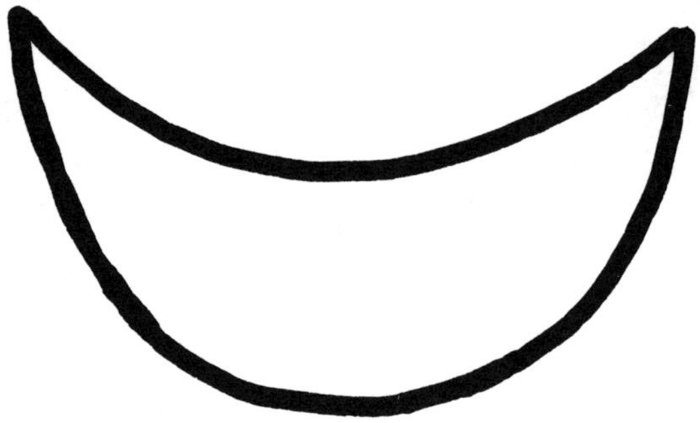

Skill 7
Step 3—Level #2 Worksheet (dancing crescent)

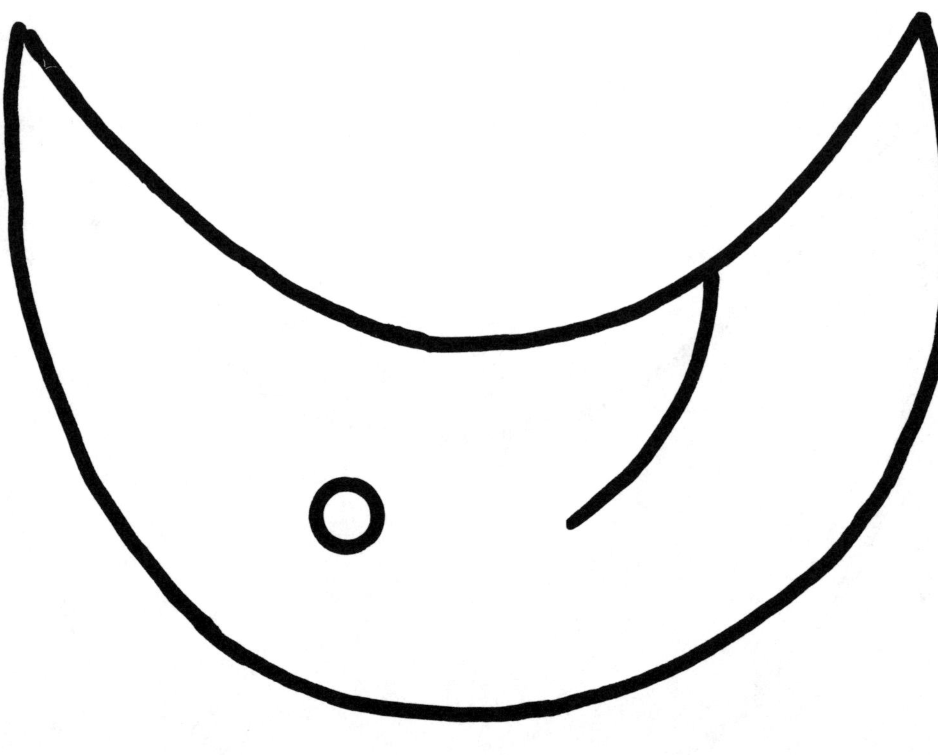

Skill 7
Step 3—Level #2 Worksheet (clown's smile)

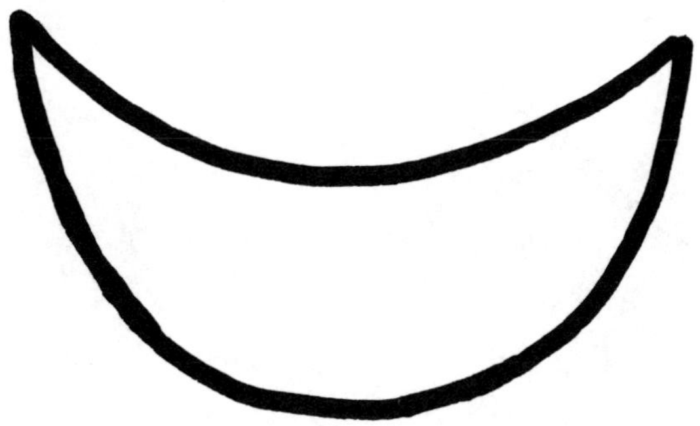

Skill 7
Step 3—Level #2 Worksheet (swing)

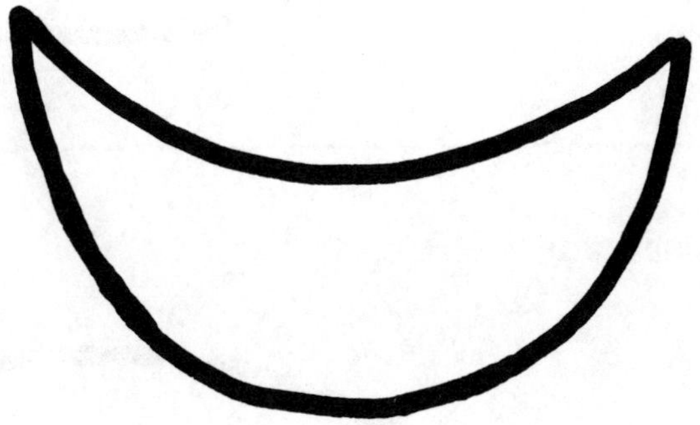

Skill 7
Step 3—Level #2 Worksheet (moon through the window)

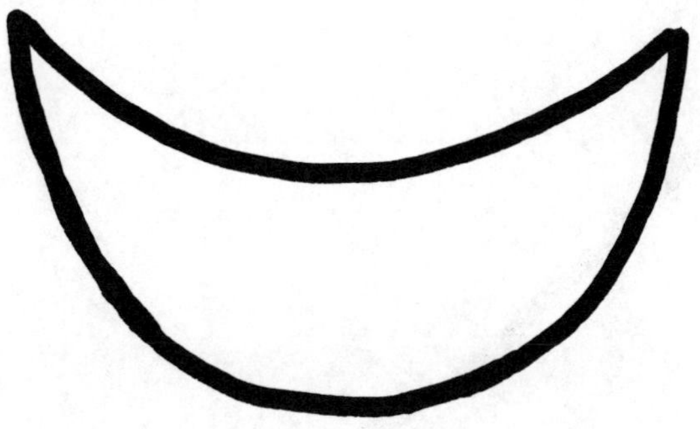

Skill 7
Step 4—Level #1 Pre/Posttest (lovebirds)

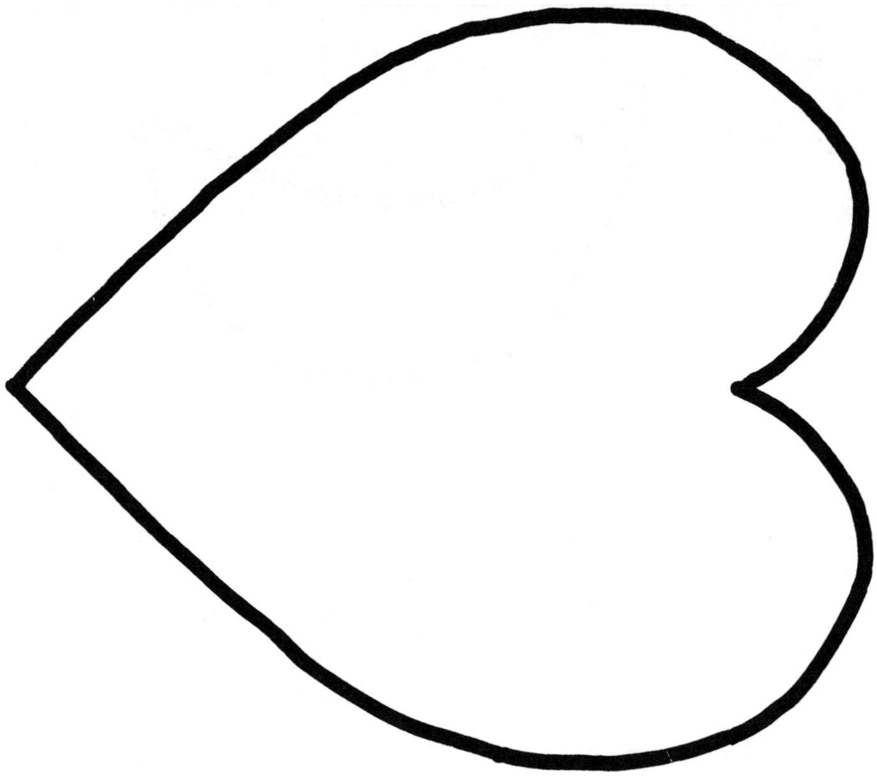

Skill 7
Step 4—Level #1 Worksheet (valentine card)

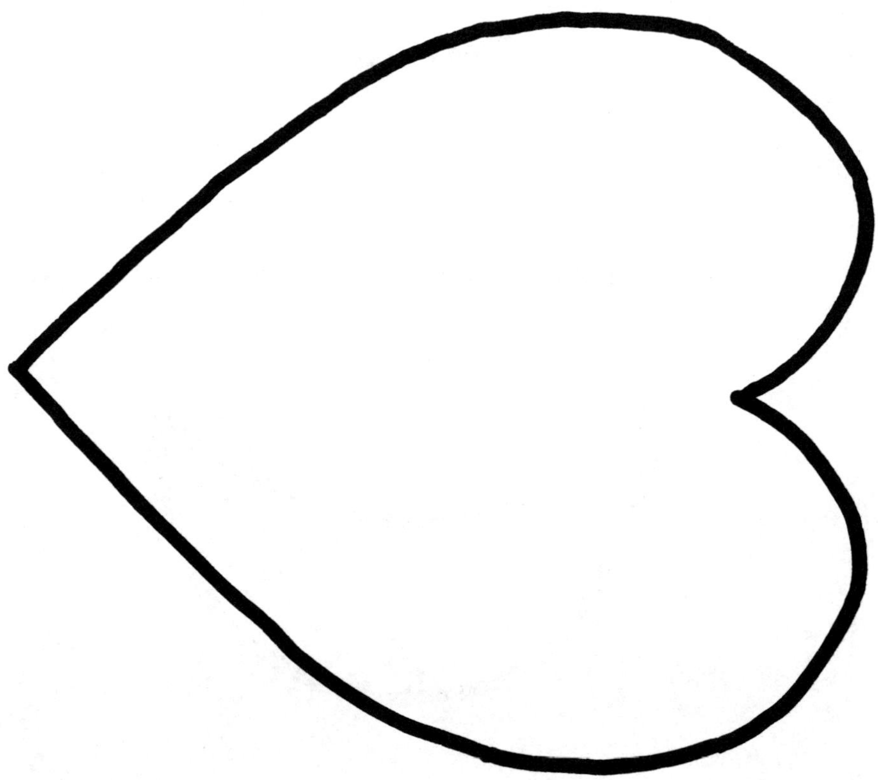

Skill 7
Step 4—Level #1 Worksheet (balloon heart)

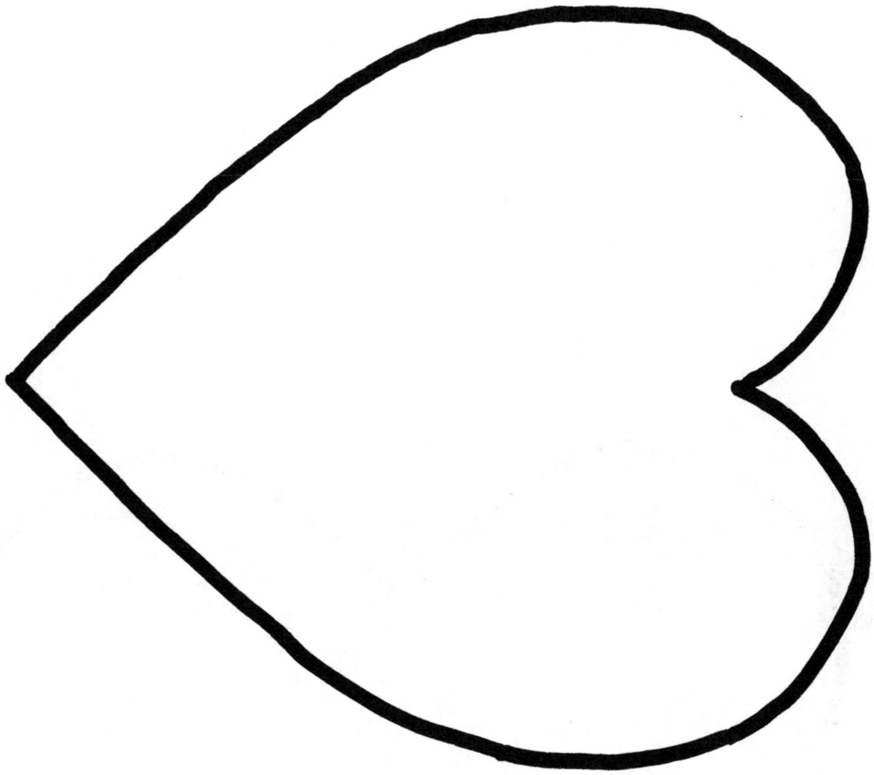

Skill 7
Step 4—Level #1 Worksheet (girl holding heart)

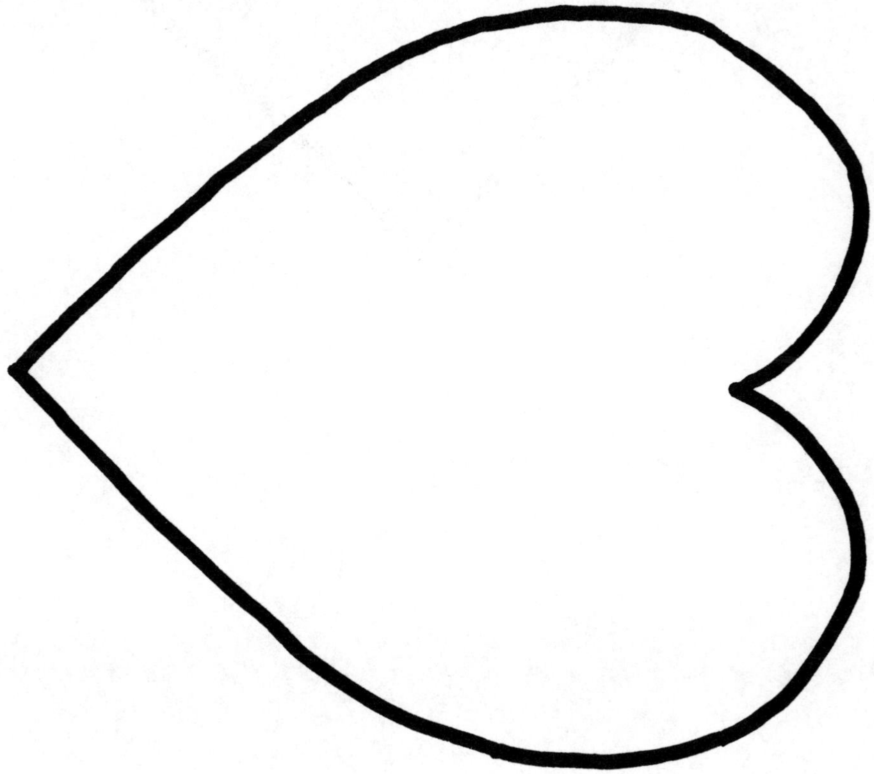

Skill 7
Step 4—Level #1 Worksheet (three hearts)

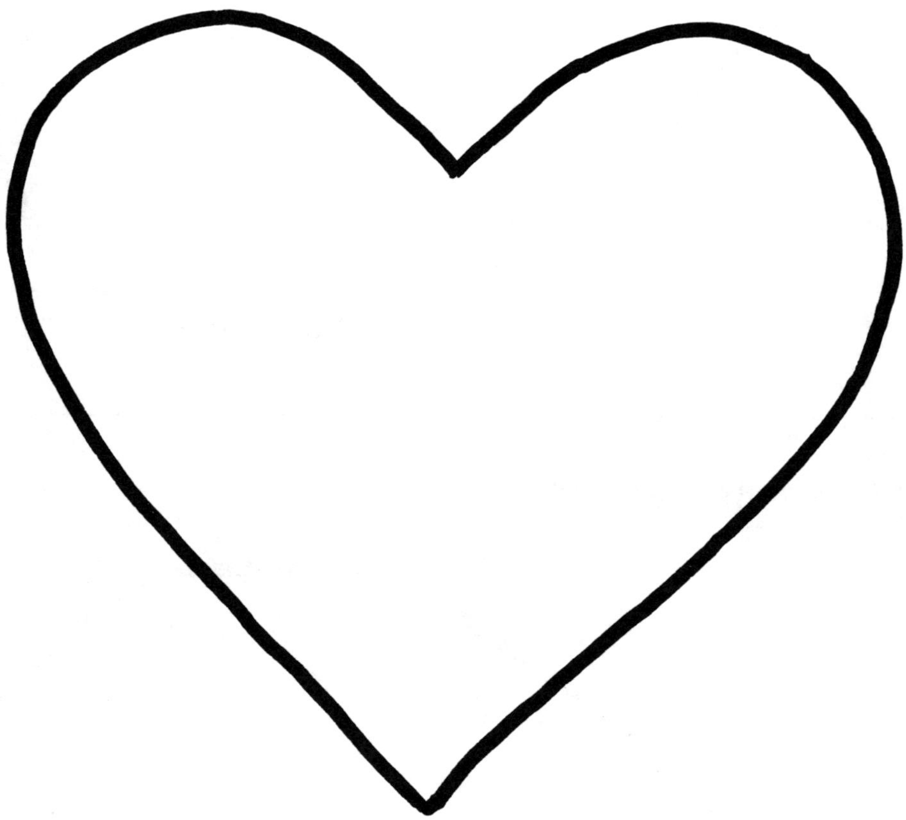

Skill 7
Step 4—Level #2 Pre/Posttest (elephant)

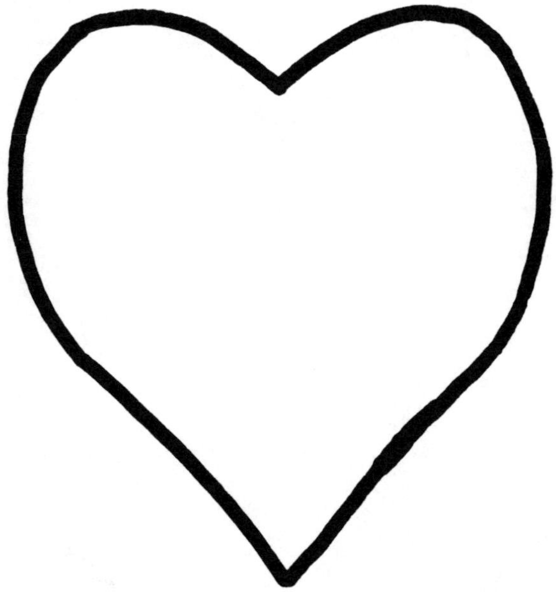

Skill 7
Step 4—Level #2 Worksheet (girl heart)

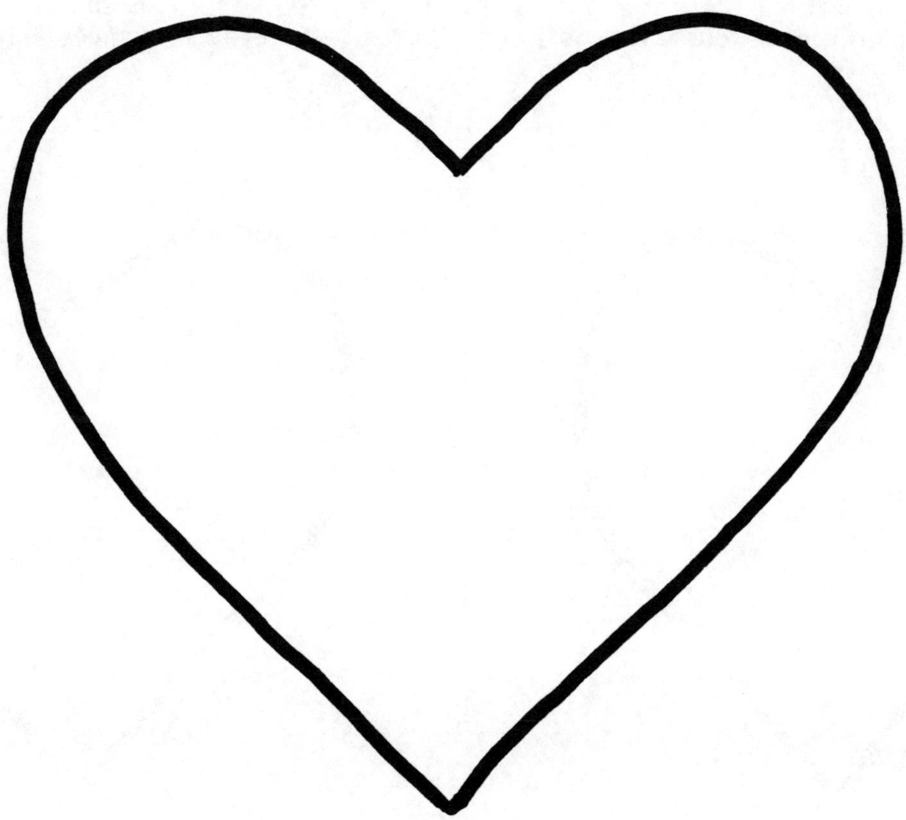

Skill 7
Step 4—Level #2 Worksheet (boy heart)

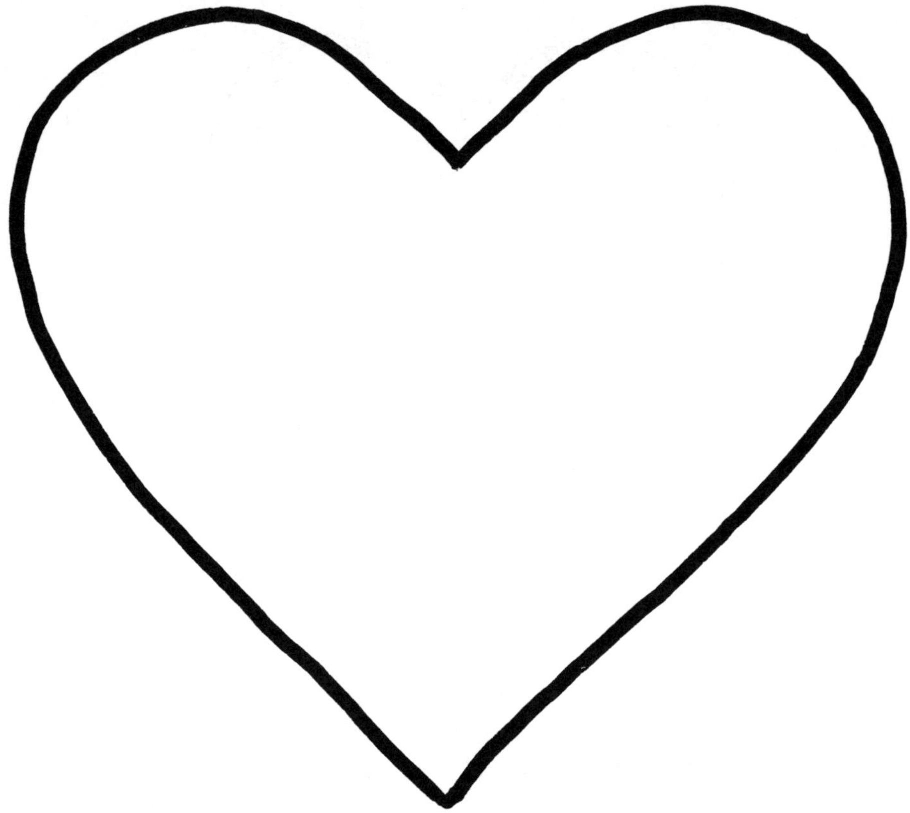

Skill 7
Step 4—Level #2 Worksheet (four-leaf clover)

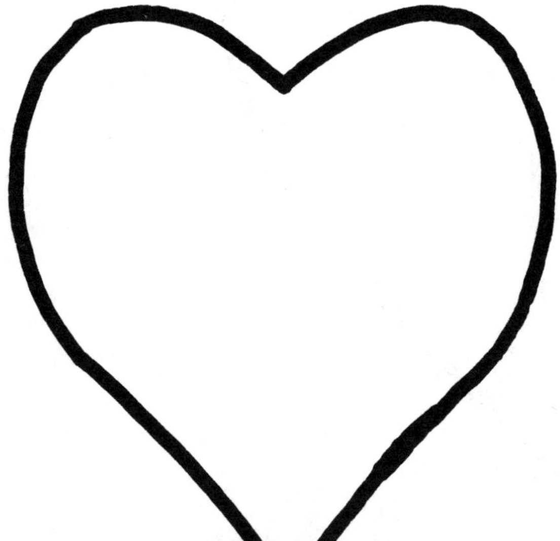

Skill 7
Step 4—Level #2 Worksheet (kitten holding heart)

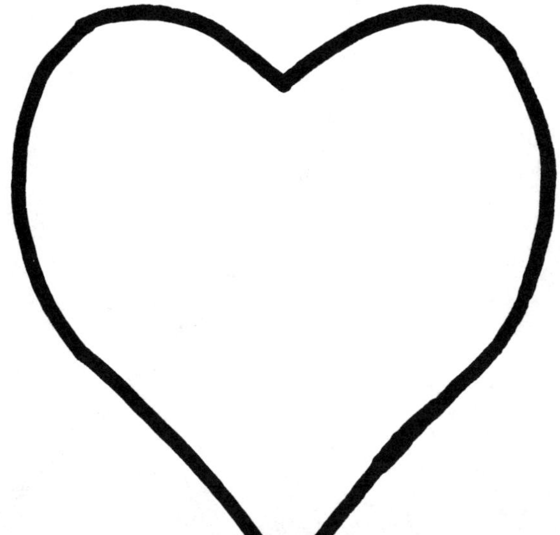

Skill 7
Step 5—Level #1 Pre/Posttest (star on door)

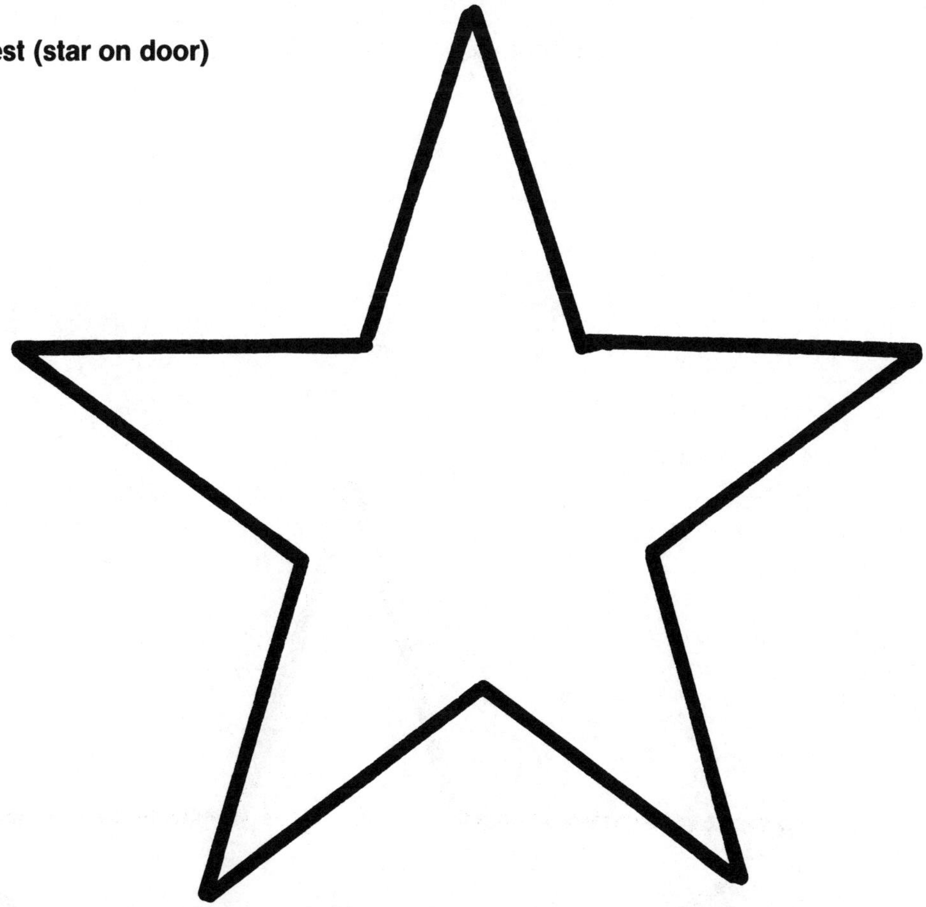

Skill 7
Step 5—Level #1 Worksheet (cloud and star)

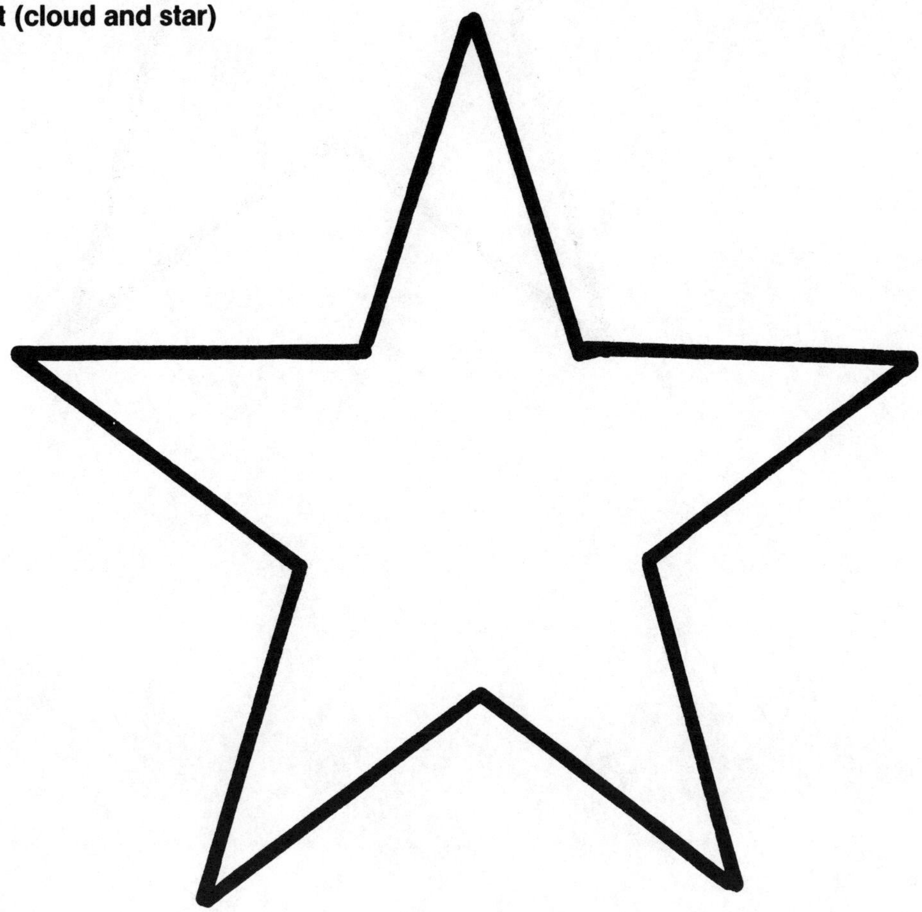

Skill 7
Step 5—Level #1 Worksheet (magic wand)

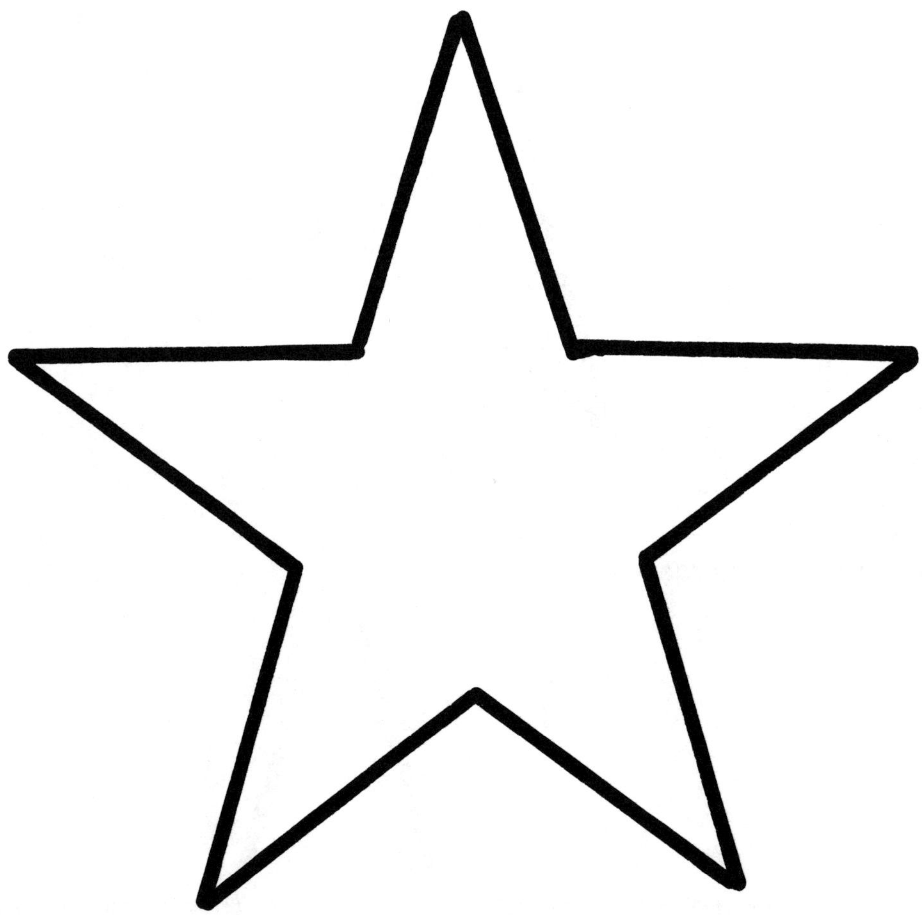

Skill 7
Step 5—Level #2 Pre/Posttest (star on flag)

Skill 7
Step 5—Level #2 Worksheet (football helmet)

Skill 7
Step 5—Level #2 Worksheet (star on box)

Skill 7
Step 5—Level #2 Worksheet (star on easel)

Skill 7
Step 5—Level #2 Worksheet (star on ball)

Skill 7
Step 5—Level #2 Worksheet (star on baby's bib)

Skill 7
Step 5—Level #2 Worksheet (star on clown)

Skill 8—Cutting Combined Circles and Complex Shapes—1/8" Line

Objective: Student cuts out two familiar shapes with a line 1/8" wide, and pastes them on the corresponding fixed outlines, with 80% accuracy.

SKILL 8—STEP 1—COMBINED SHAPES

Pretest: Student takes Step 1 Pretest (grapevine—1¼" circle and 2½" crescent).

If criterion met: Student advances to Step 2.

If criterion not met:

1. Student cuts Step 1 worksheets:
   balloon and moon—5" circle and 2¾" crescent
   beetle and mushroom—2" circle and 4" oval
   train—1¾" circle and 3¼" oval
   doll with lollipop—2" circle and 2½" oval
2. Student takes Step 1 Posttest (grapevine).

   If criterion met: Student advances to Step 2.

   If criterion not met: Student repeats Step 1 worksheets and Posttest.

Skill 8
Step 1 Pre/Posttest

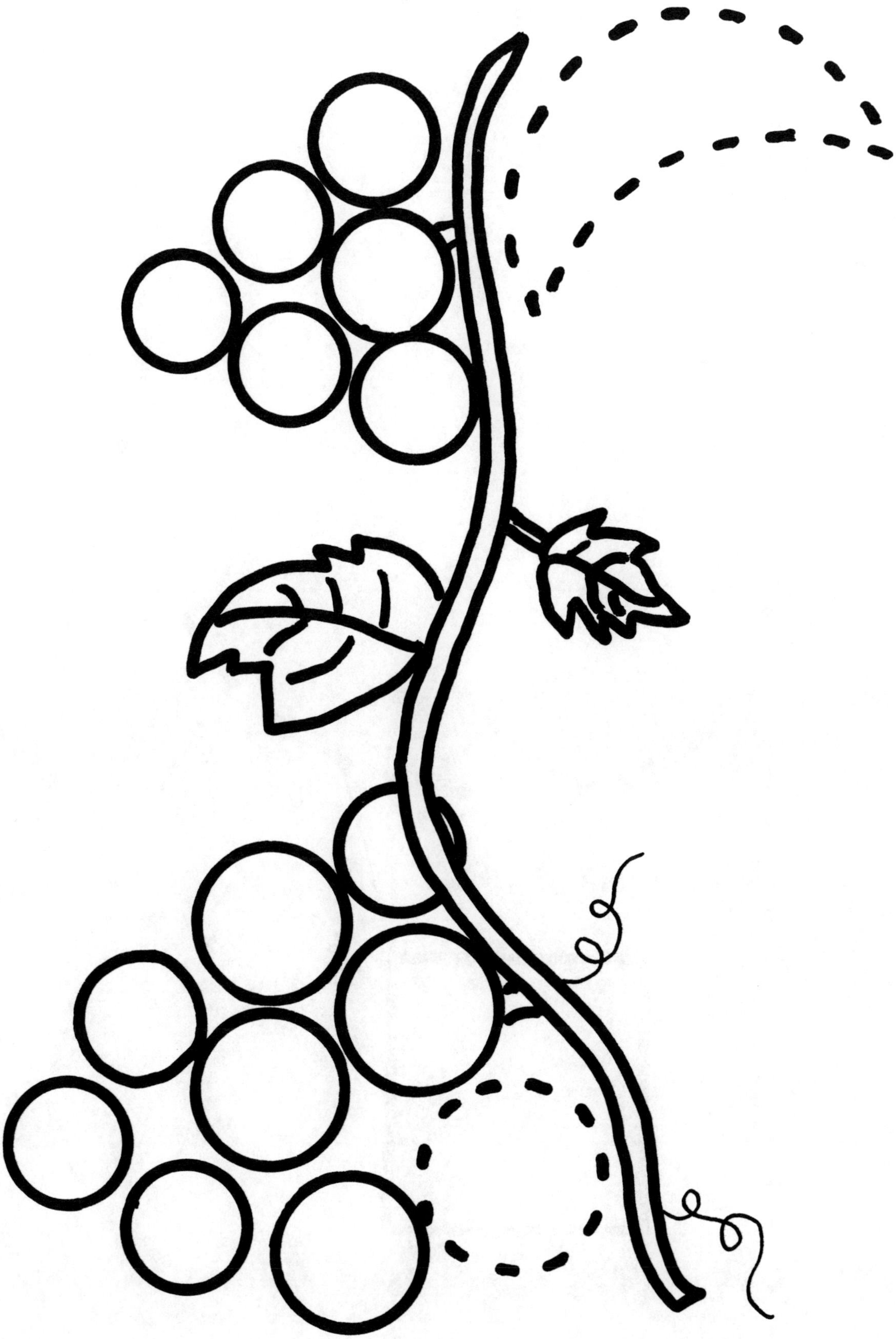

Skill 8
Step 1 Worksheet

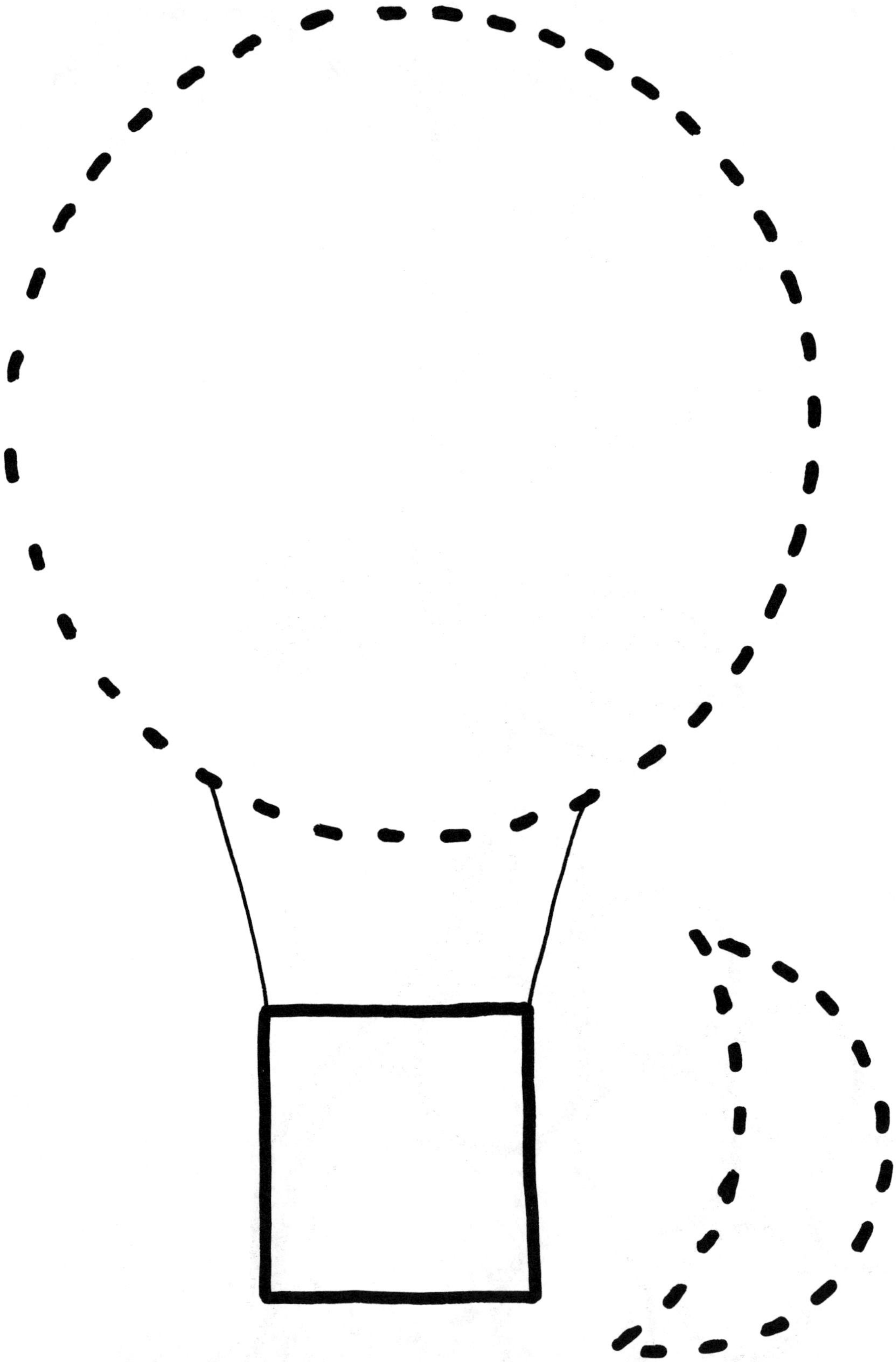

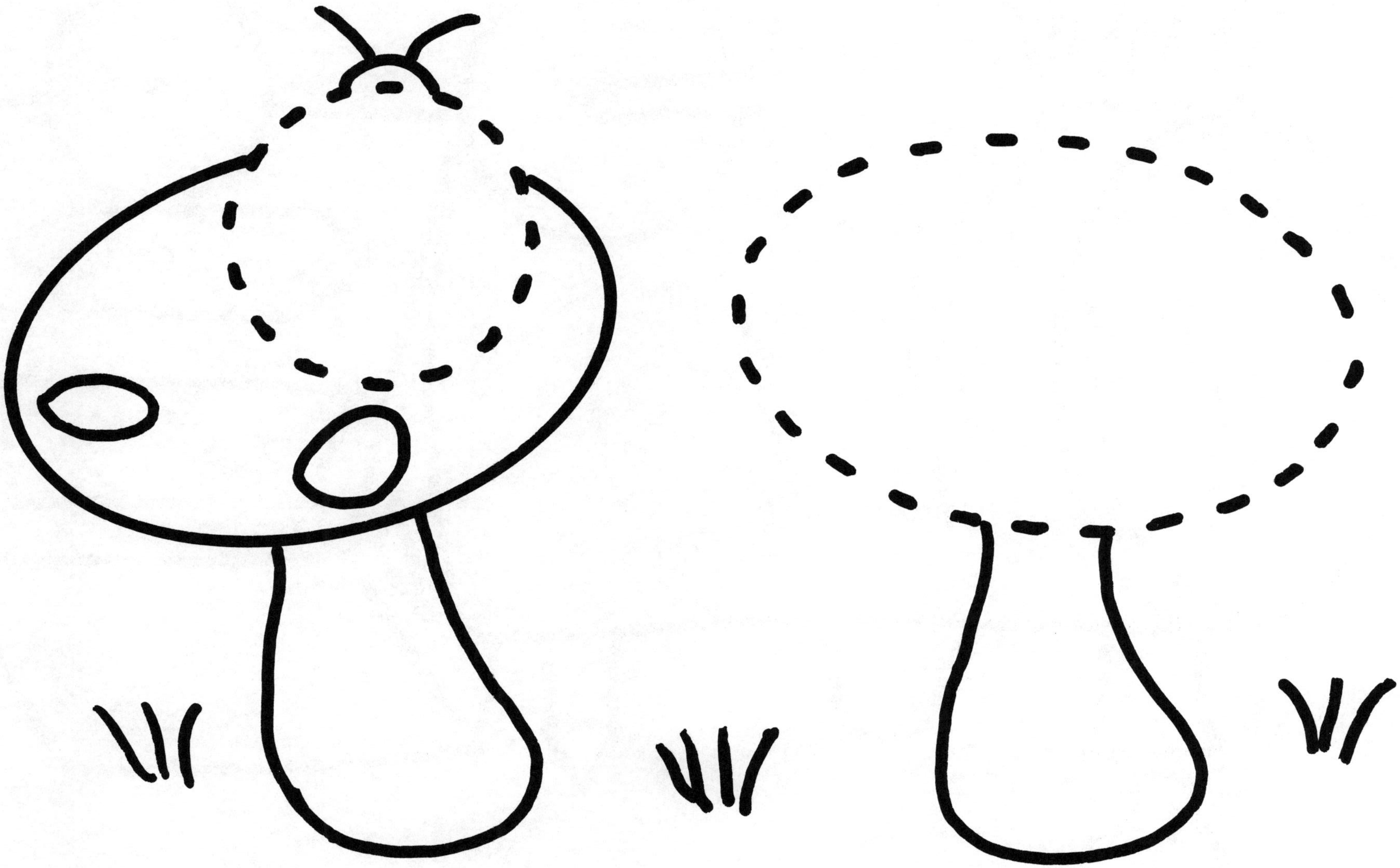

Skill 8
Step 1 Worksheet

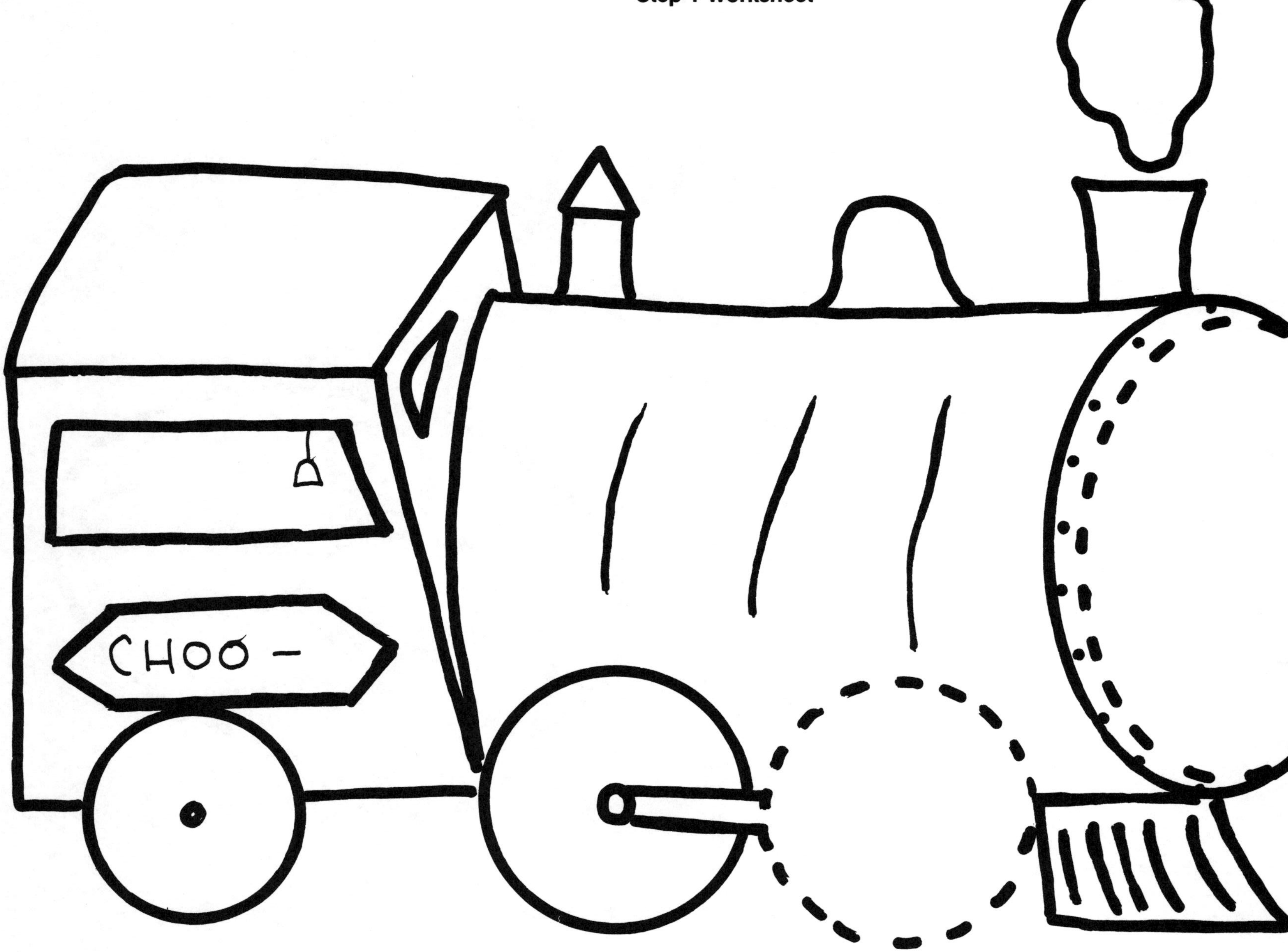

Skill 8
Step 1 Worksheet

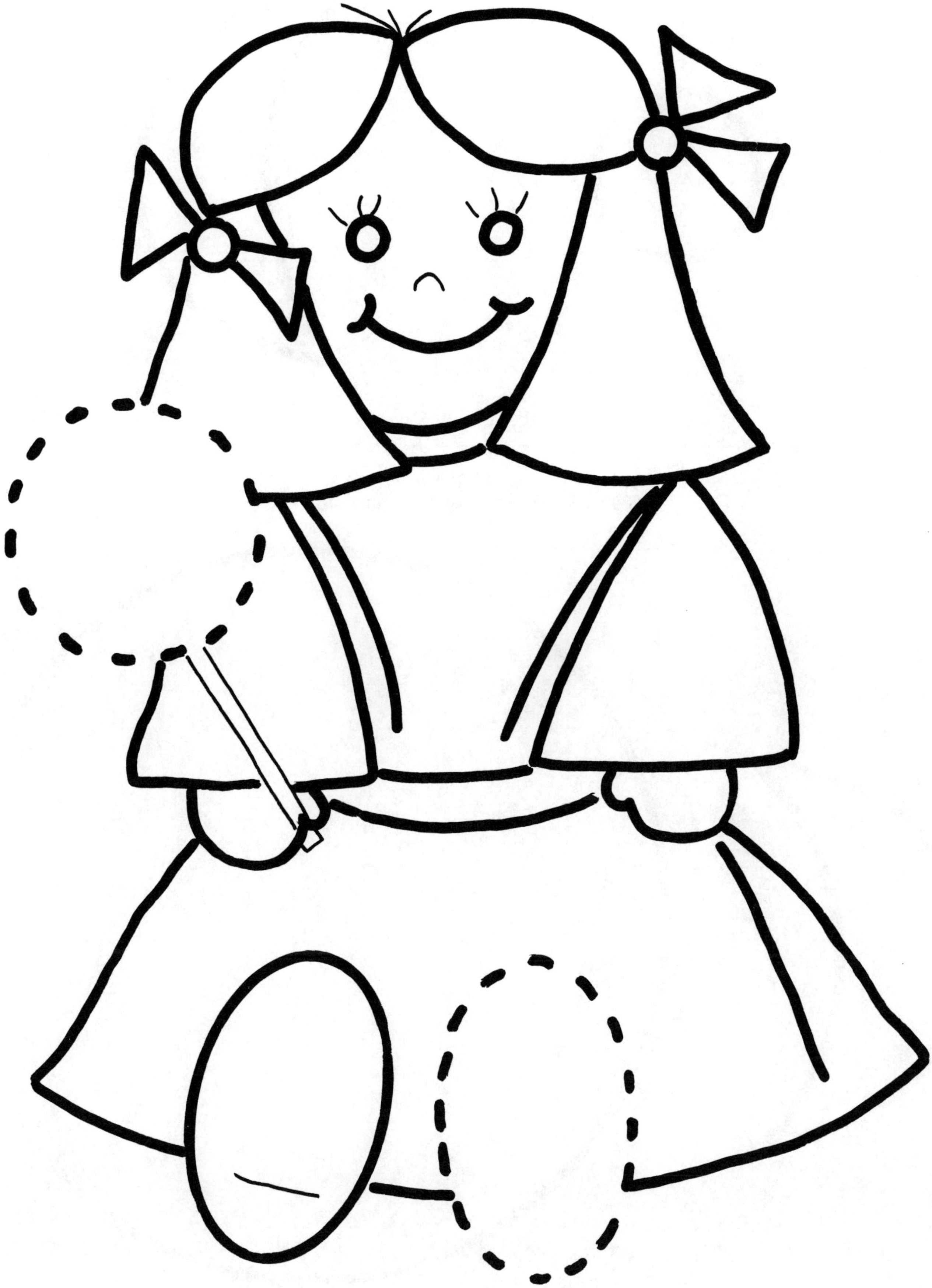

Skill 8
Step 1 Pre/Posttest (grapevine)

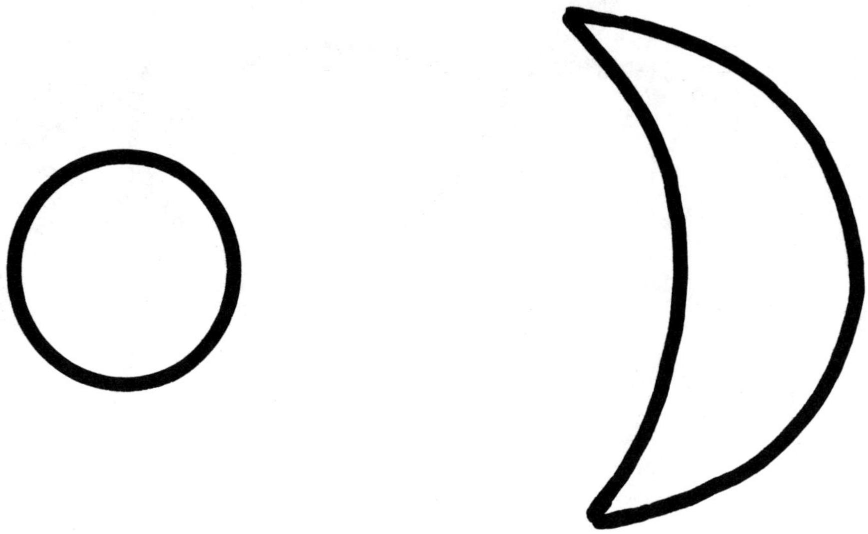

Skill 8
Step 1 Worksheet (balloon and moon)

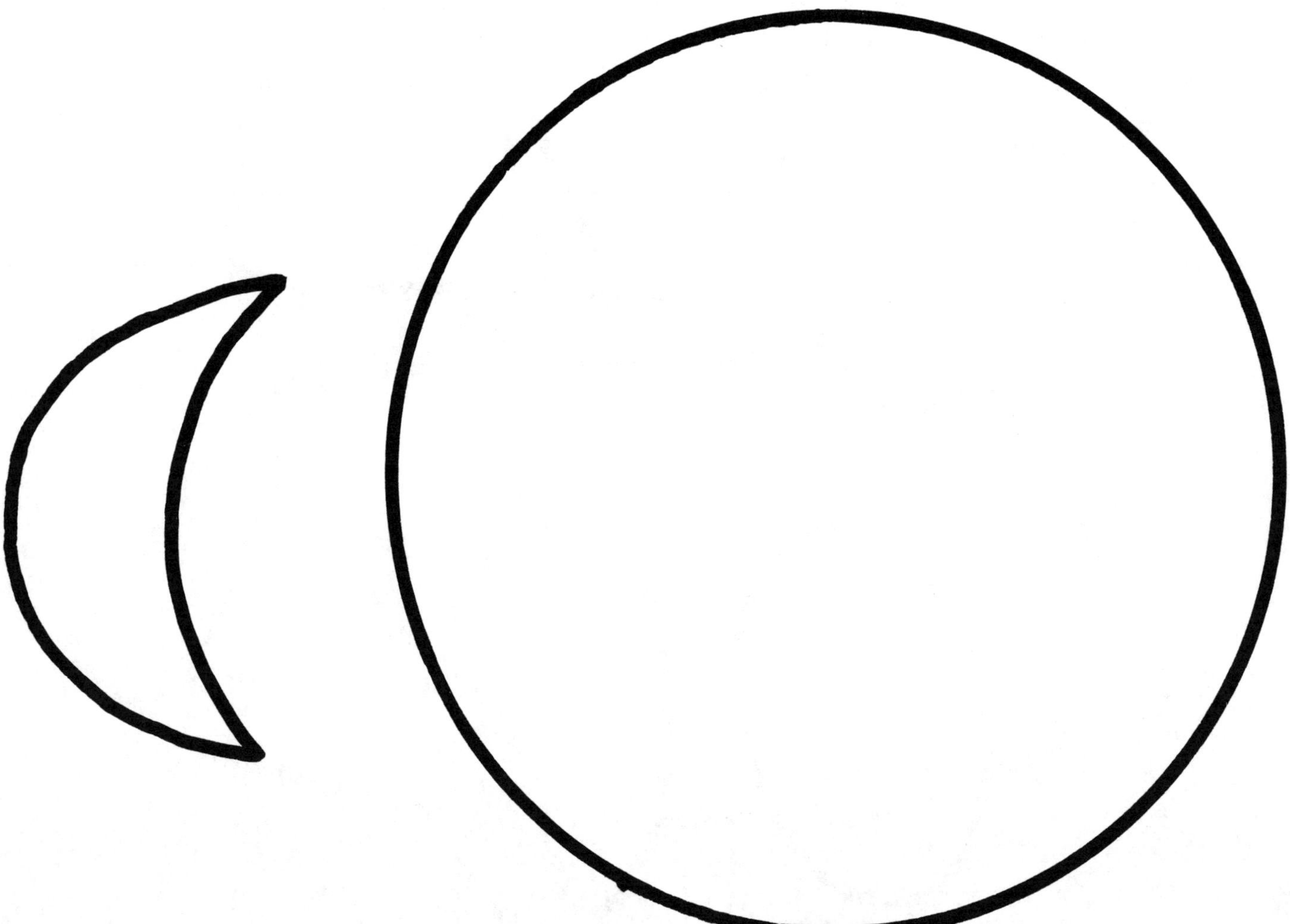

Skill 8
Step 1 Worksheet (beetle and mushroom)

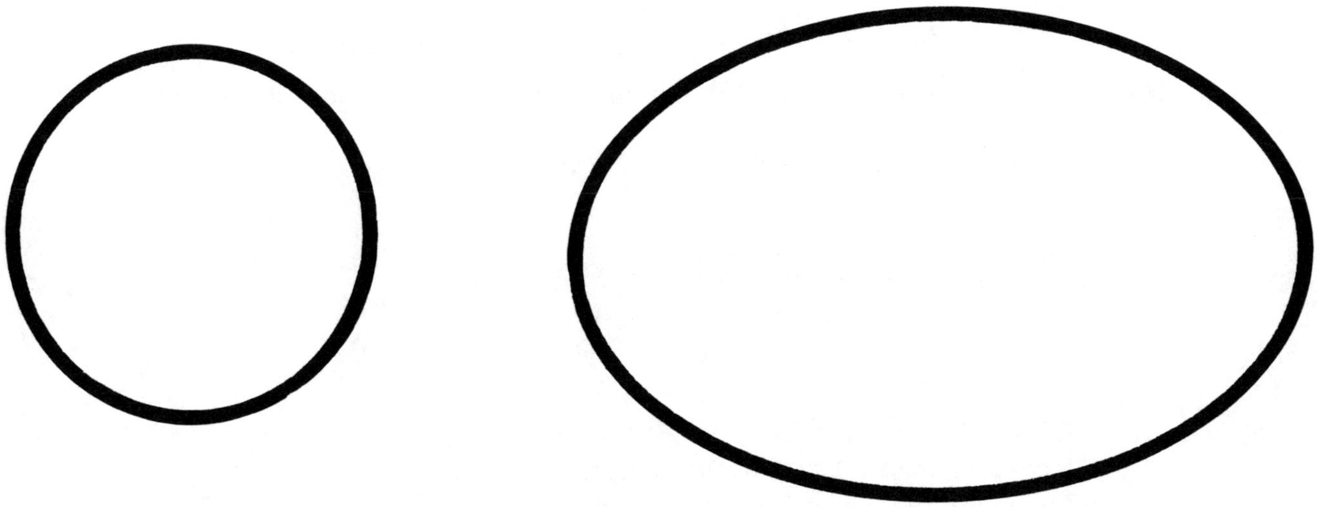

Skill 8
Step 1 Worksheet (train)

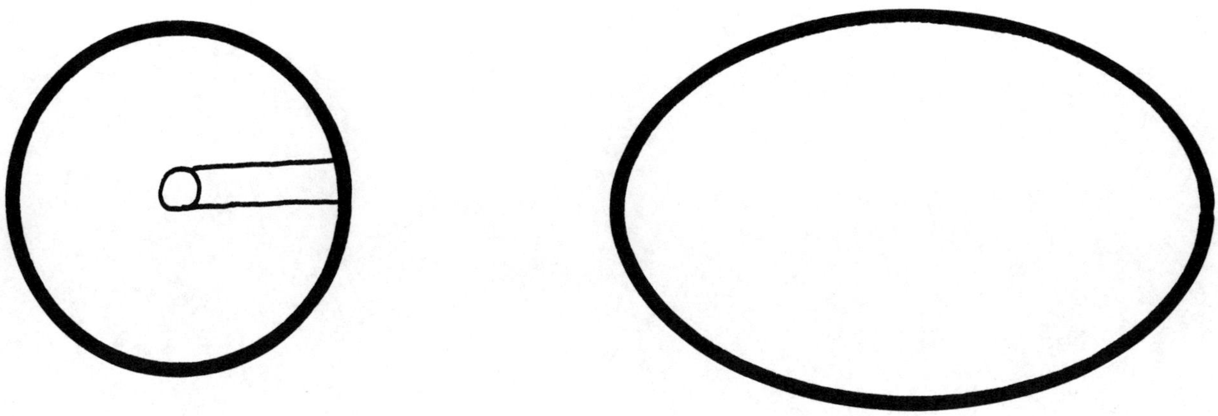

Skill 8
Step 1 Worksheet (doll with lollipop)

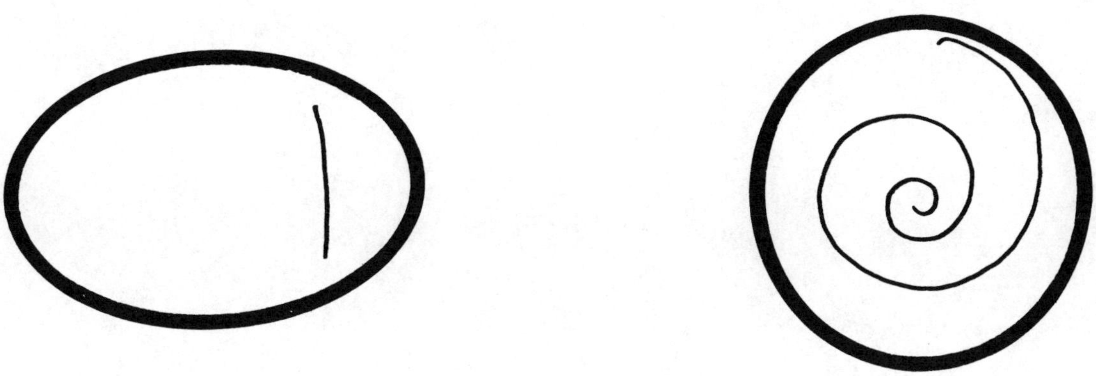

SKILL 8—STEP 2—SMALLER COMBINED SHAPES

Pretest: Student takes Step 2 Pretest (shape balloons—3″ star and 2½″ crescent).

If criterion met: Student works independently on art projects.

If criterion not met:

1. Student cuts Step 2 worksheets:
   tree and moon—1″ circle and 2½″ crescent
   butterfly—2¼″ circle and 3″ heart
   bird and star 2¼″ circle and 4½″ star
   at the beach—3″ star and 3″ circle
2. Student takes Step Posttest (shape balloons).

   If criterion met: Student works independently on art projects.

   If criterion not met: Student repeats Step 2 worksheets and Posttest.

Skill 8
Step 2 Pre/Posttest

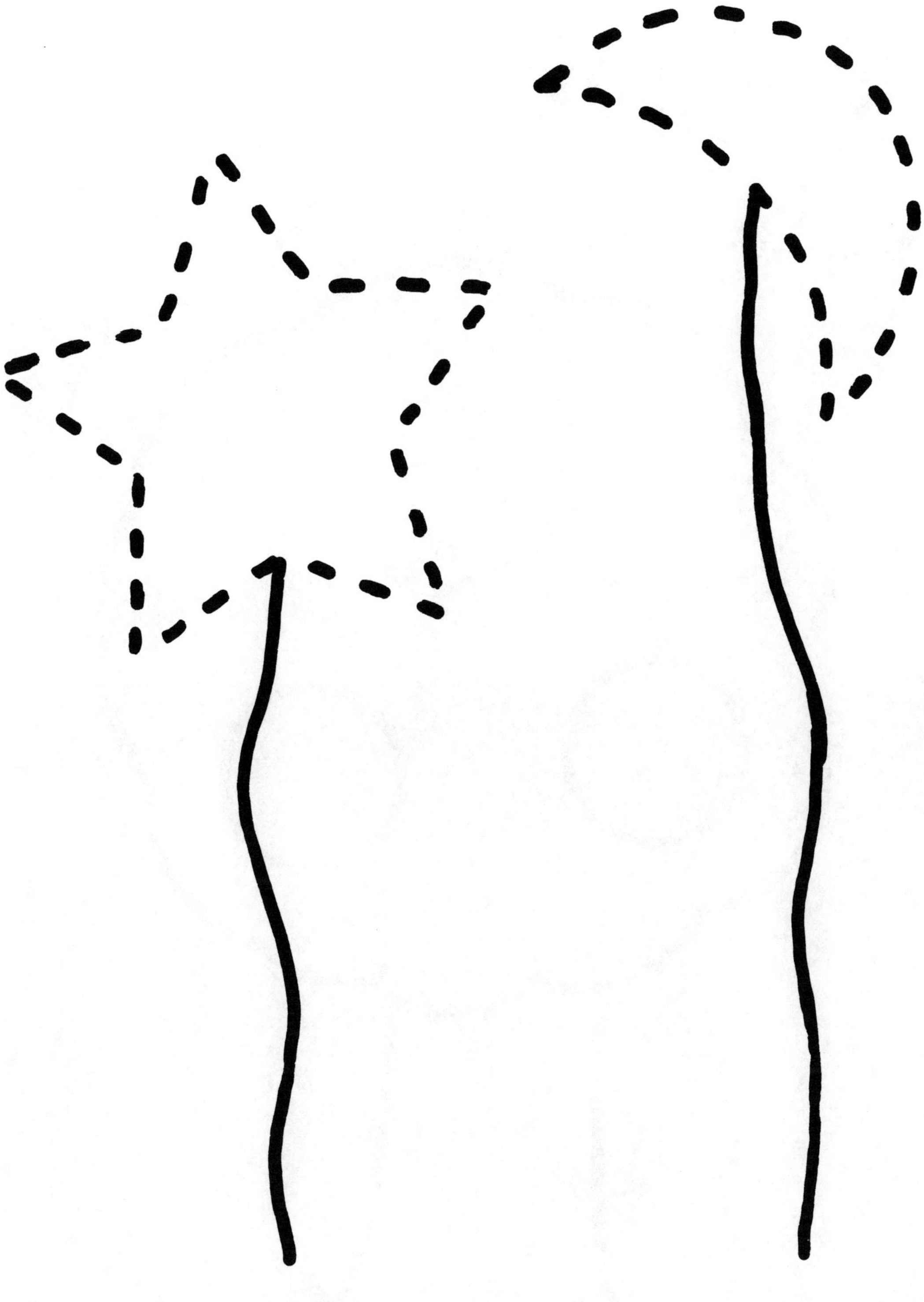

Skill 8
Step 2 Worksheet

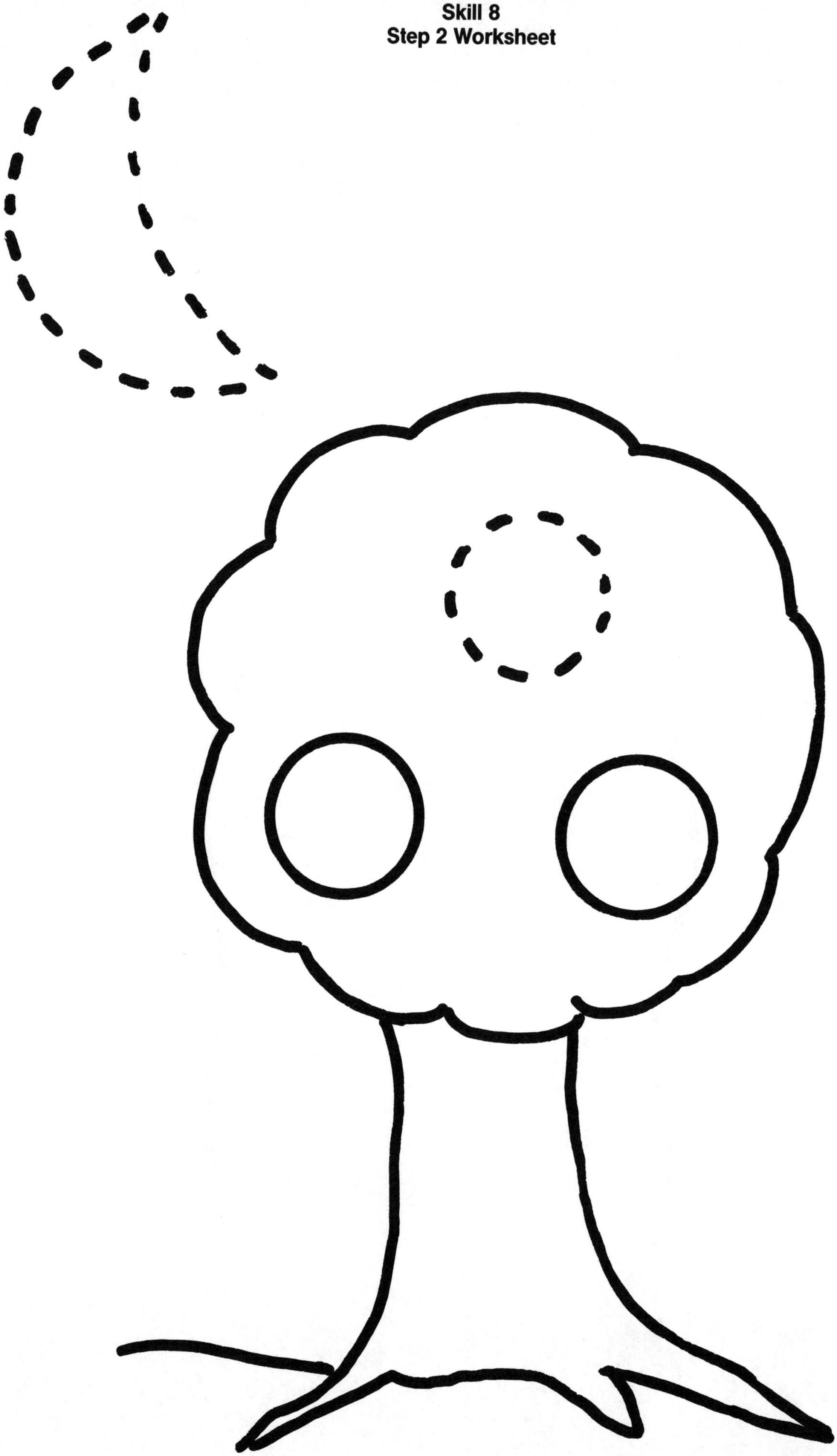

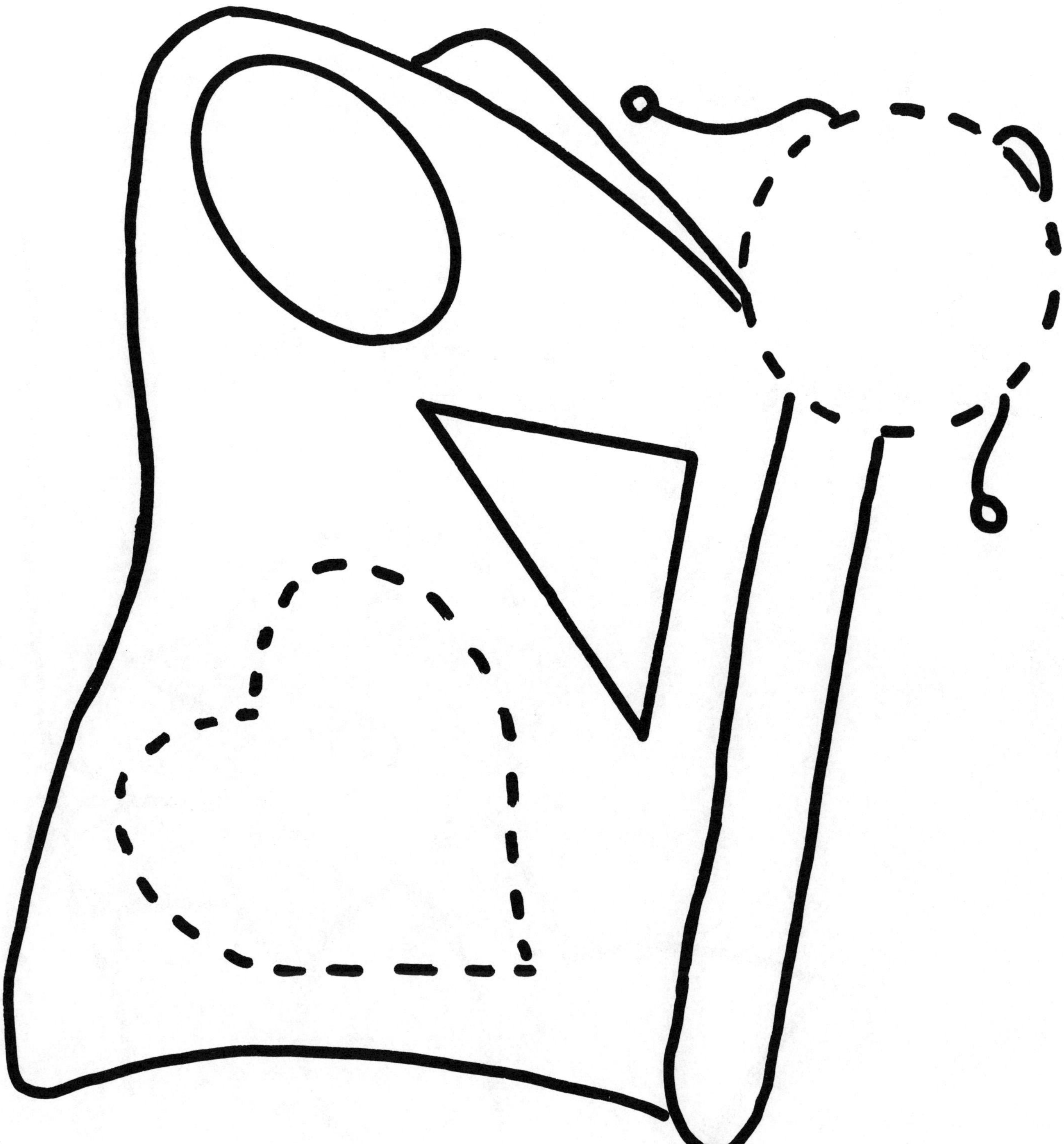

Skill 8
Step 2 Worksheet

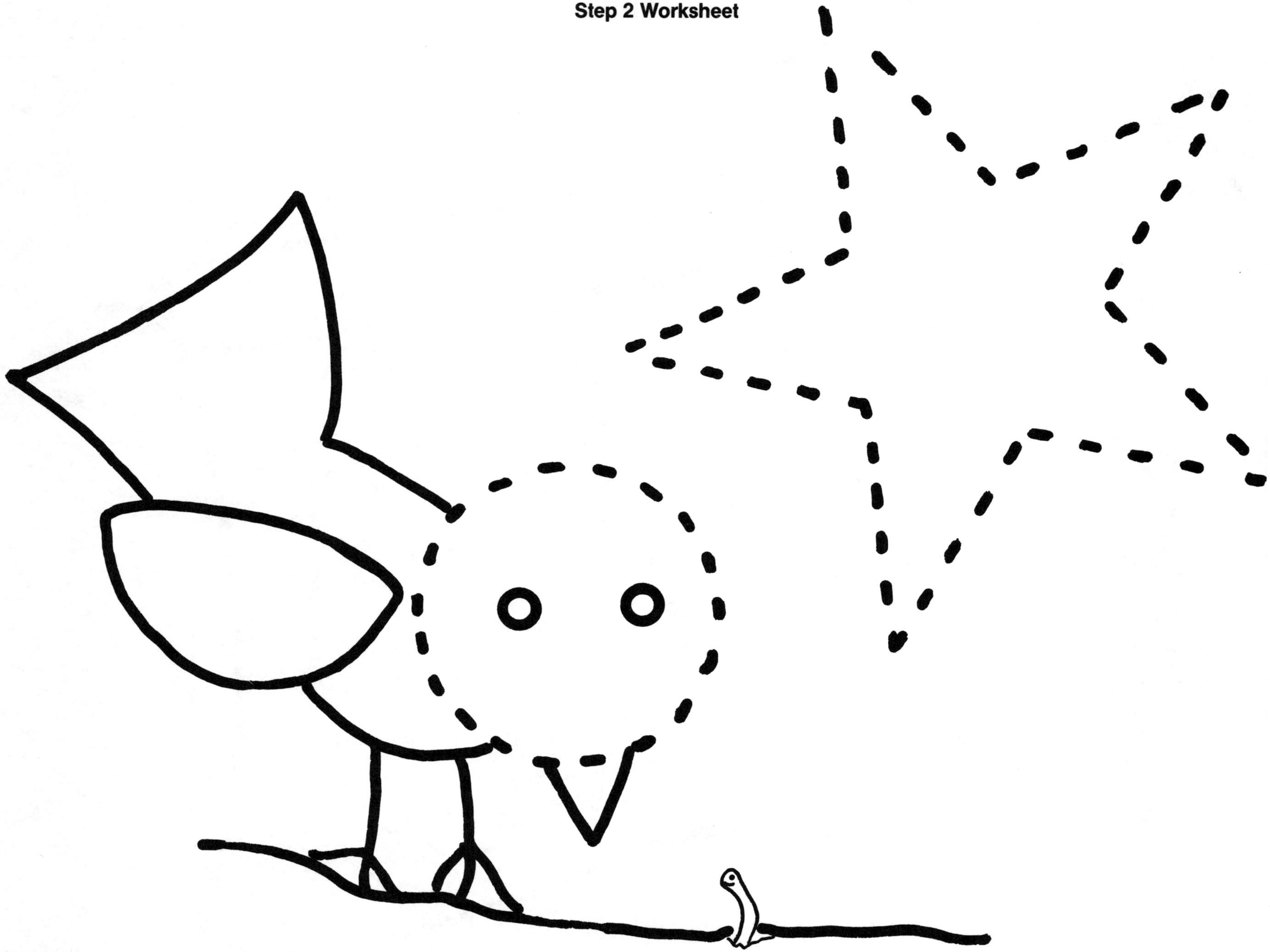

Skill 8
Step 2 Worksheet

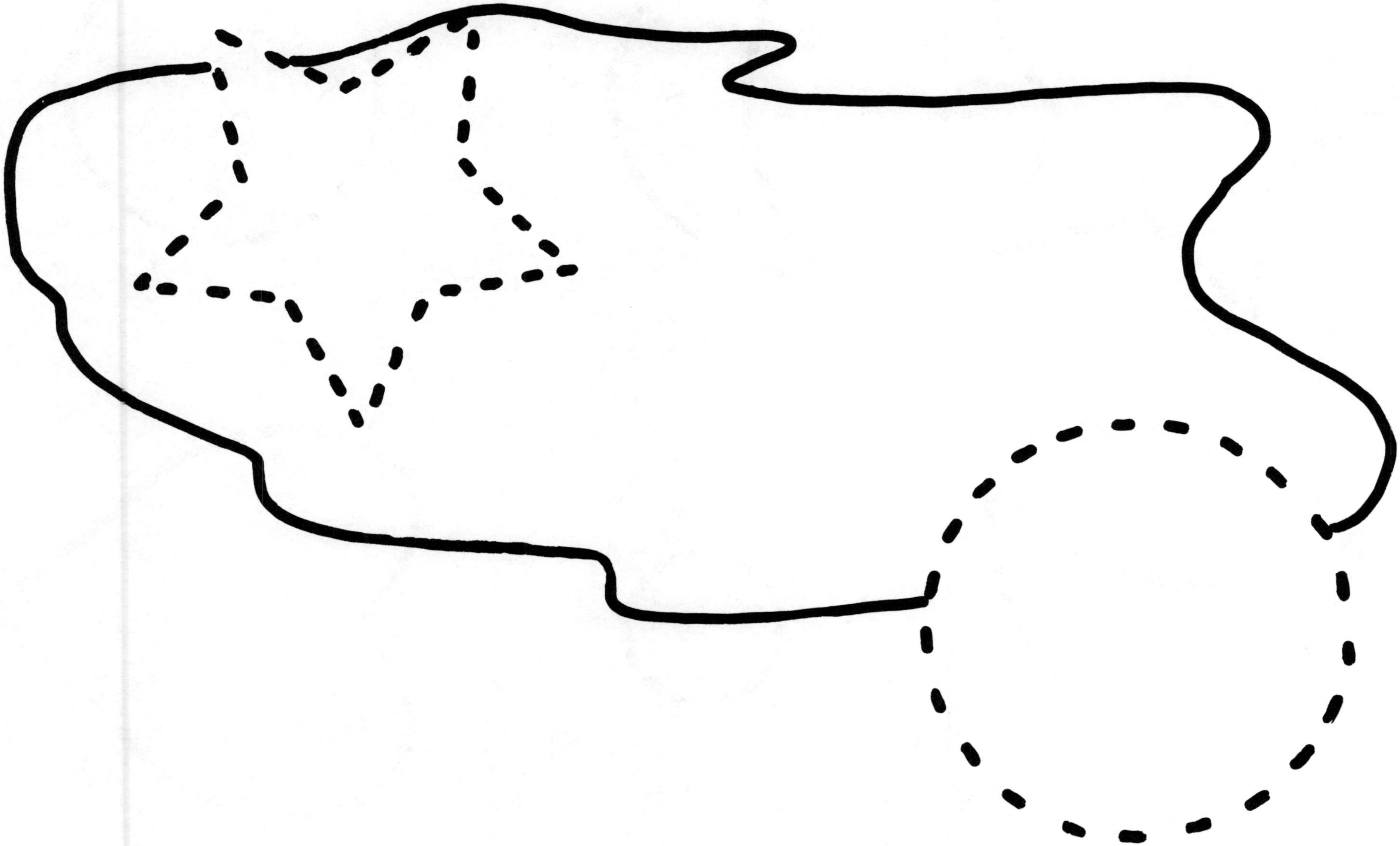

Skill 8
Step 2 Pre/Posttest (shape balloons)

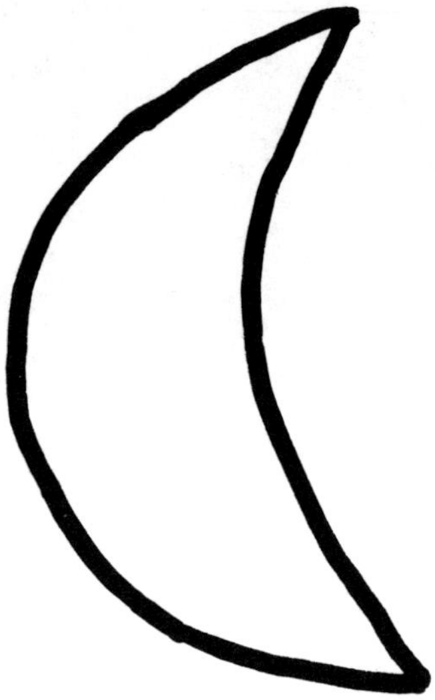

Skill 8
Step 2 Worksheet (tree and moon)

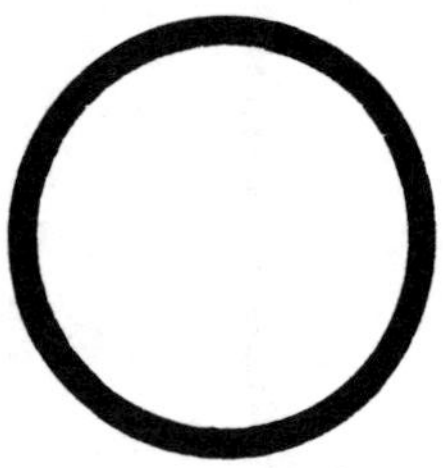

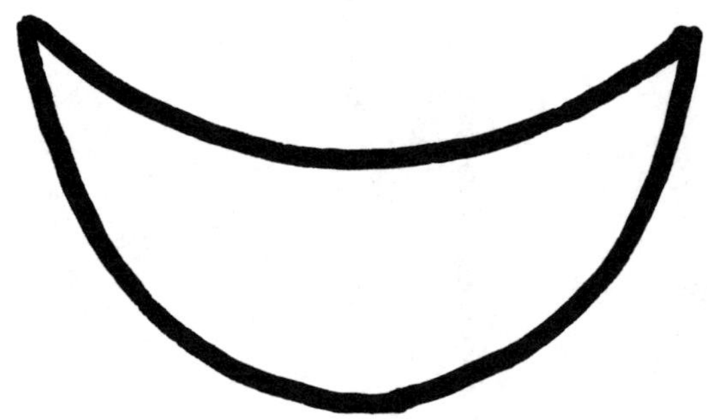

Skill 8
Step 2 Worksheet (butterfly)

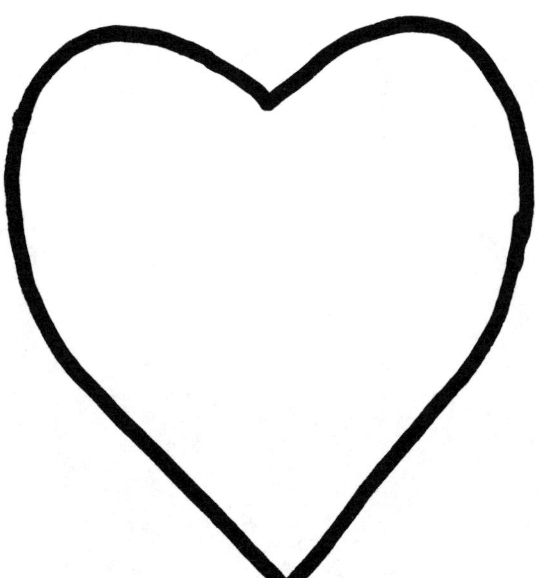

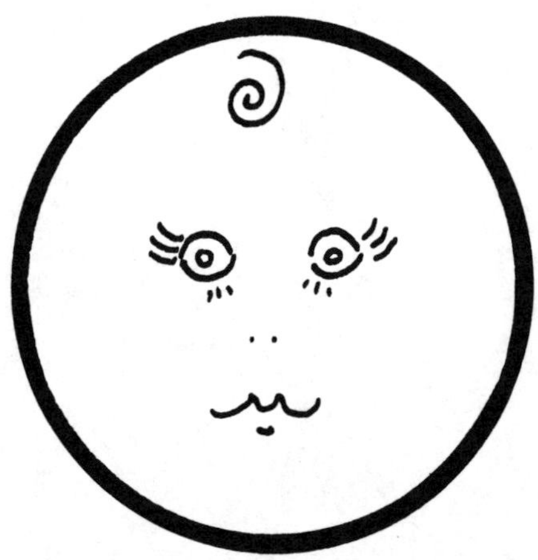

Skill 8
Step 2 Worksheet (bird and star)

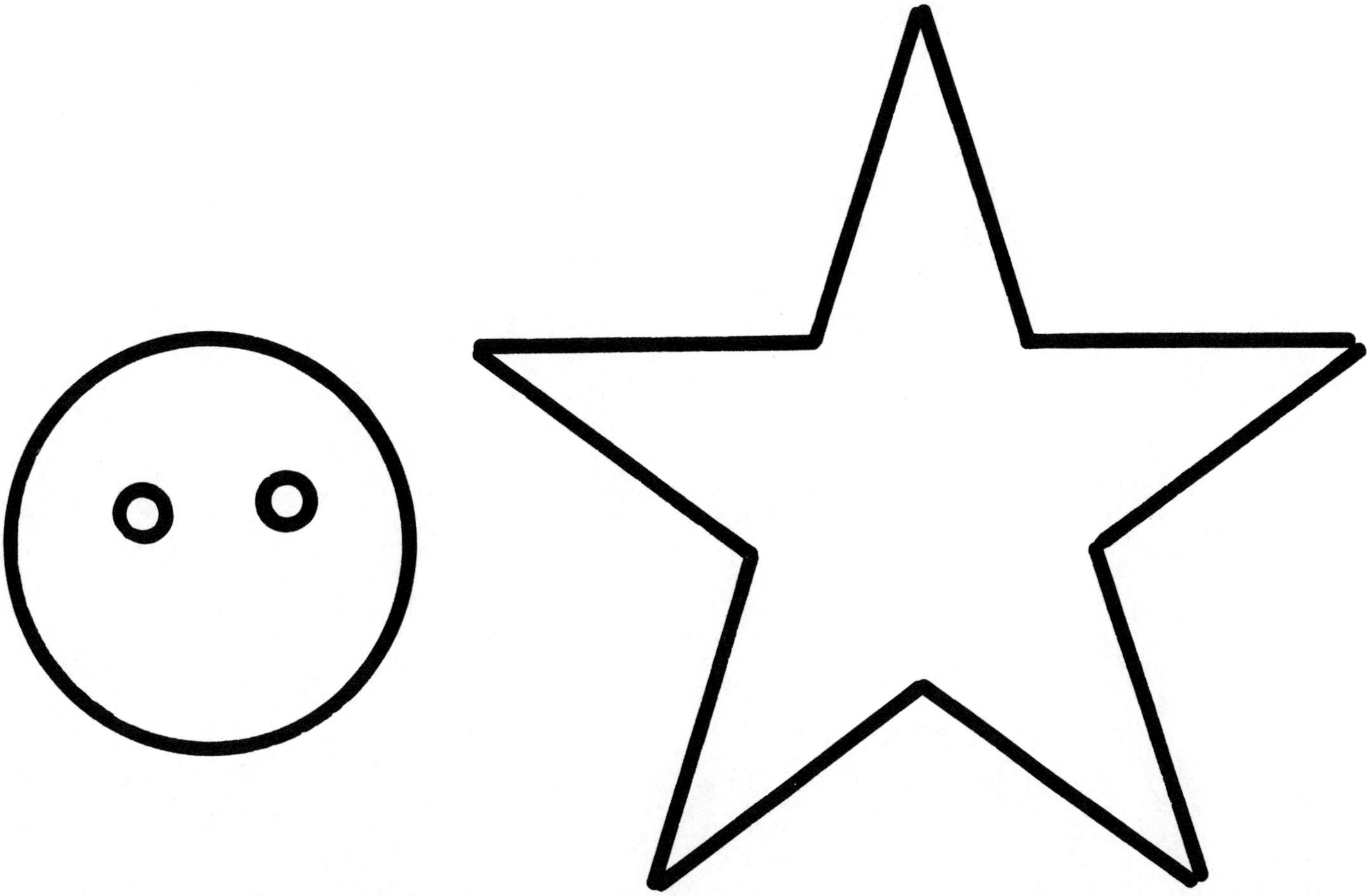

Skill 8
Step 2 Worksheet (at the beach)

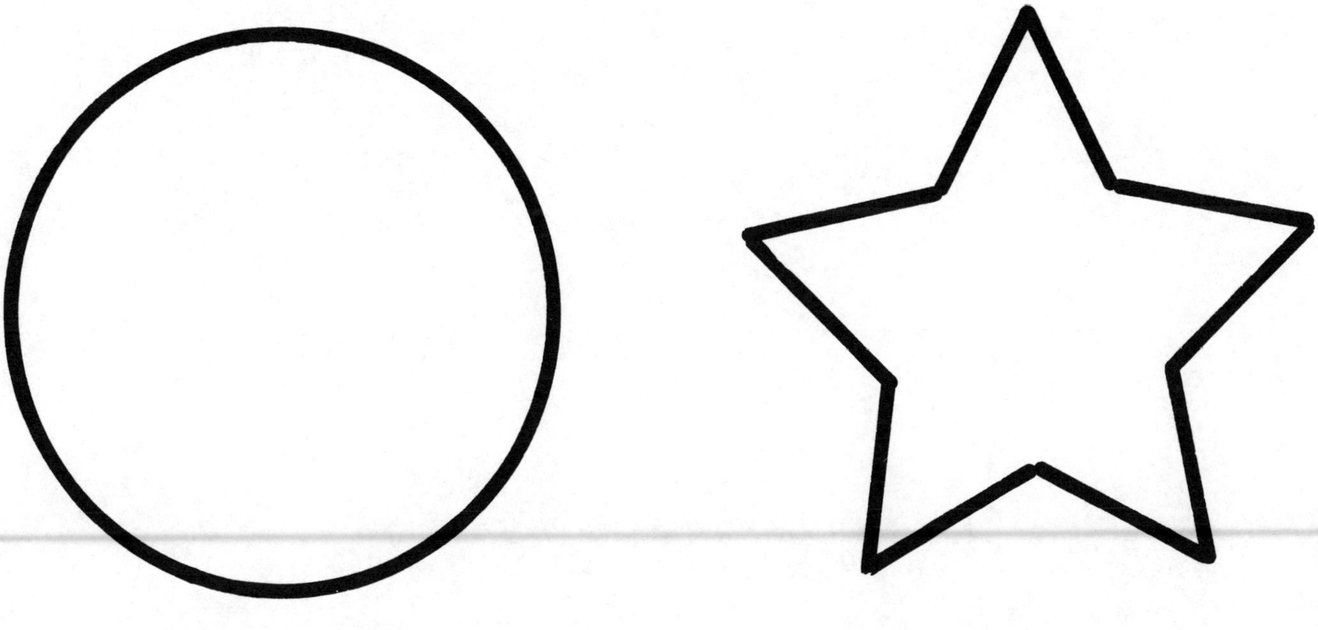

PART 2
Art Projects

This part of the *Learn to Cut* program consists of patterns for 61 cutting activities, including 25 holiday art projects. All patterns are reproducible.

For each project, a small illustration shows the completed work. You may wish to construct an actual model and tack it to the corkboard at the Art Station.

Objective: Working independently, student cuts out shapes of varying sizes with a line ⅛″ wide, and pastes them to complete the project.

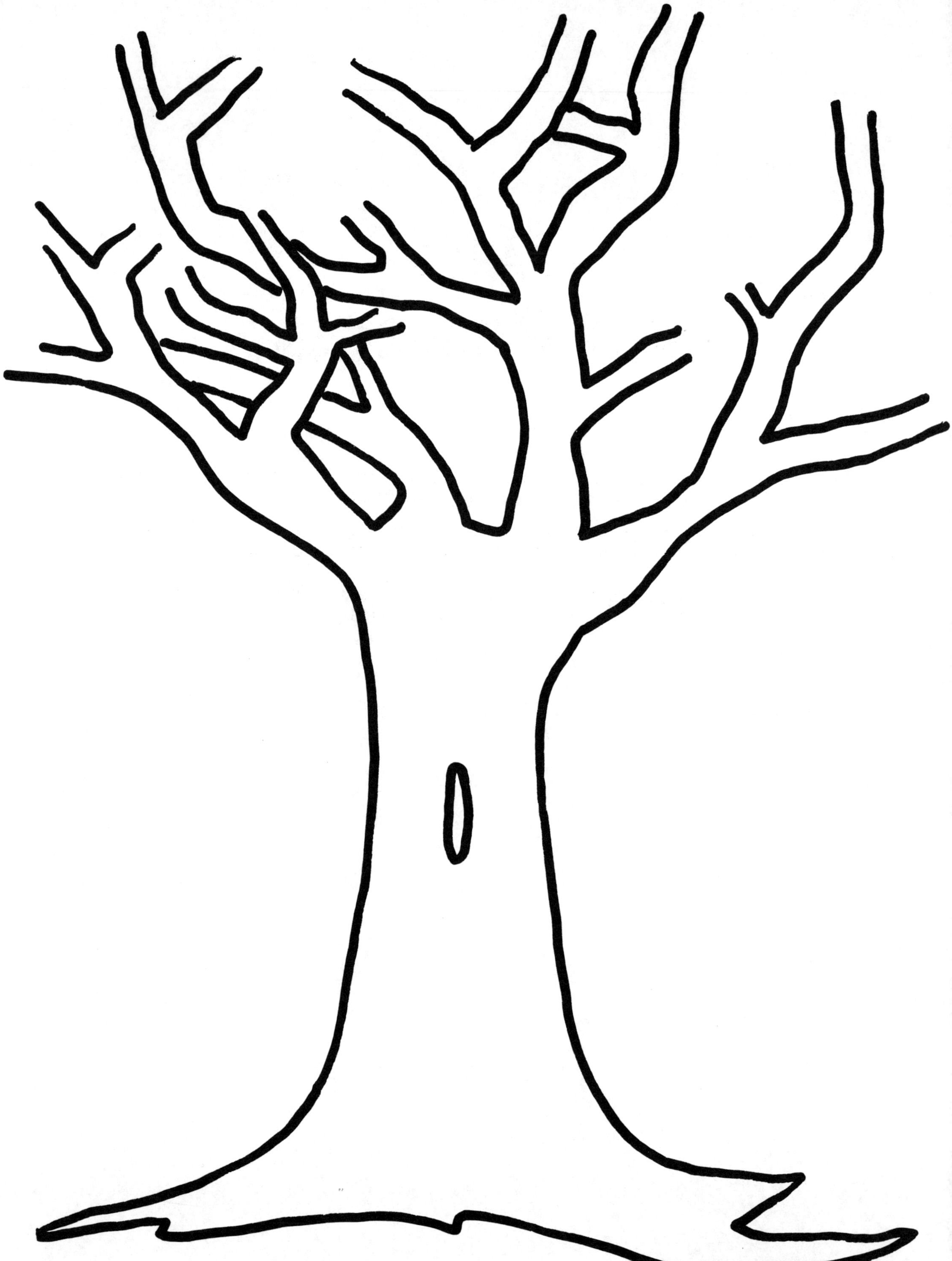

Leafy Tree

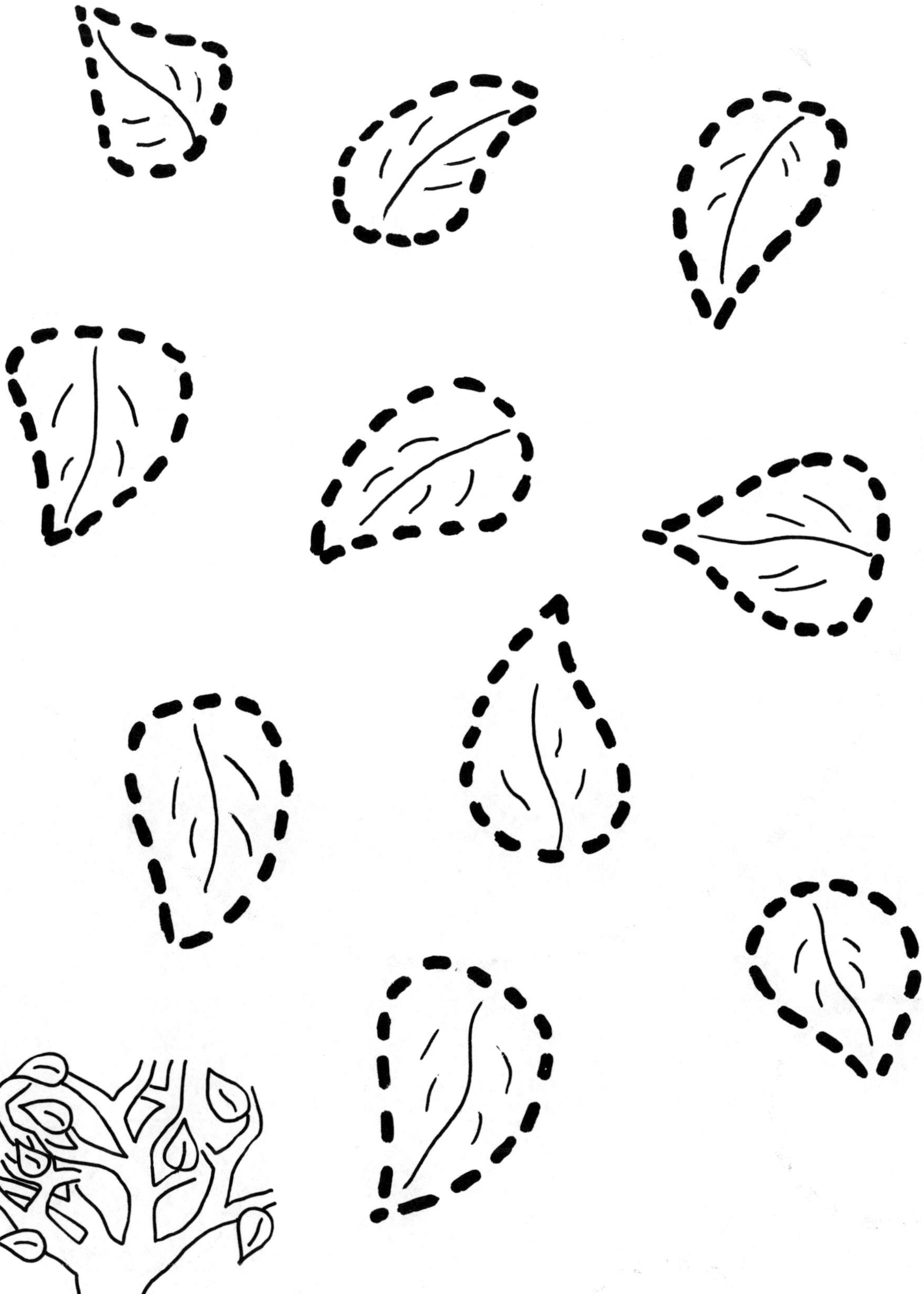

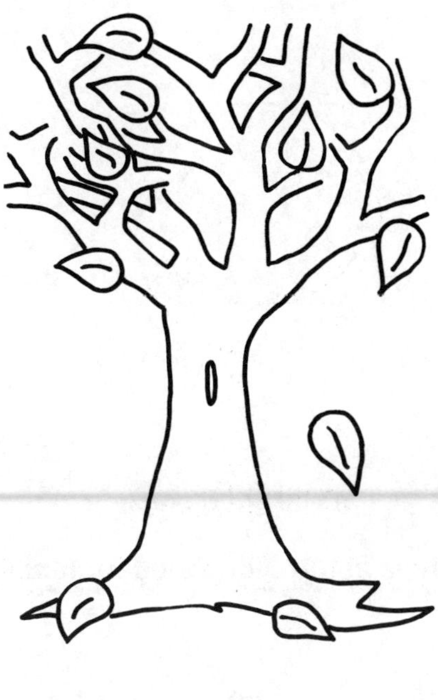

Leafy Tree

Autumn Tree—Use yellow, rust, and orange construction paper for the leaves.

Spring Tree—Use light green construction paper for the leaves.

Tree trunk and branches—Use brown construction paper for the tree trunk and branches.

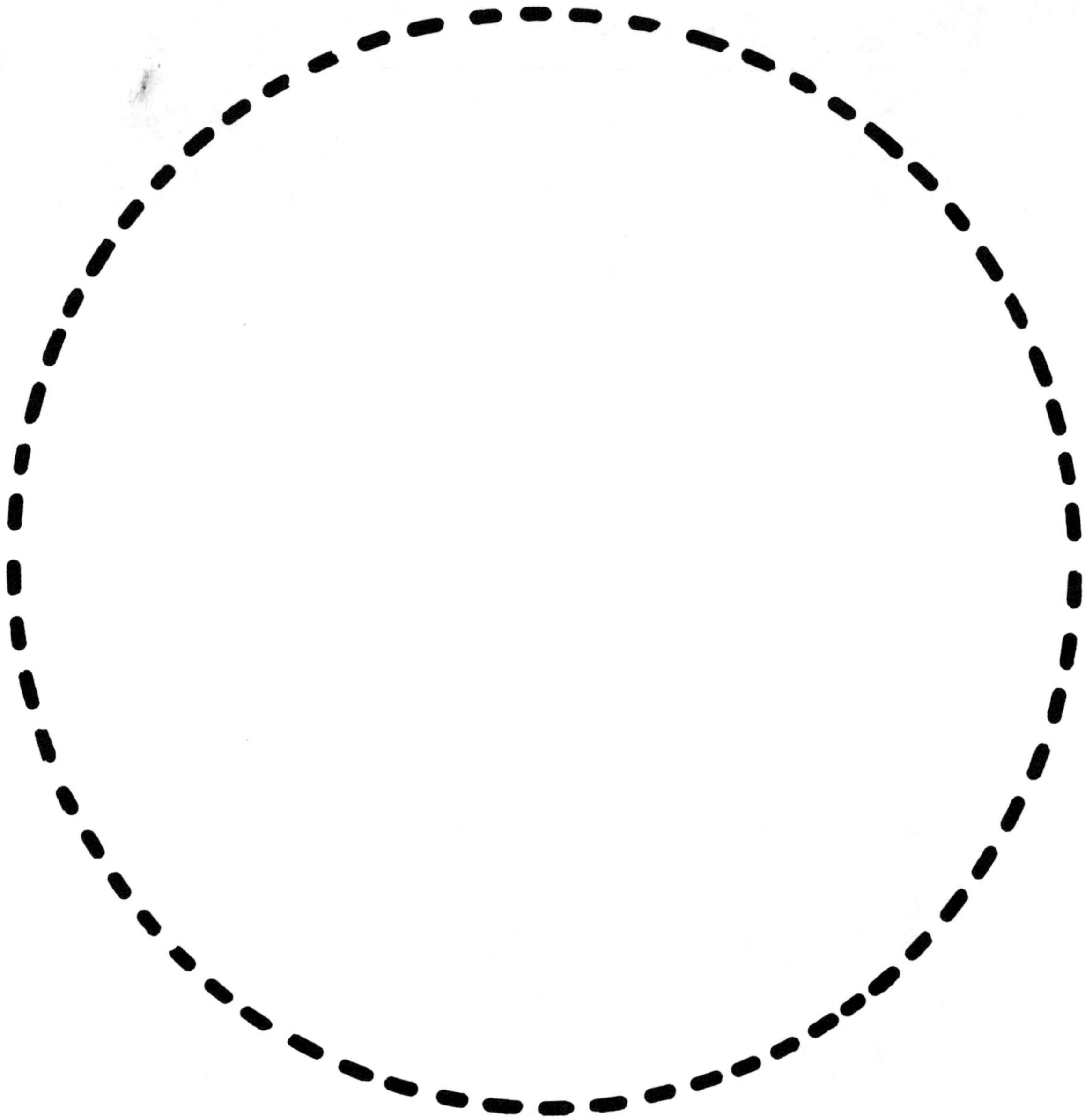

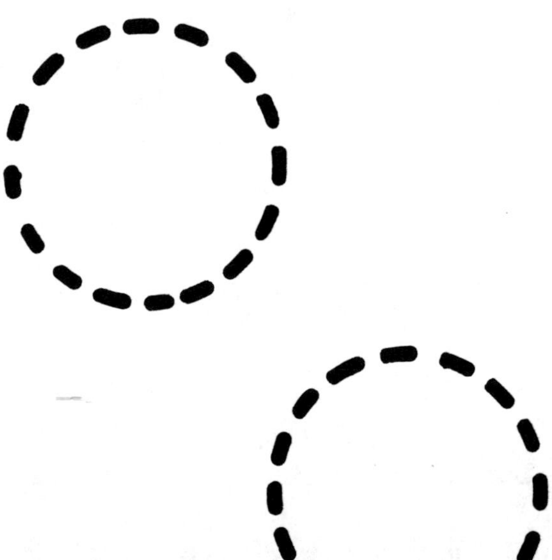

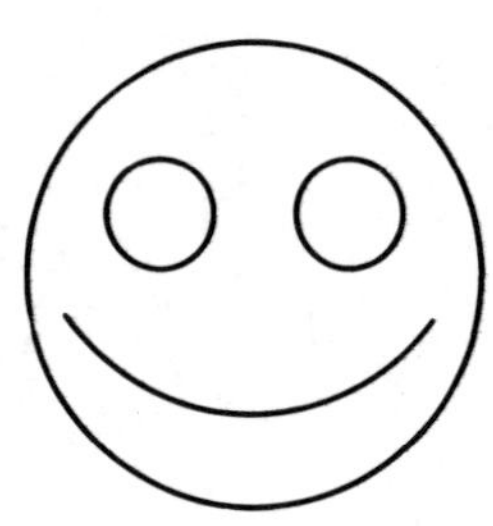

Smiling Face

Optional: Punch hole at top. Add string for mobile.

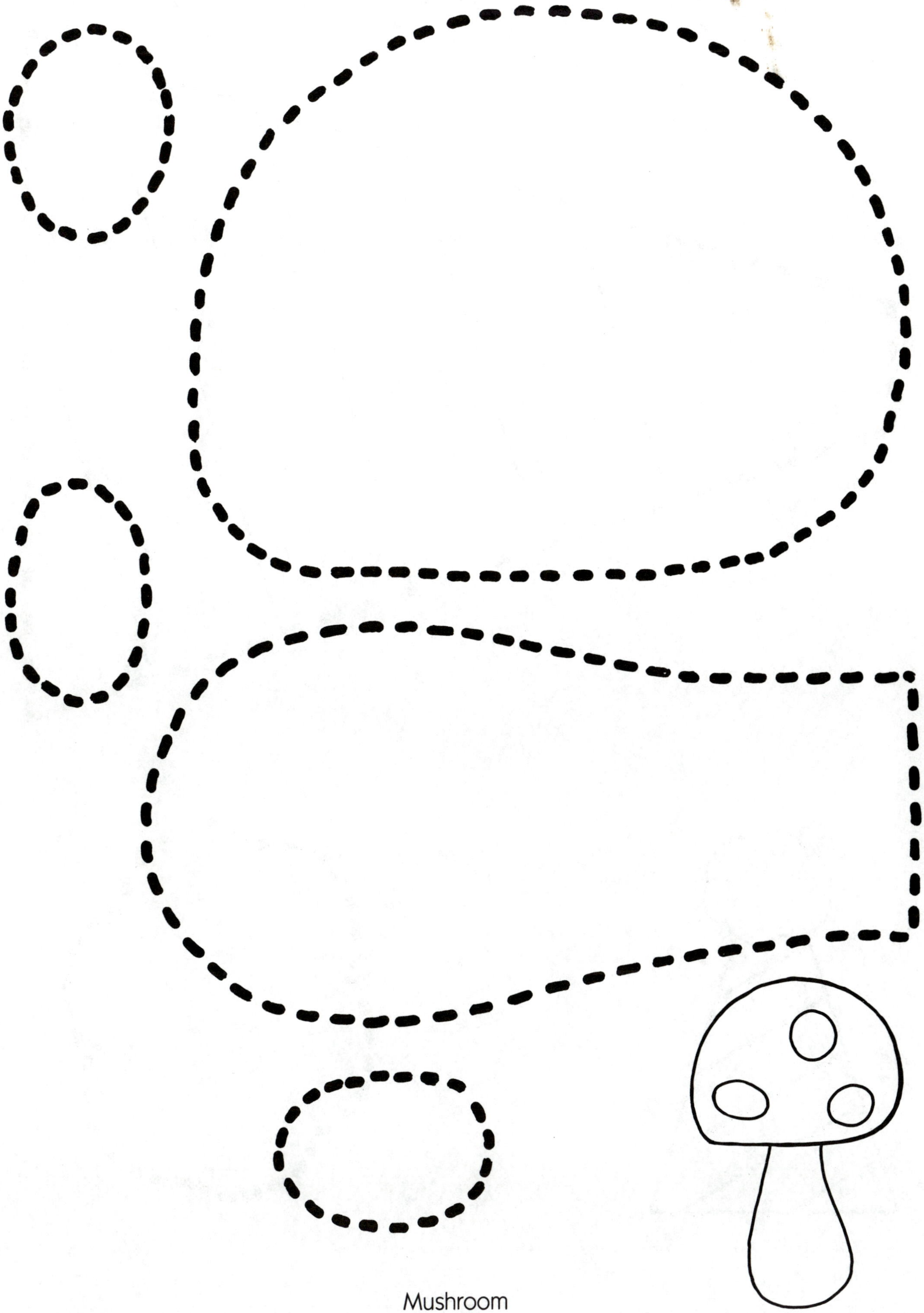

Mushroom

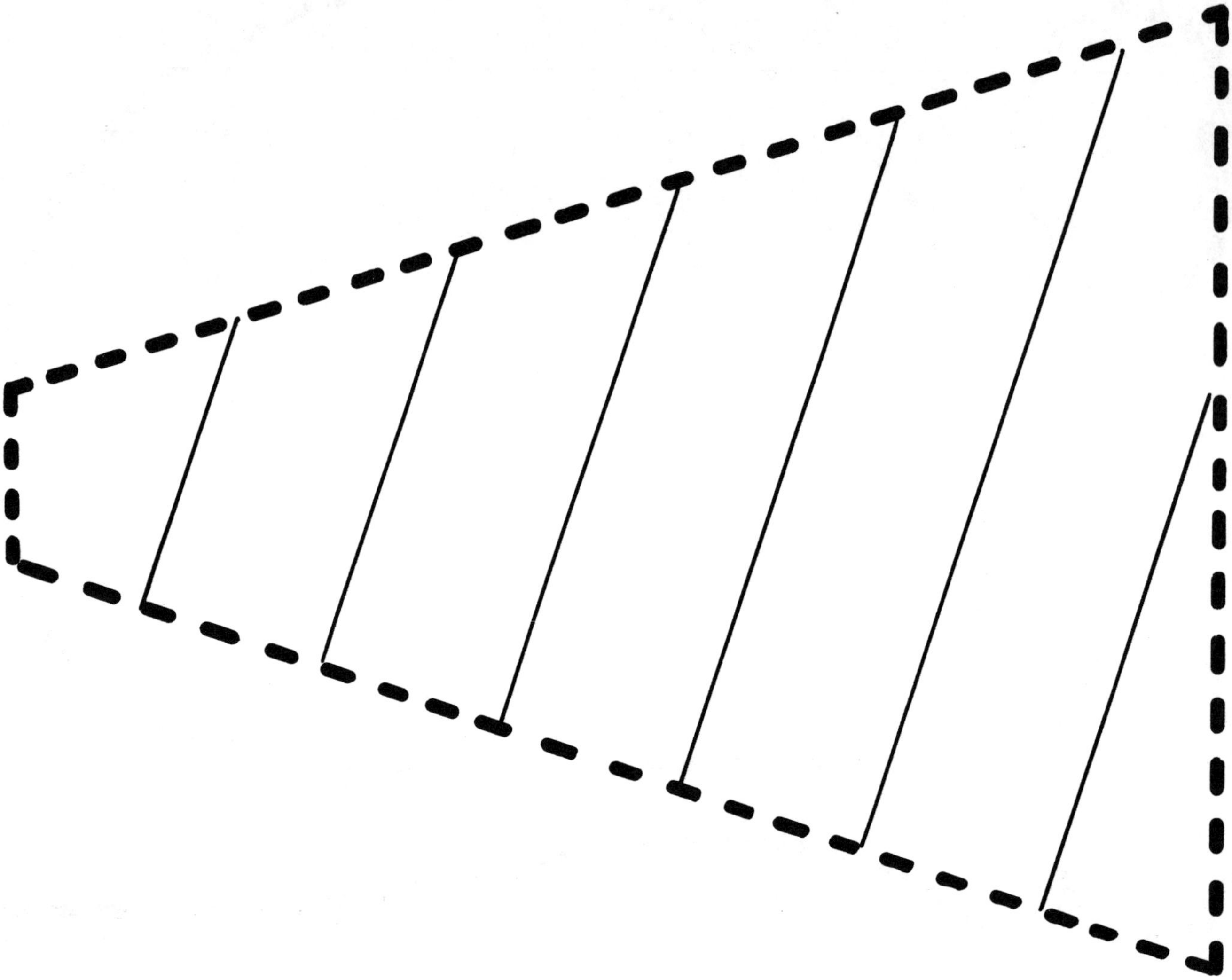

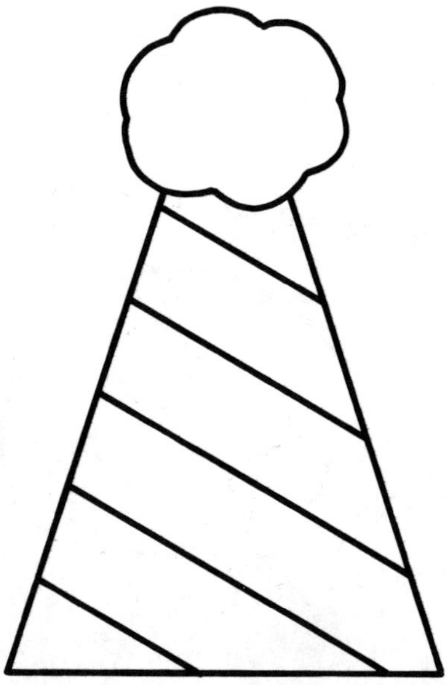

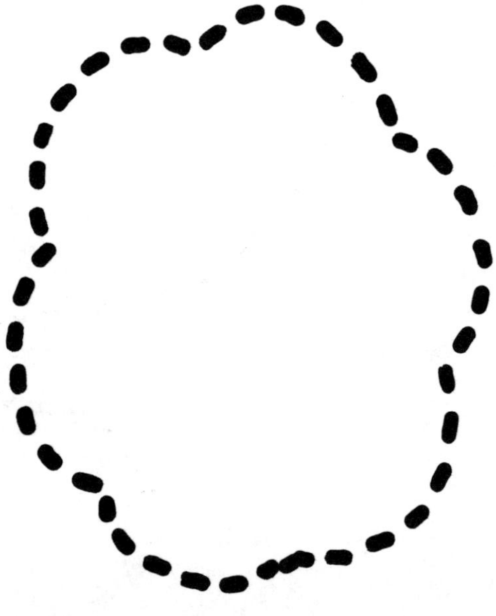

Party Hat

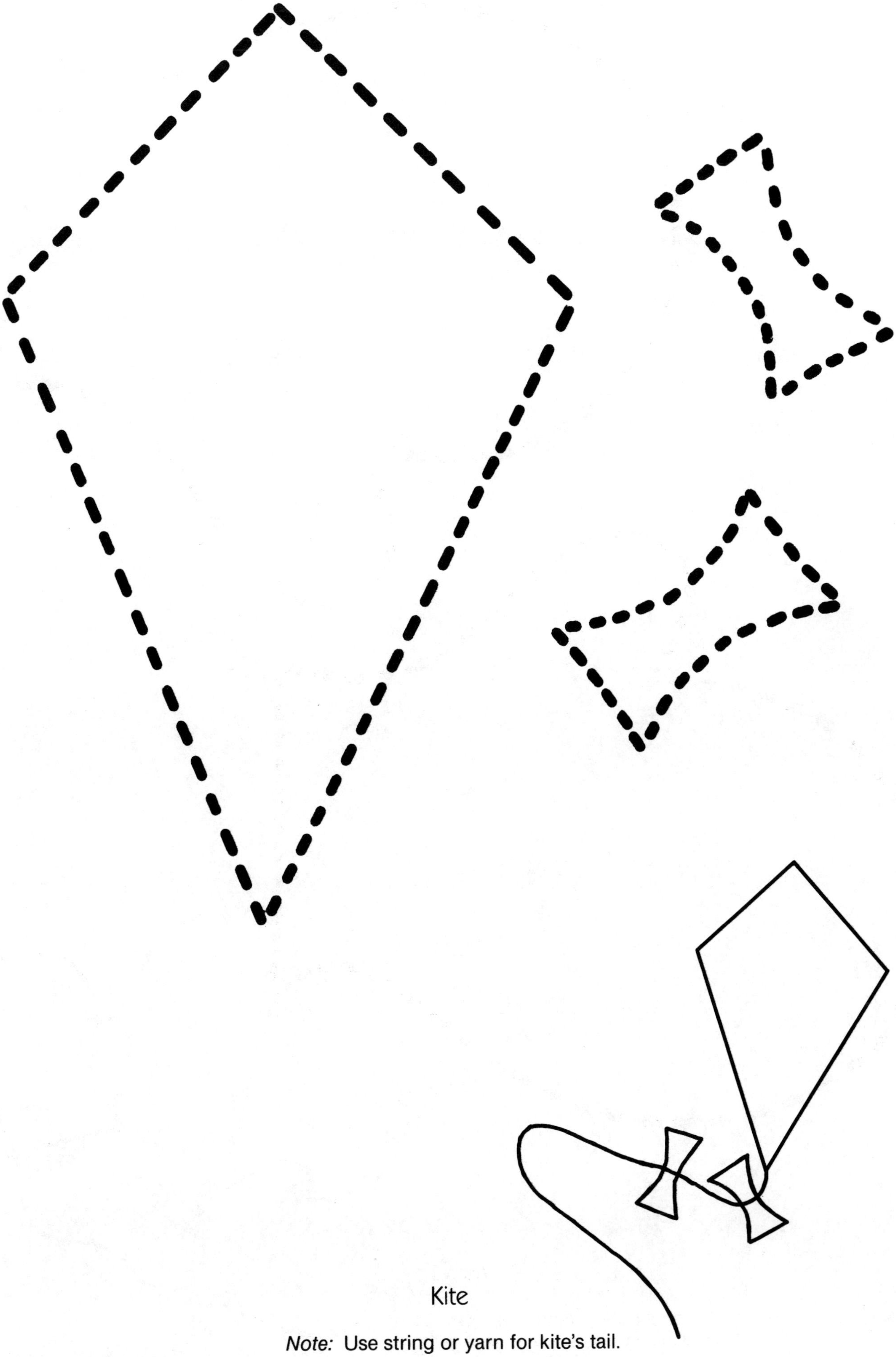

Kite

Note: Use string or yarn for kite's tail.

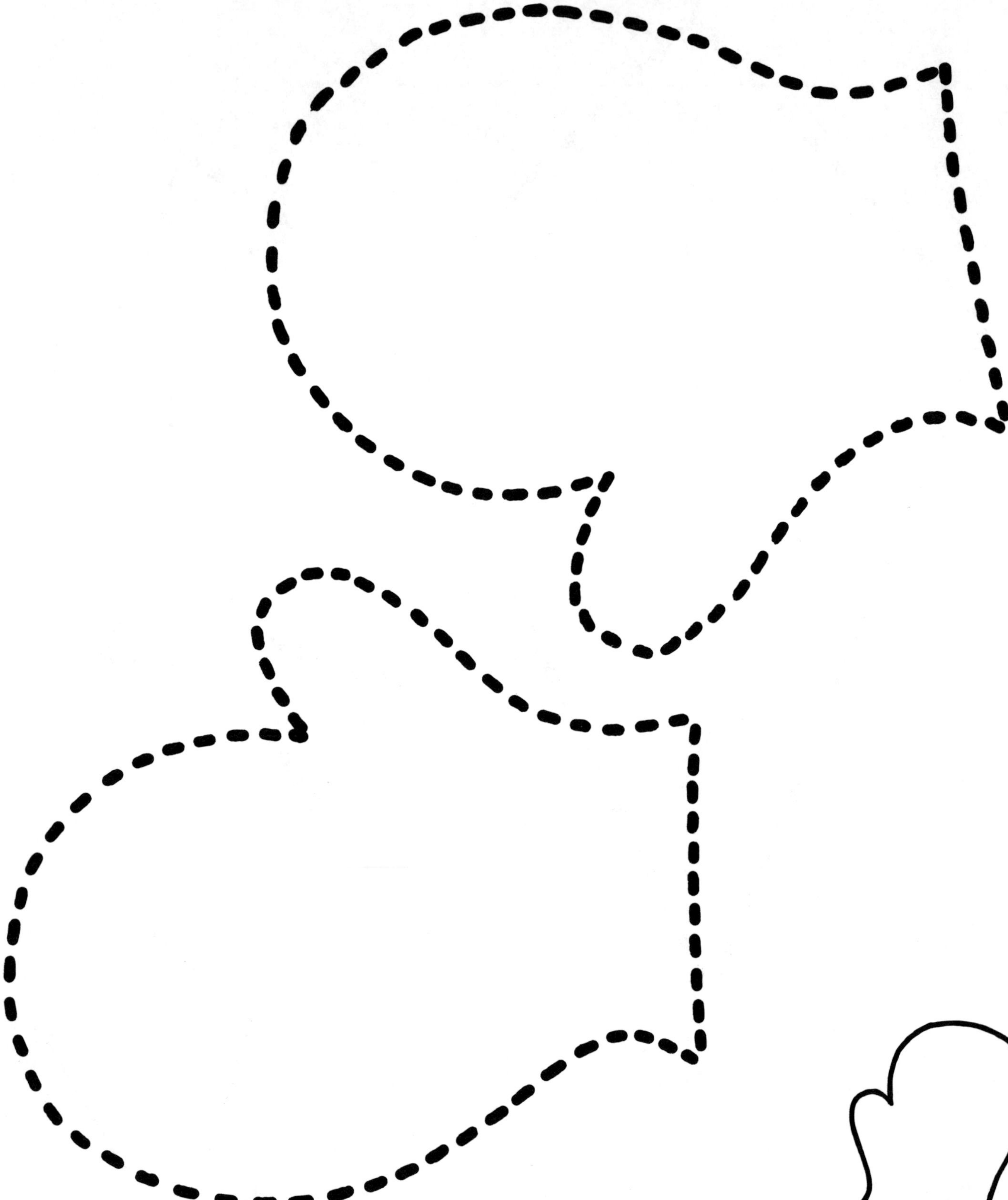

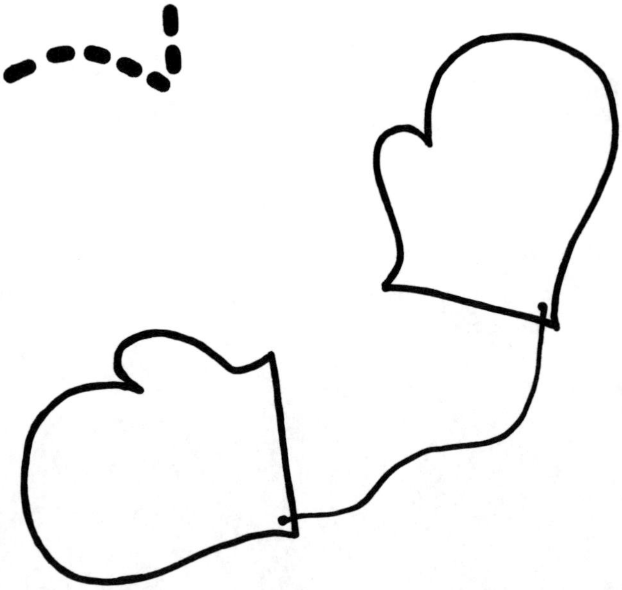

Mittens

Punch a hole in mitten corners.
Add yarn to fasten mittens together.

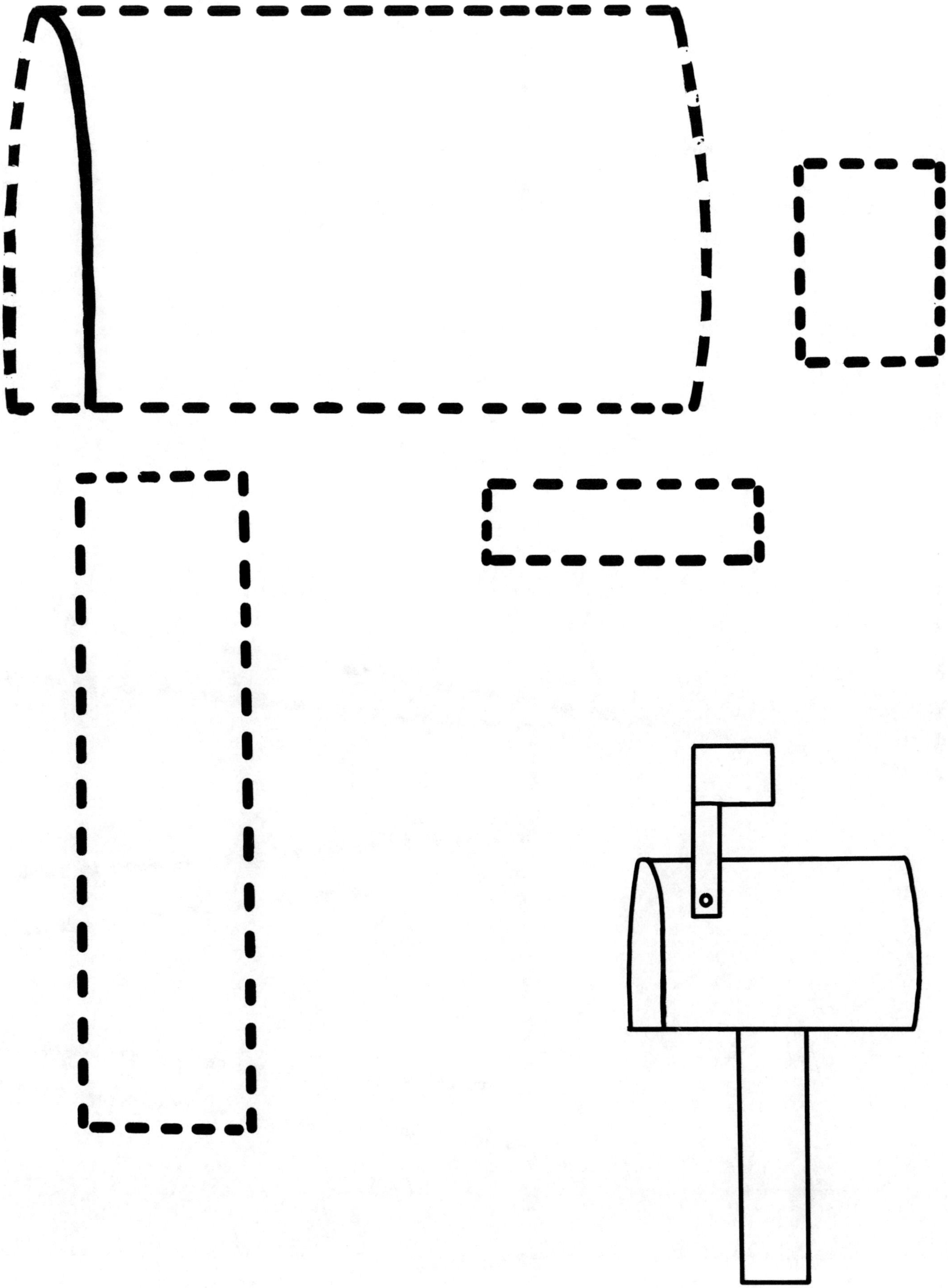

Mailbox

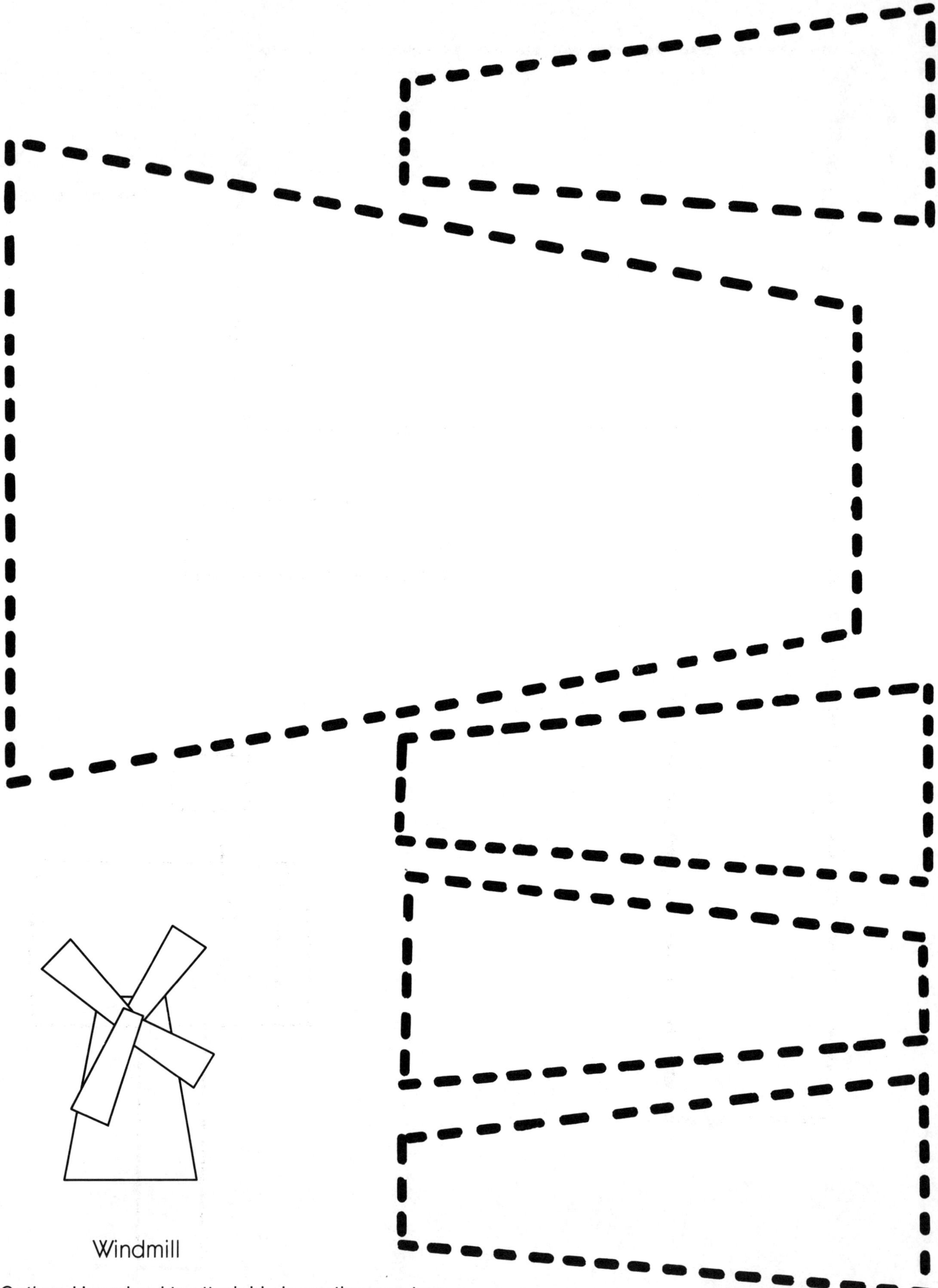

Windmill

Option: Use a brad to attach blades so they can turn.

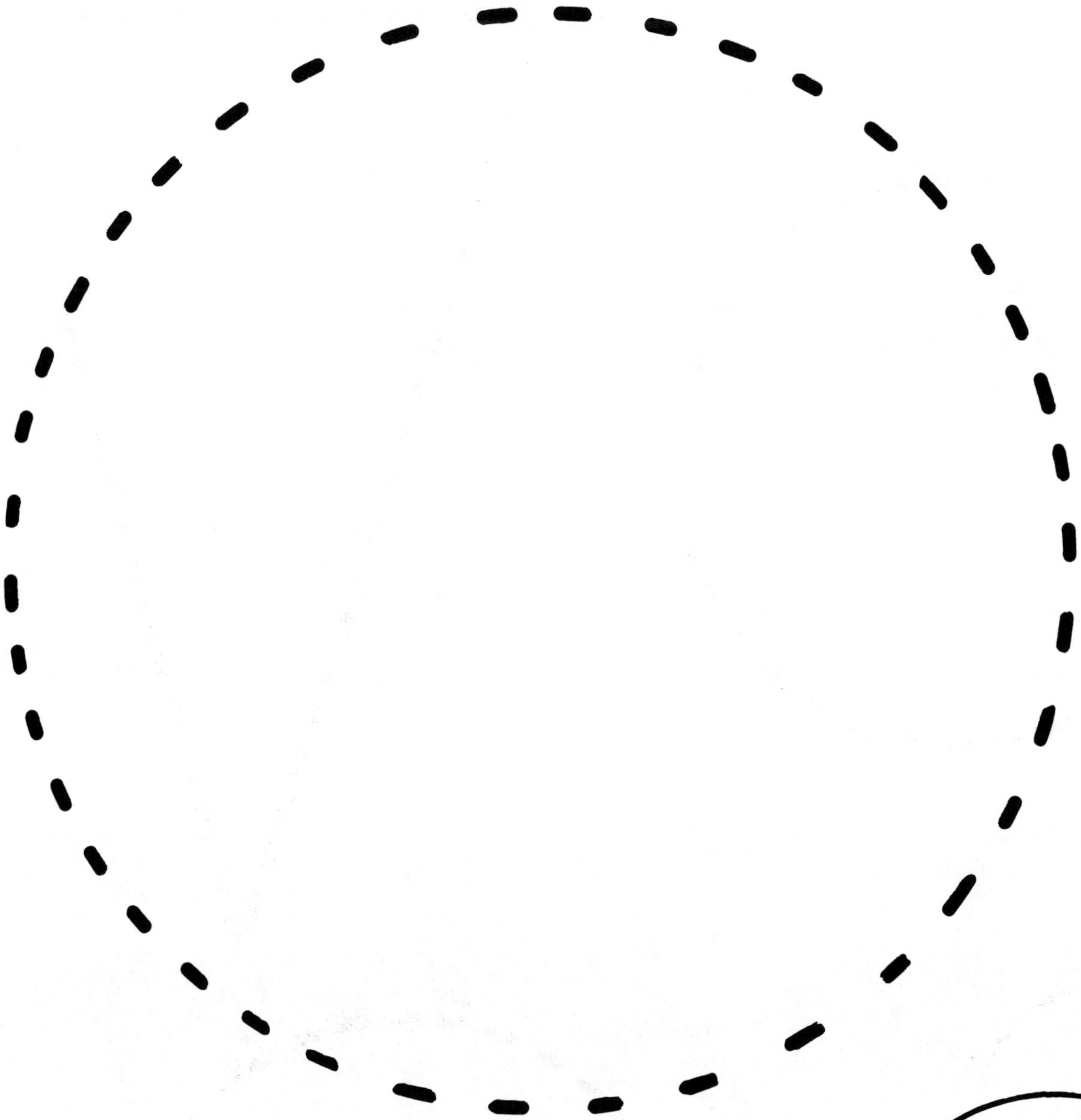

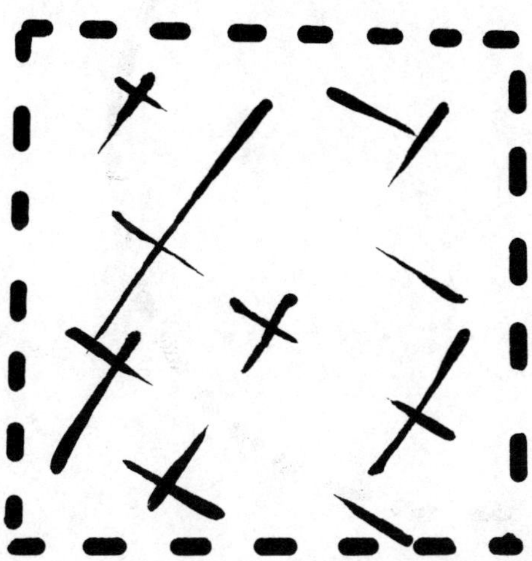

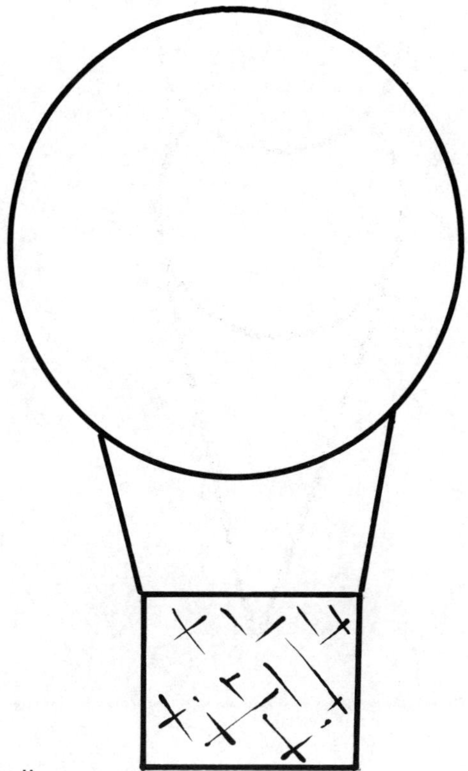

Hot Air Balloon

Use string or yarn to attach basket to balloon.

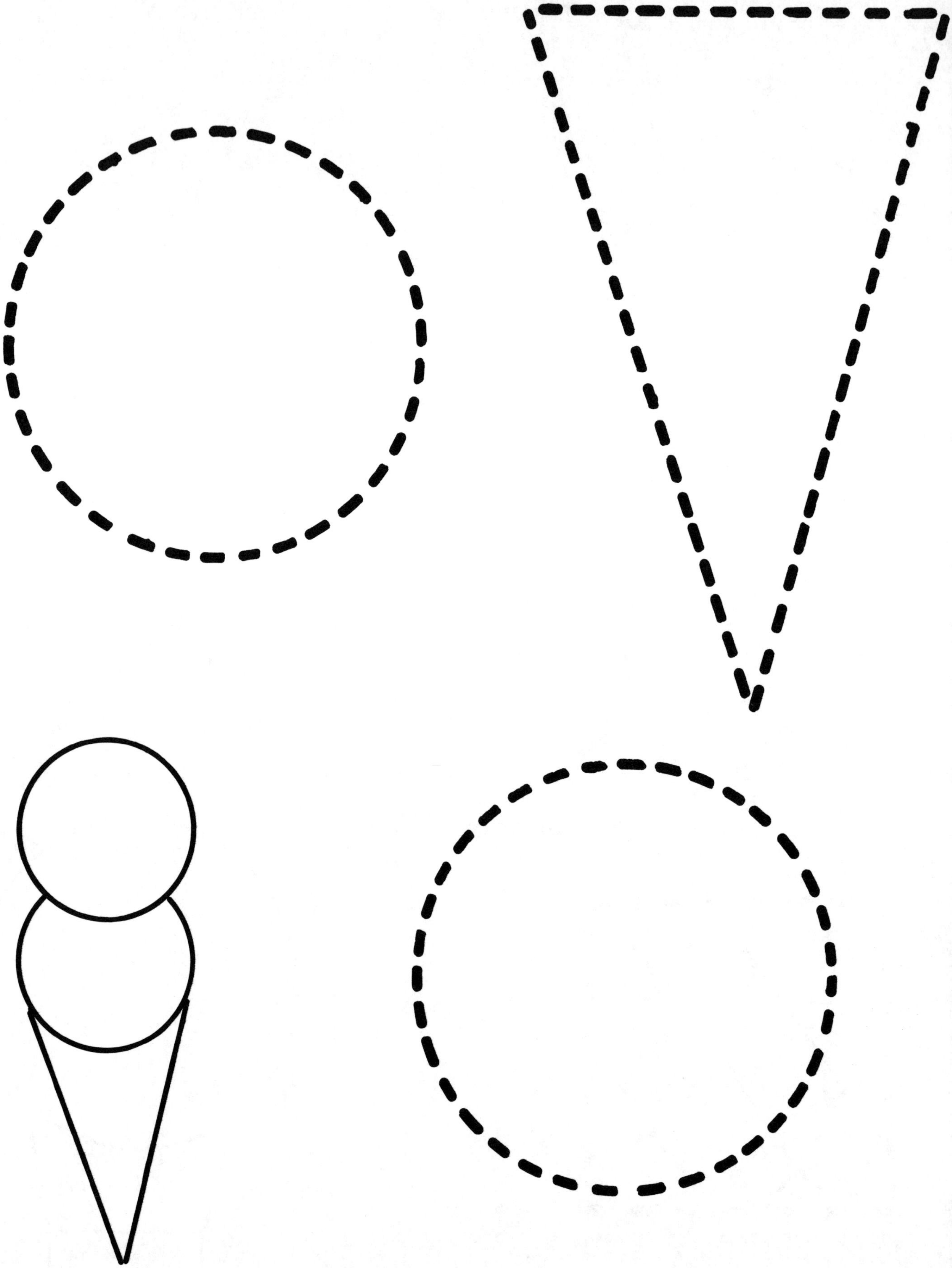

Ice-Cream Cone

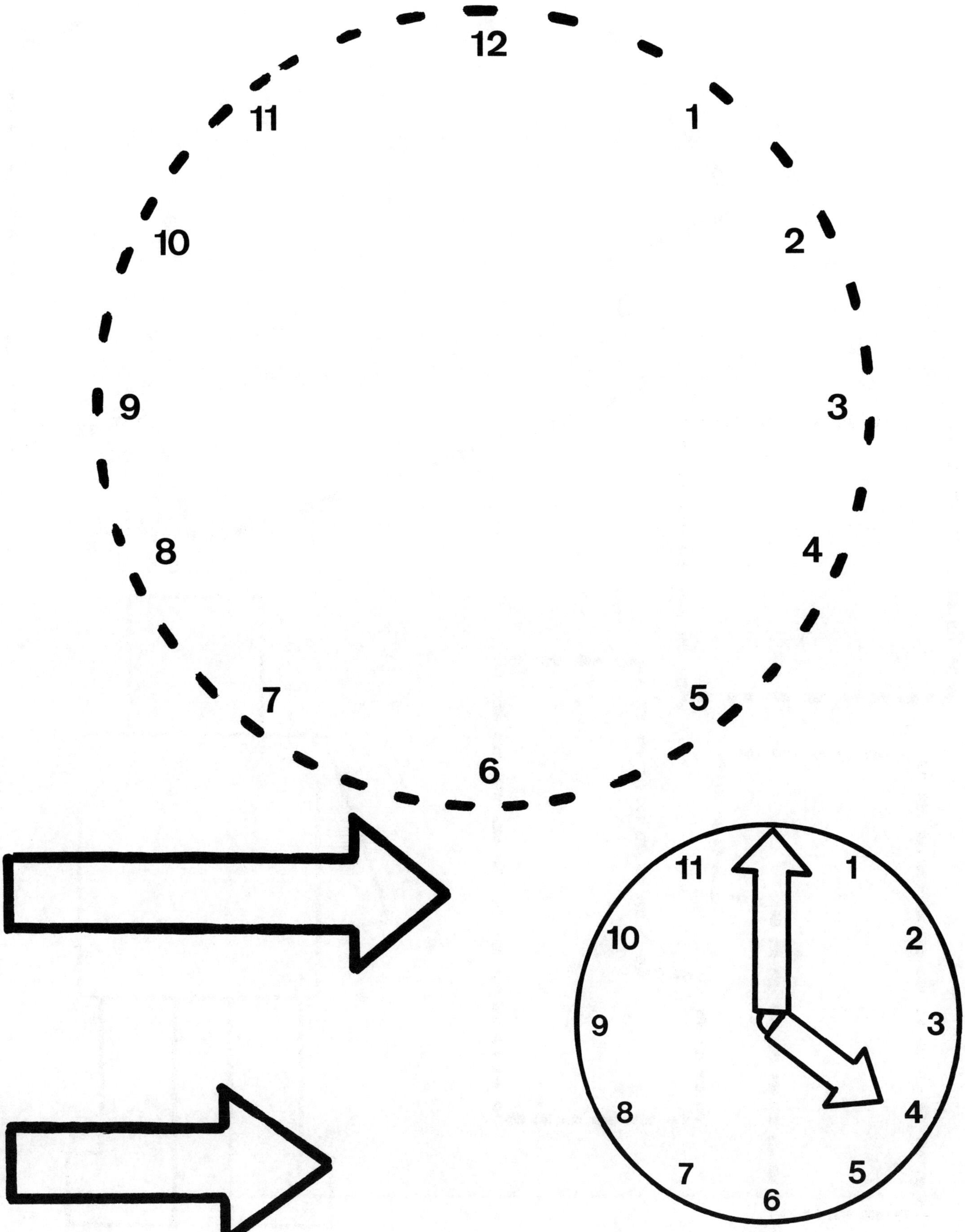

Clock

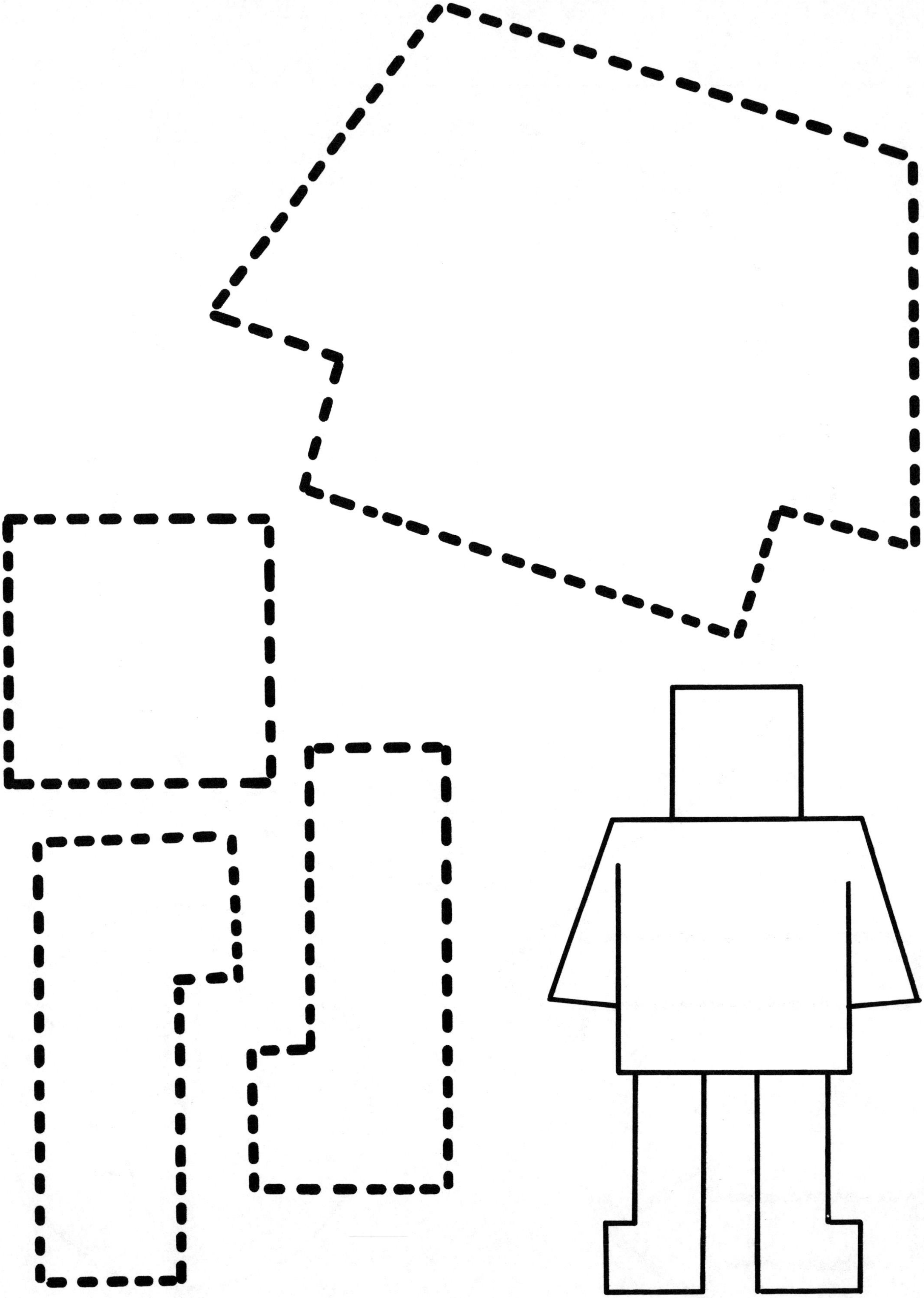

Robot

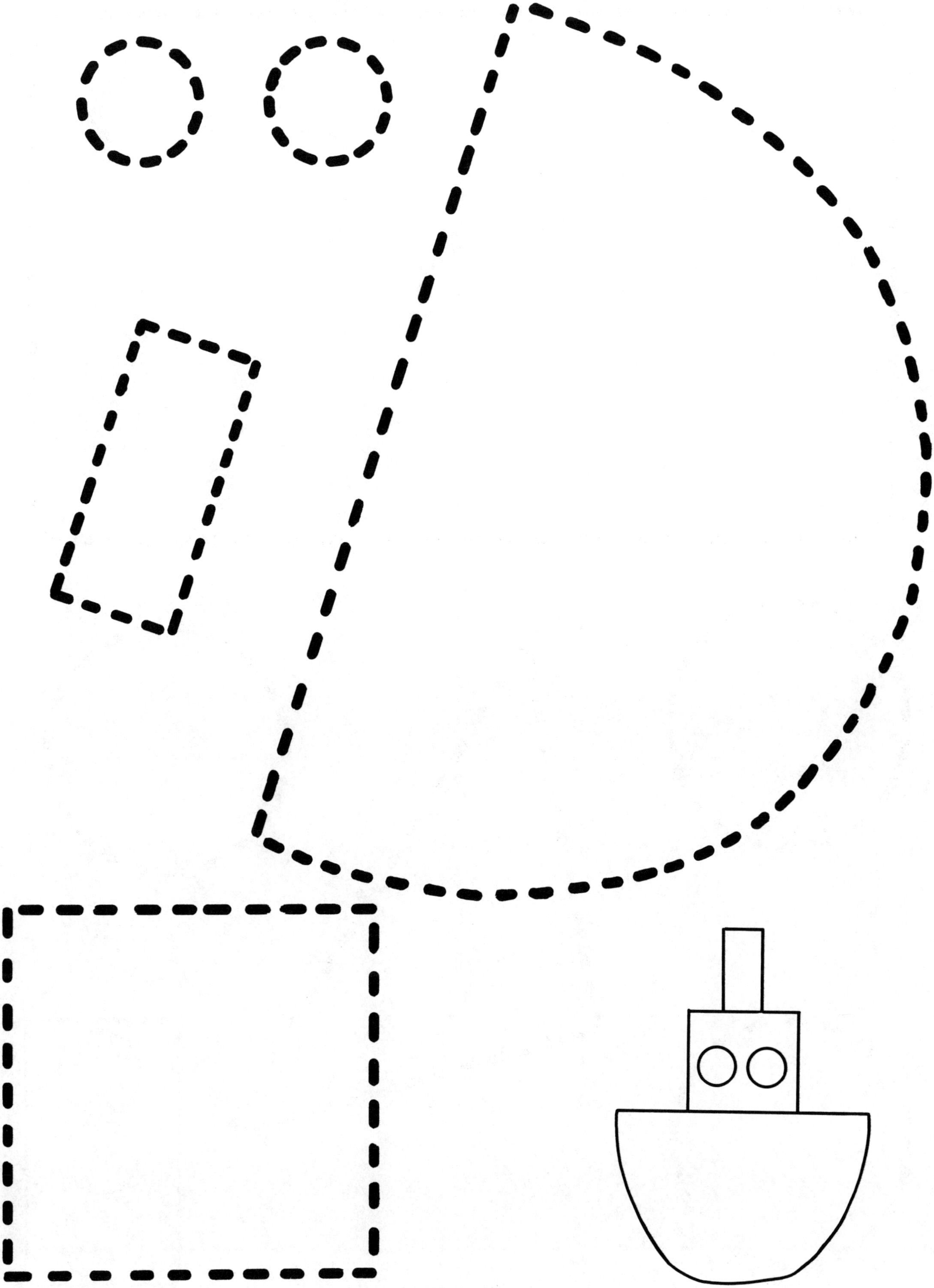

Tugboat

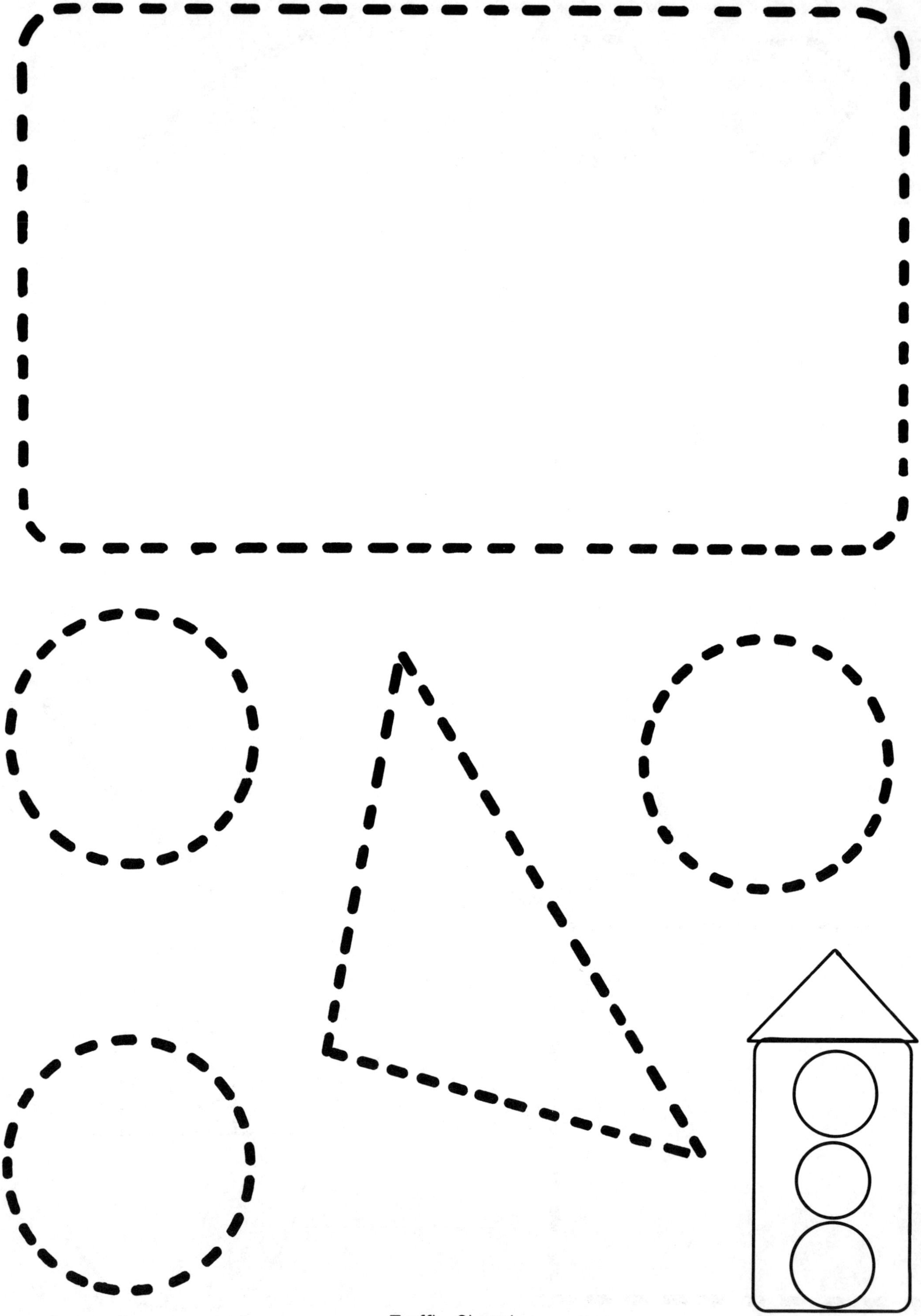

Traffic Signal

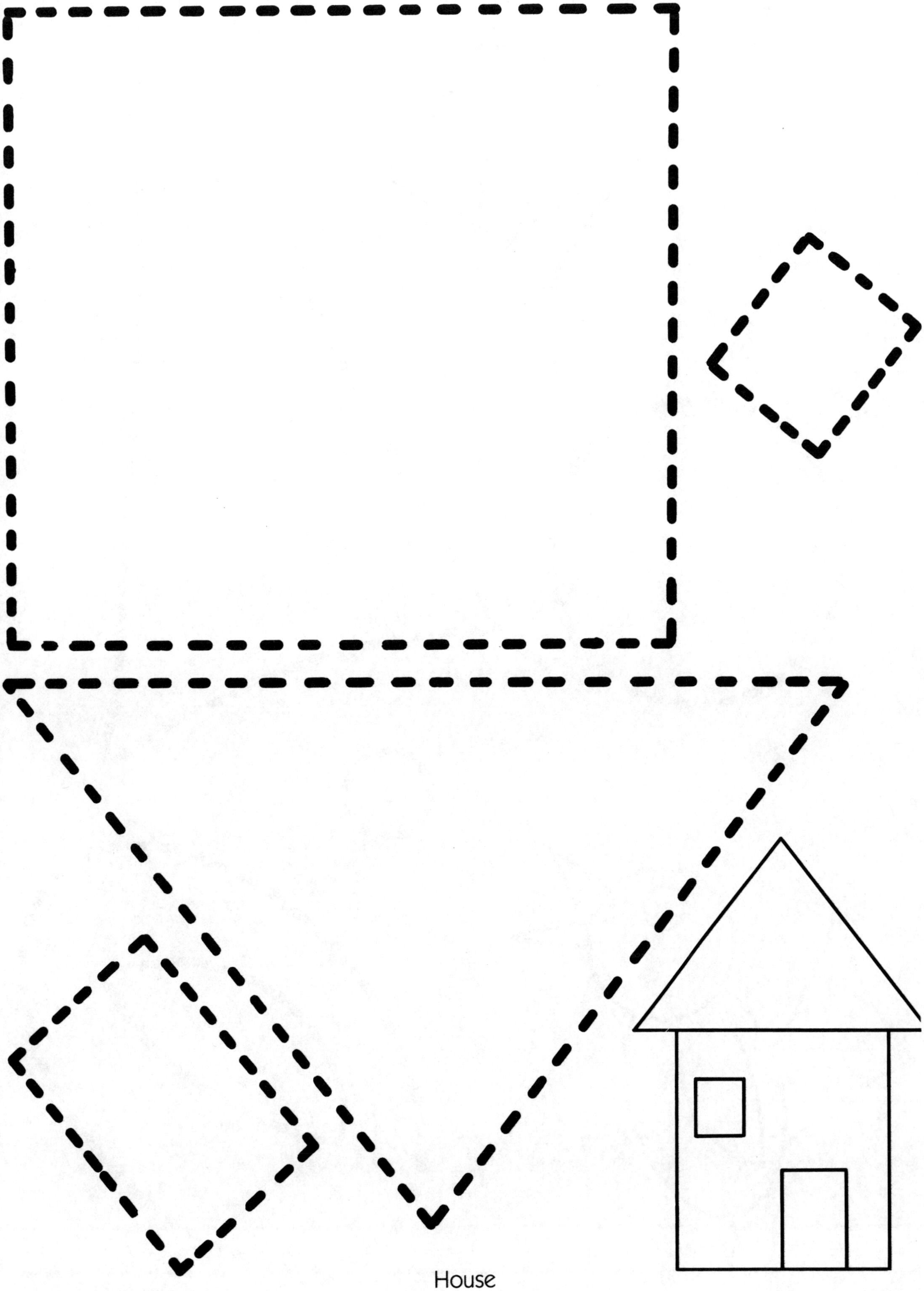

House

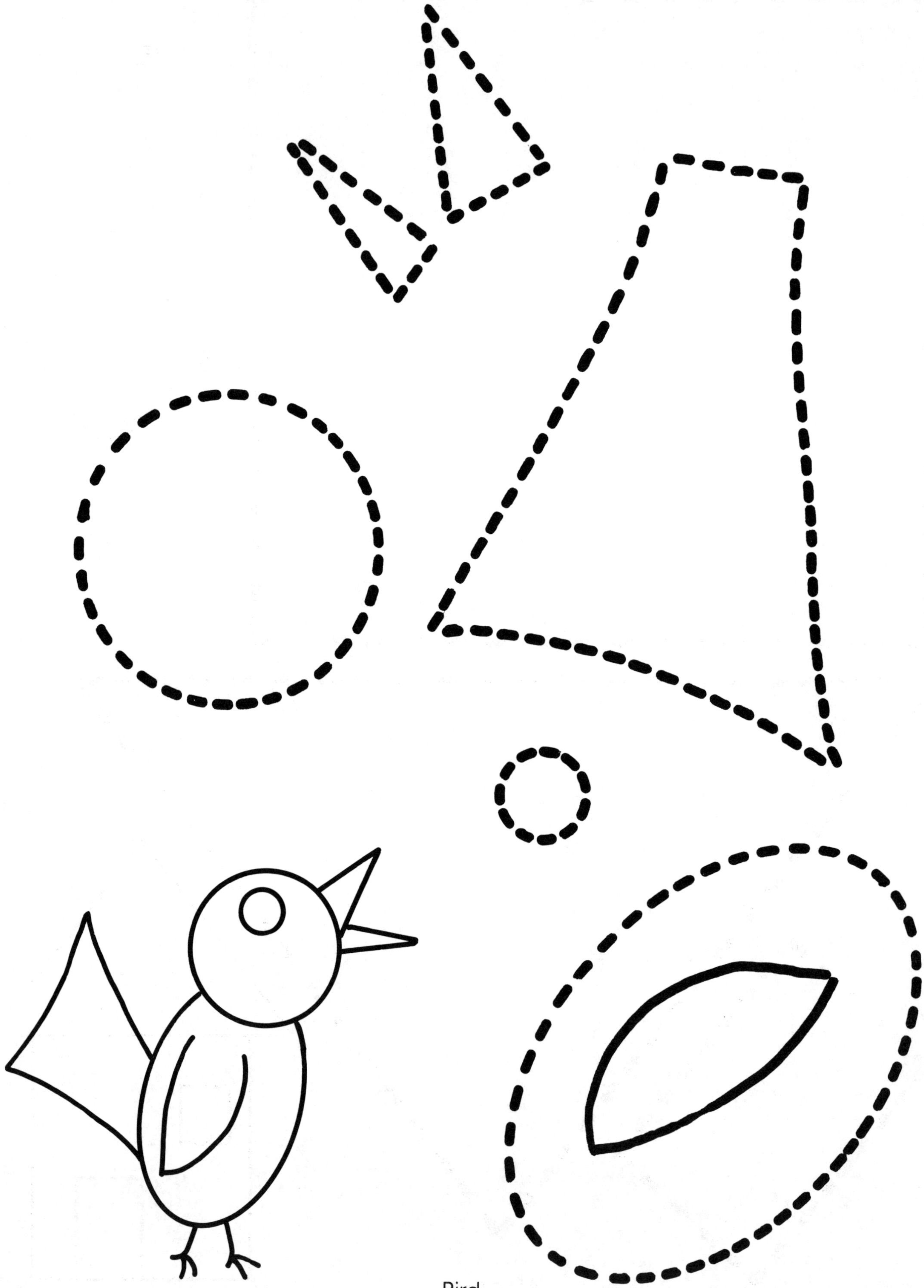

Bird

Flower

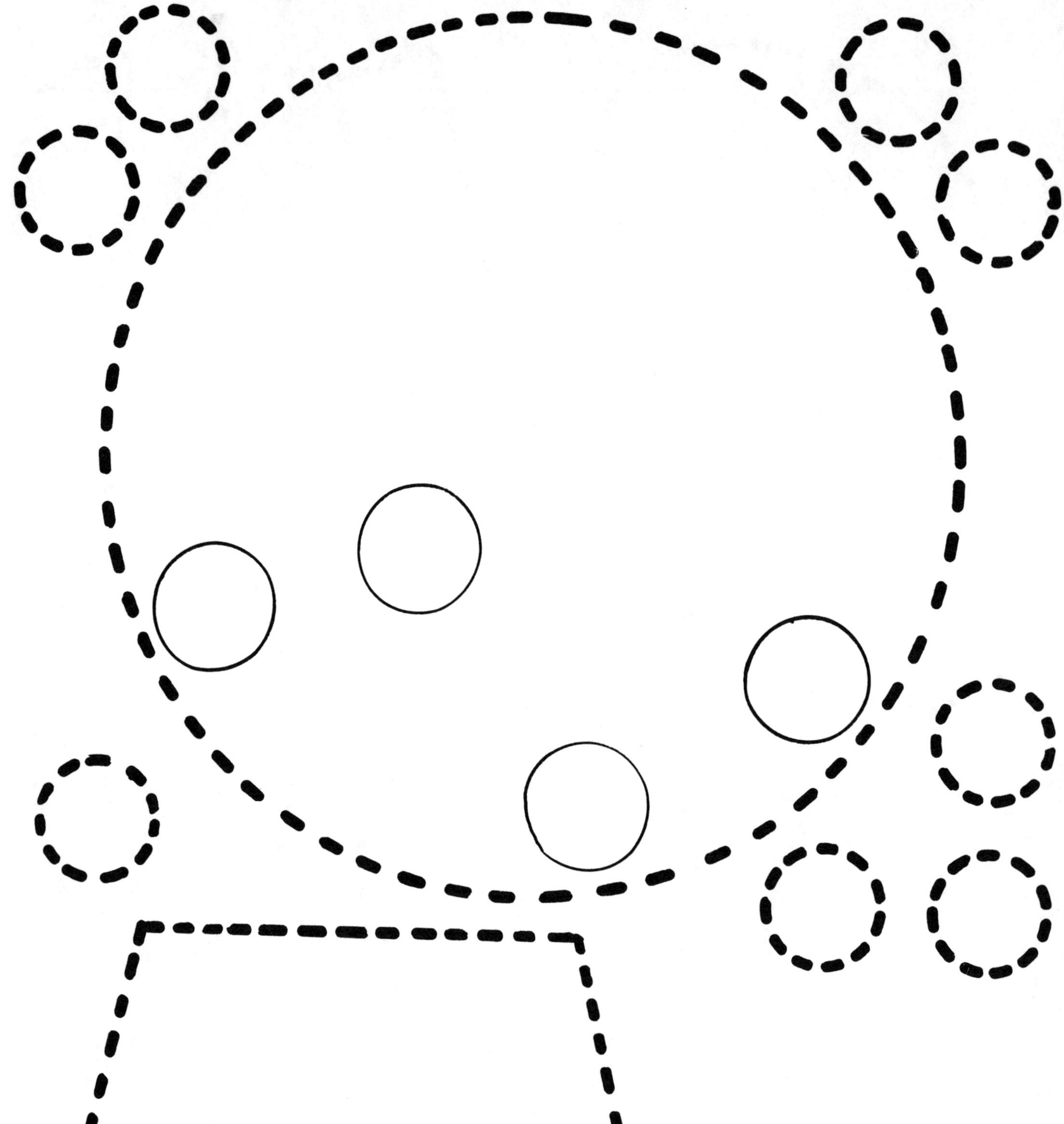

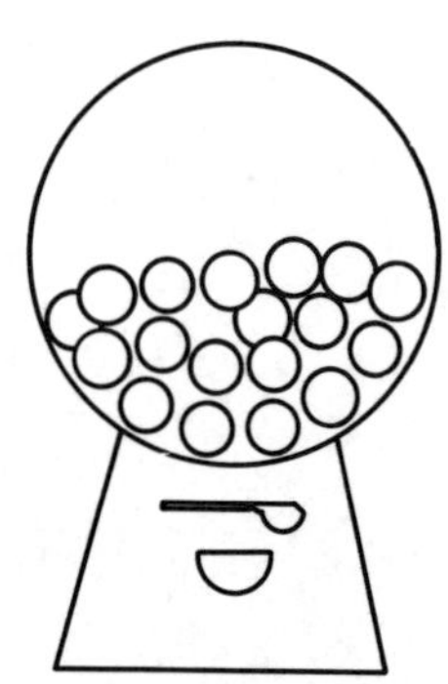

Gumball Machine

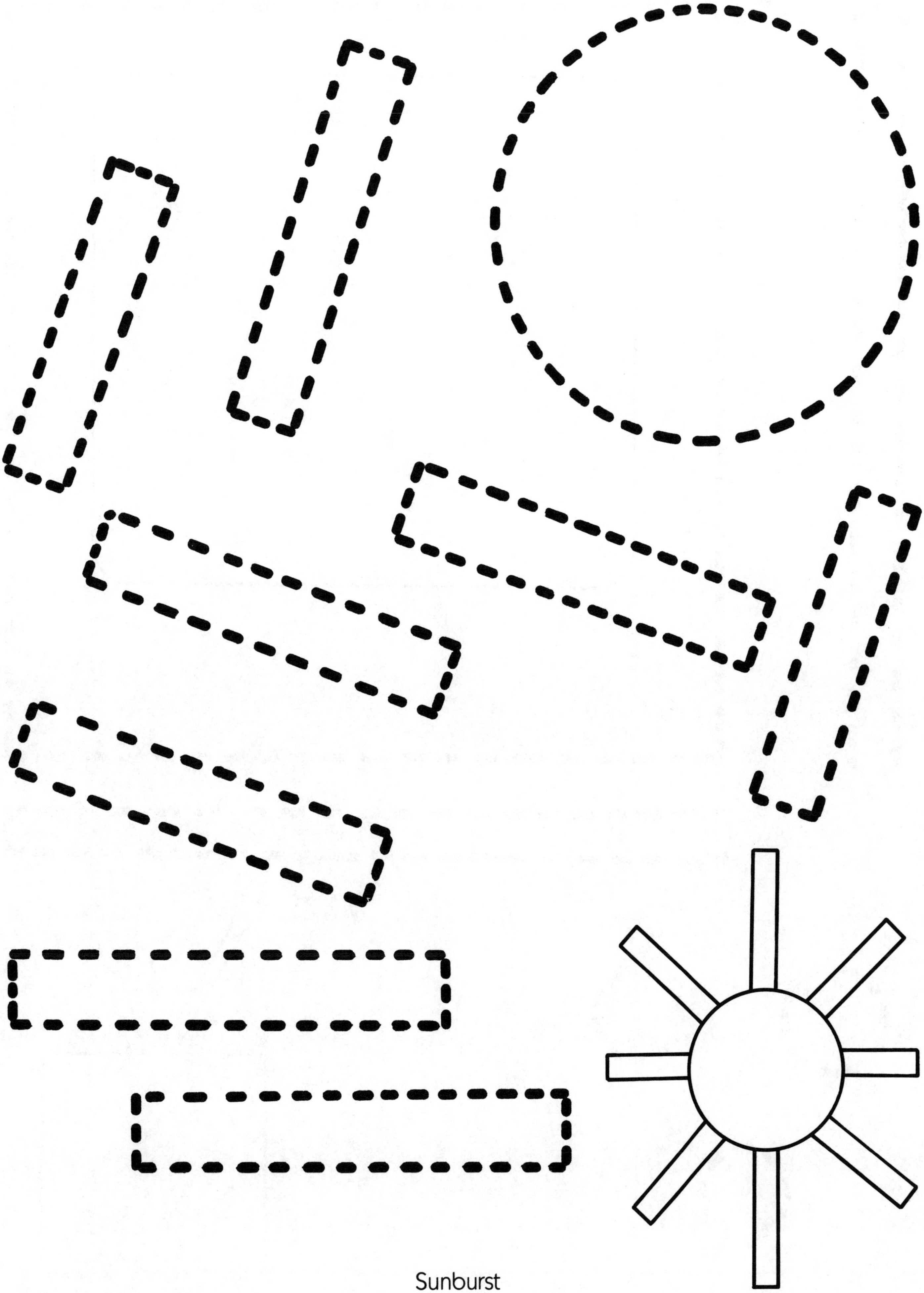

Sunburst

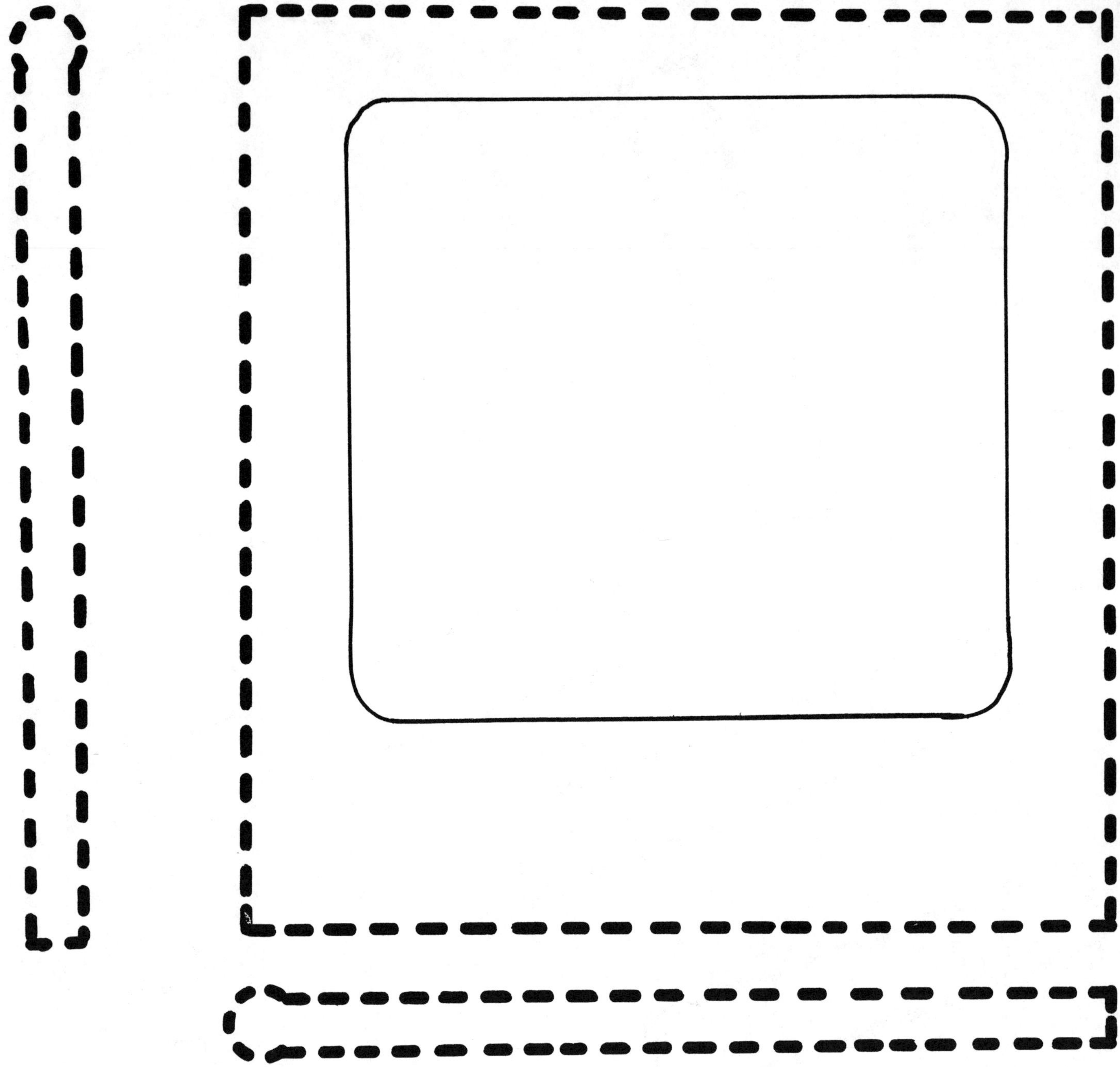

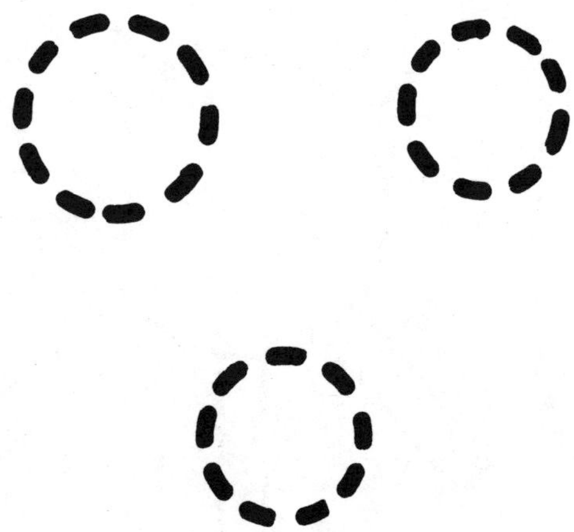

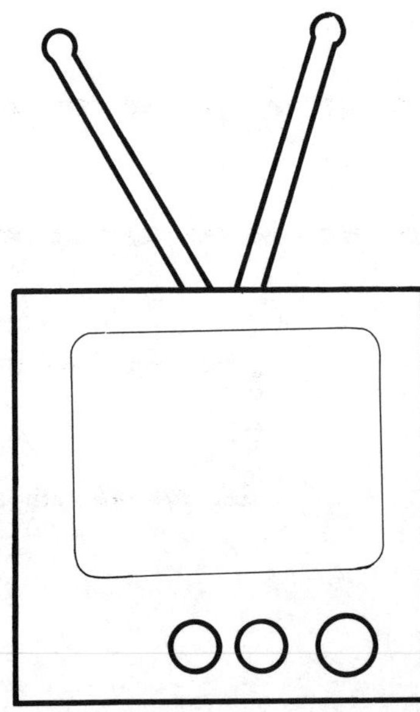

Television

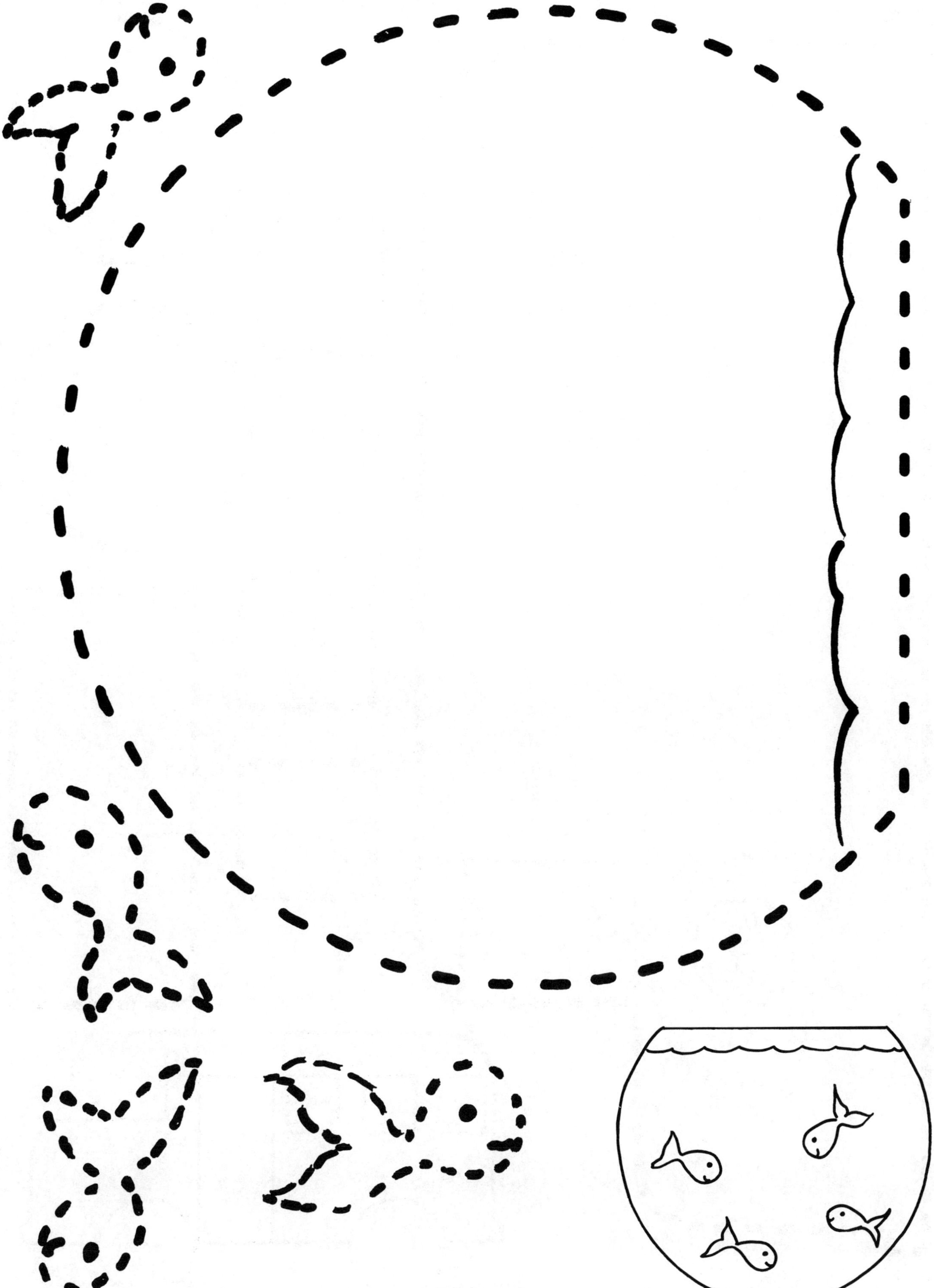

Fishbowl

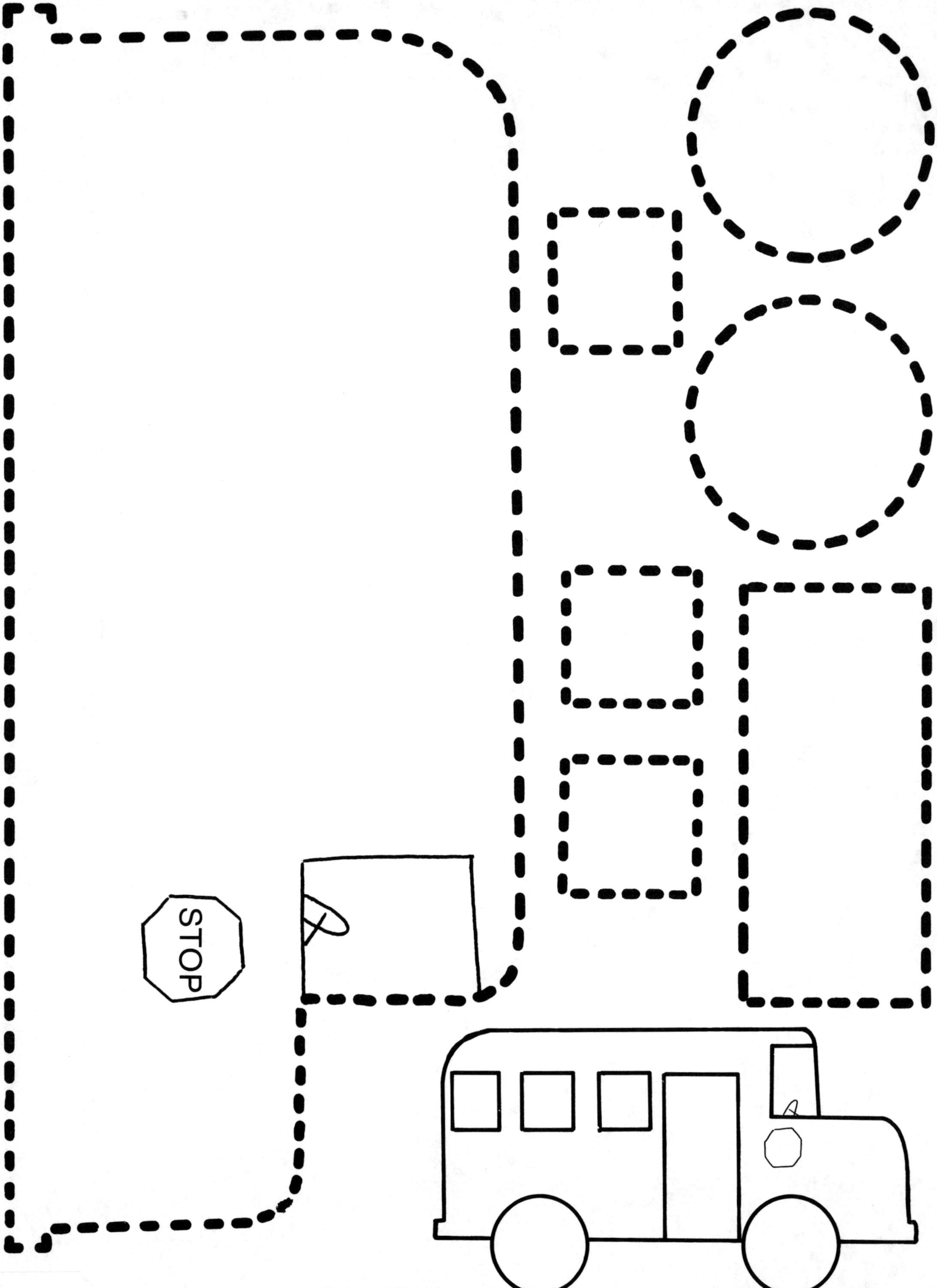

School Bus

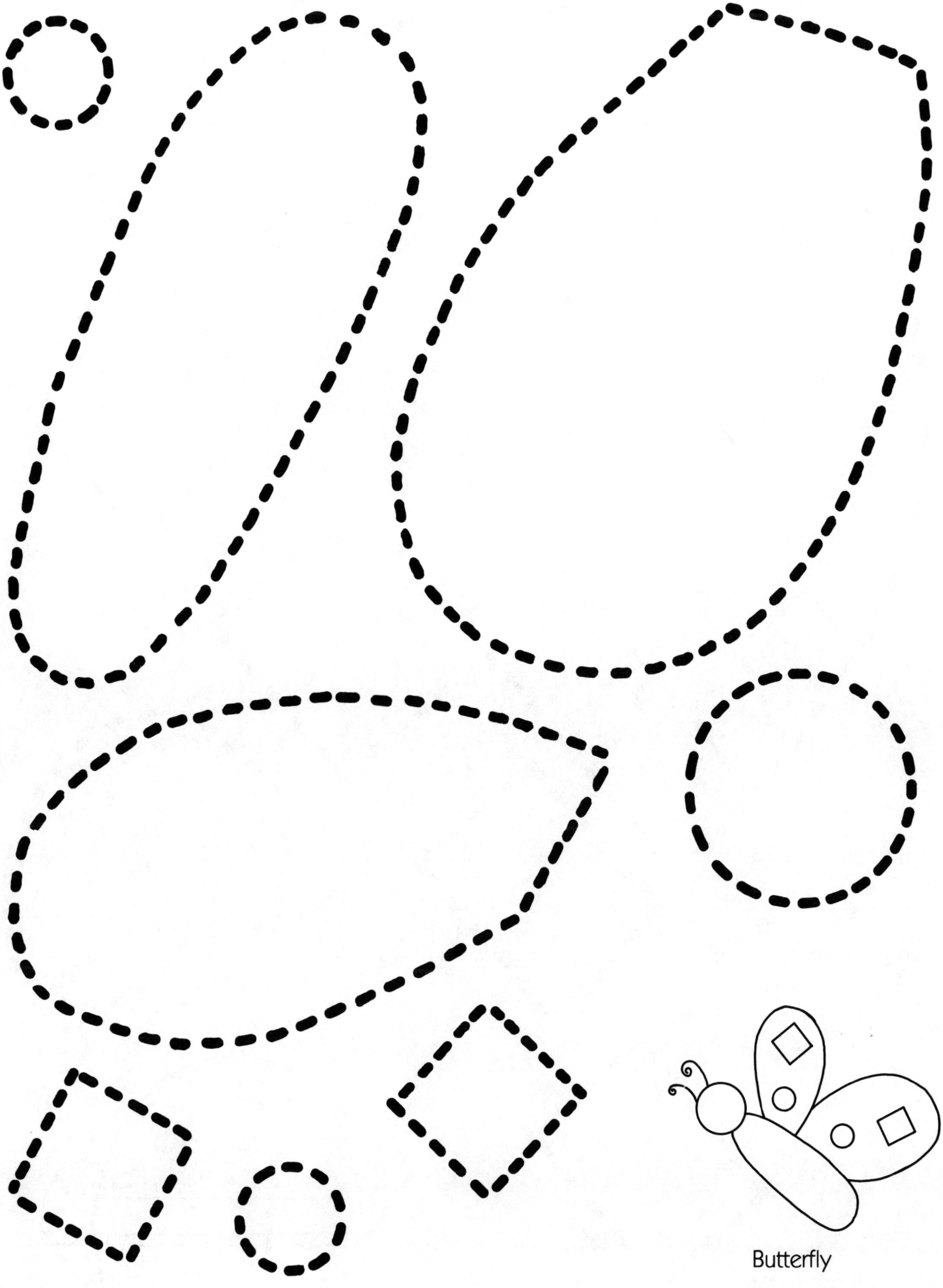

Butterfly

Use pipe cleaners for antennae.

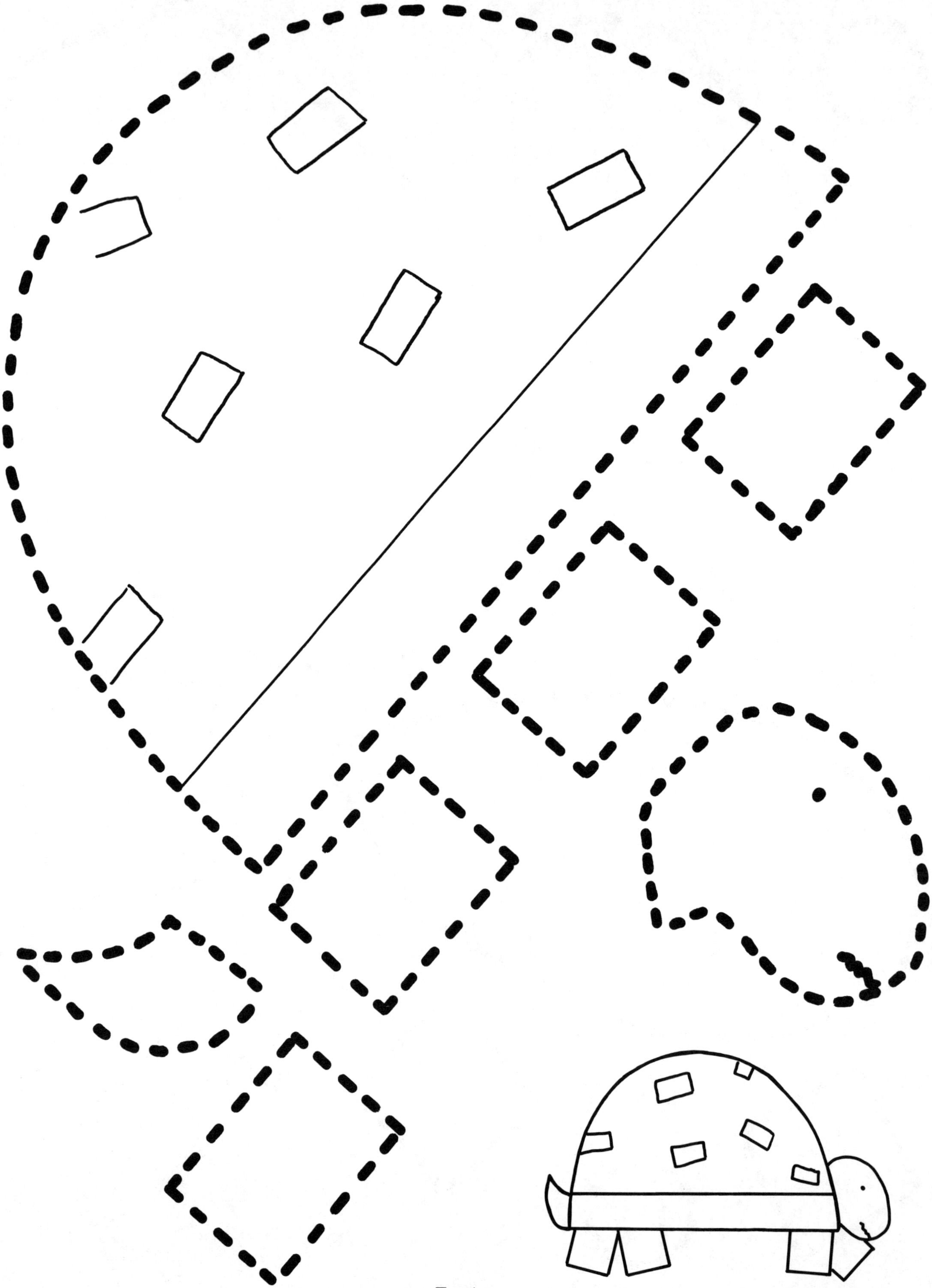

Turtle

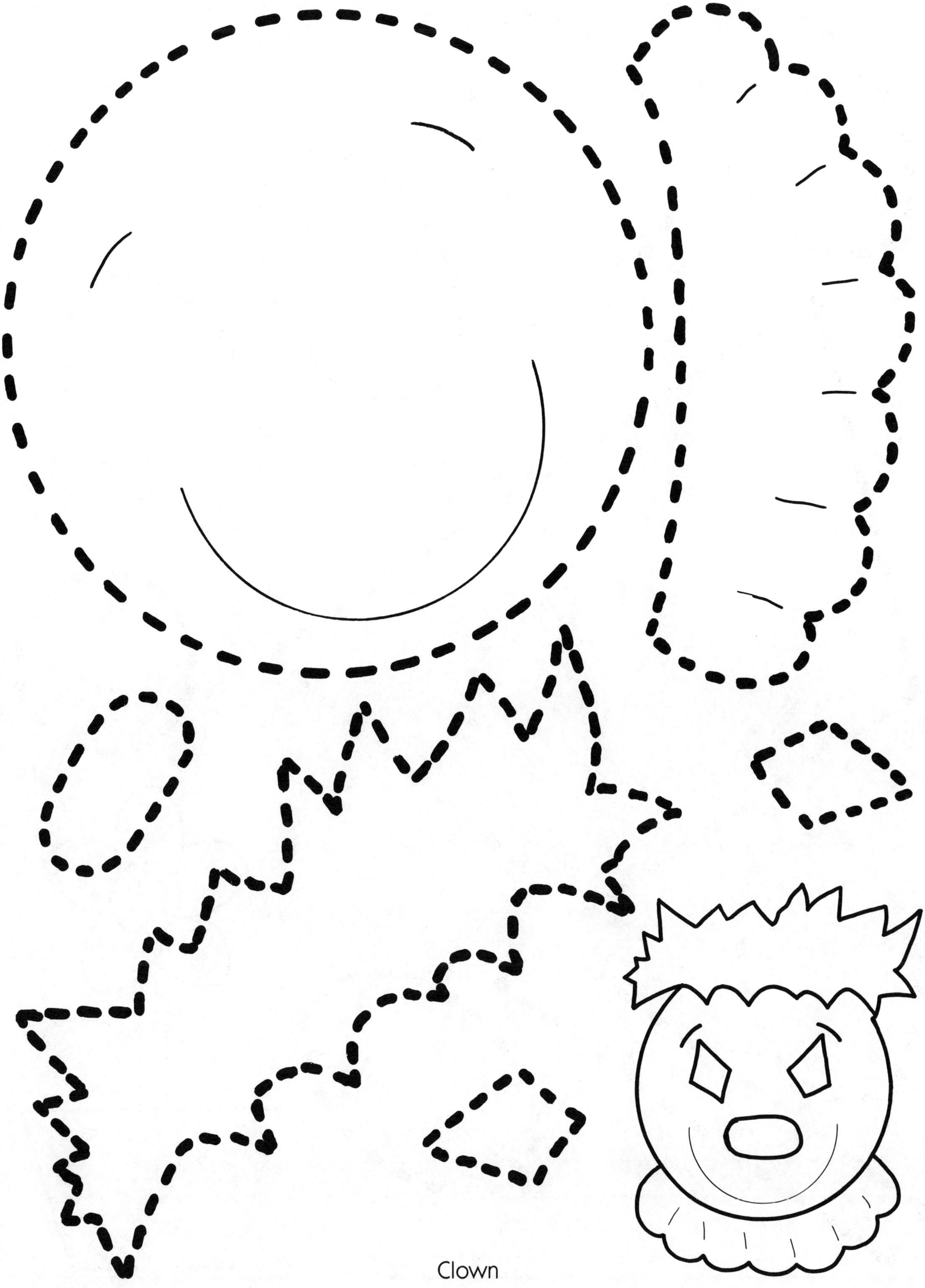

Clown

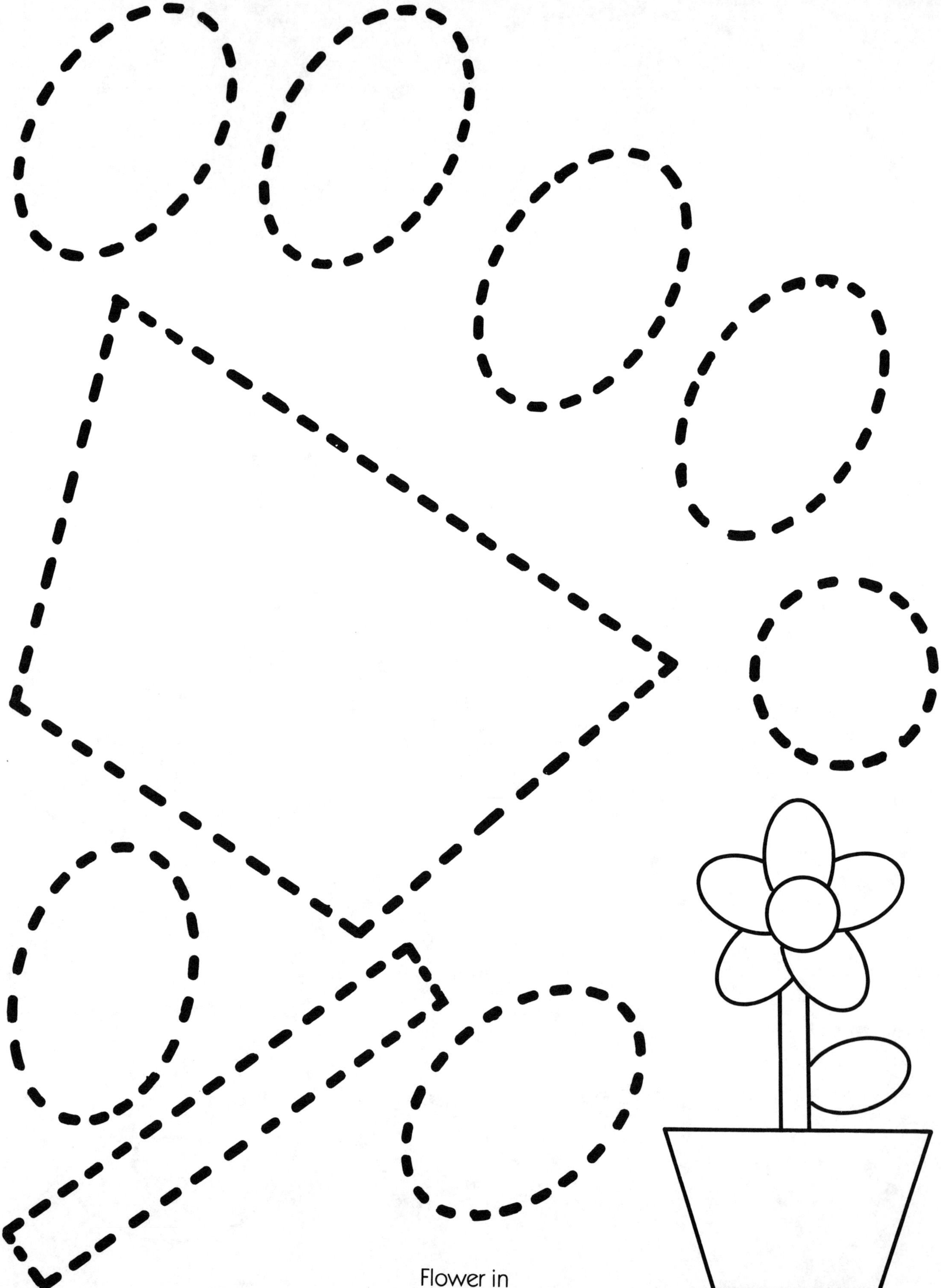

Flower in
a Flowerpot

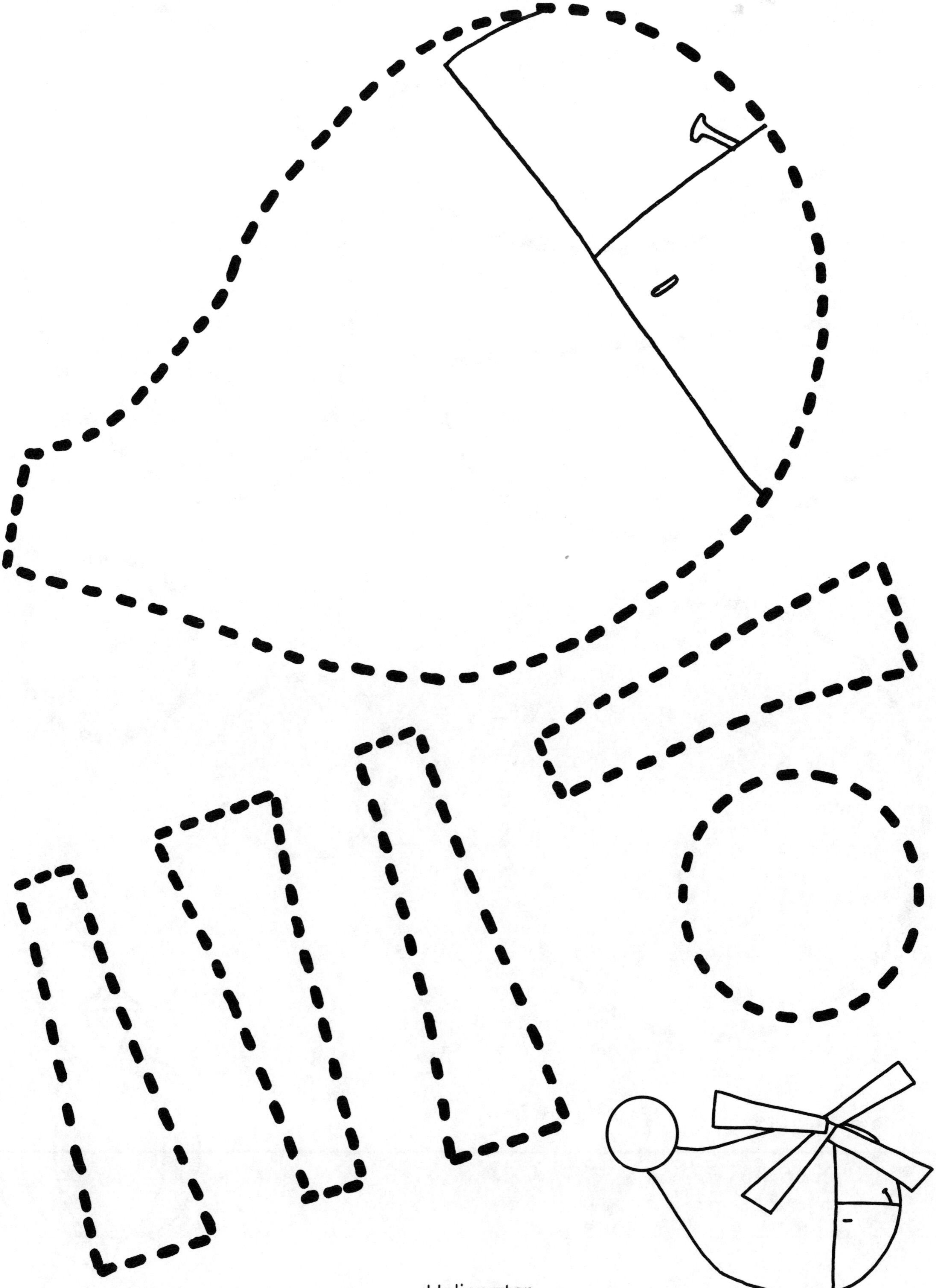

Helicopter

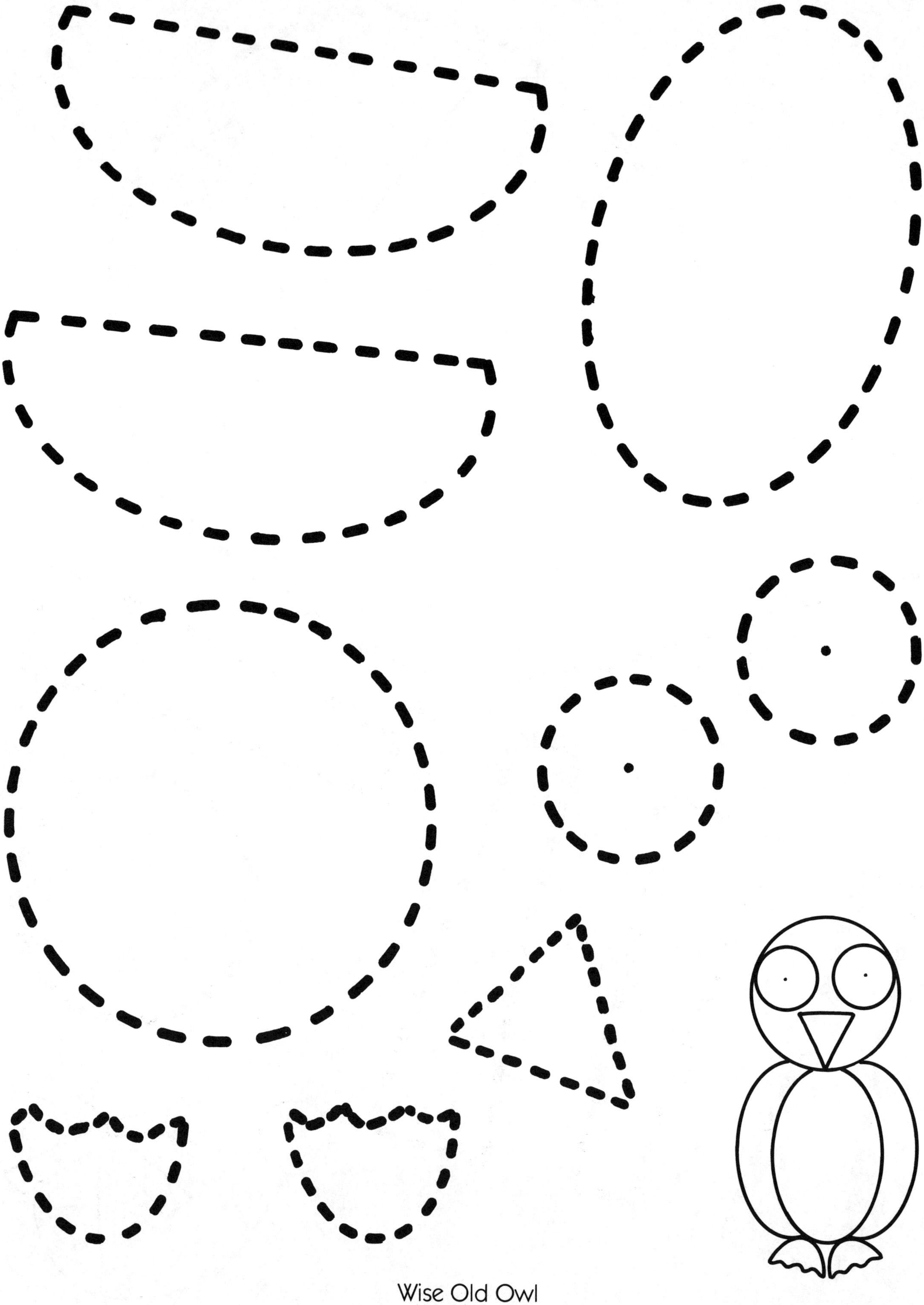

Wise Old Owl

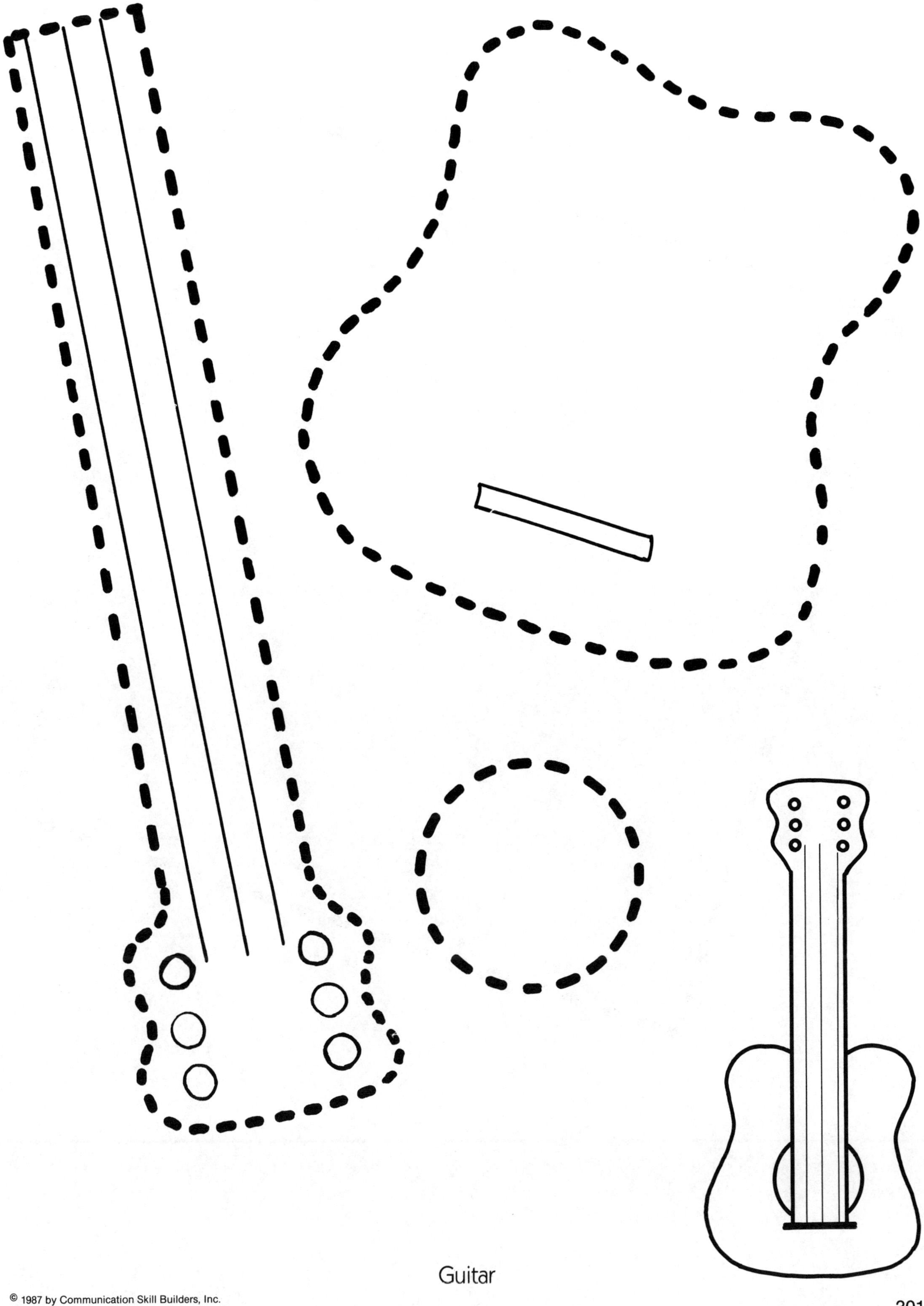

Guitar

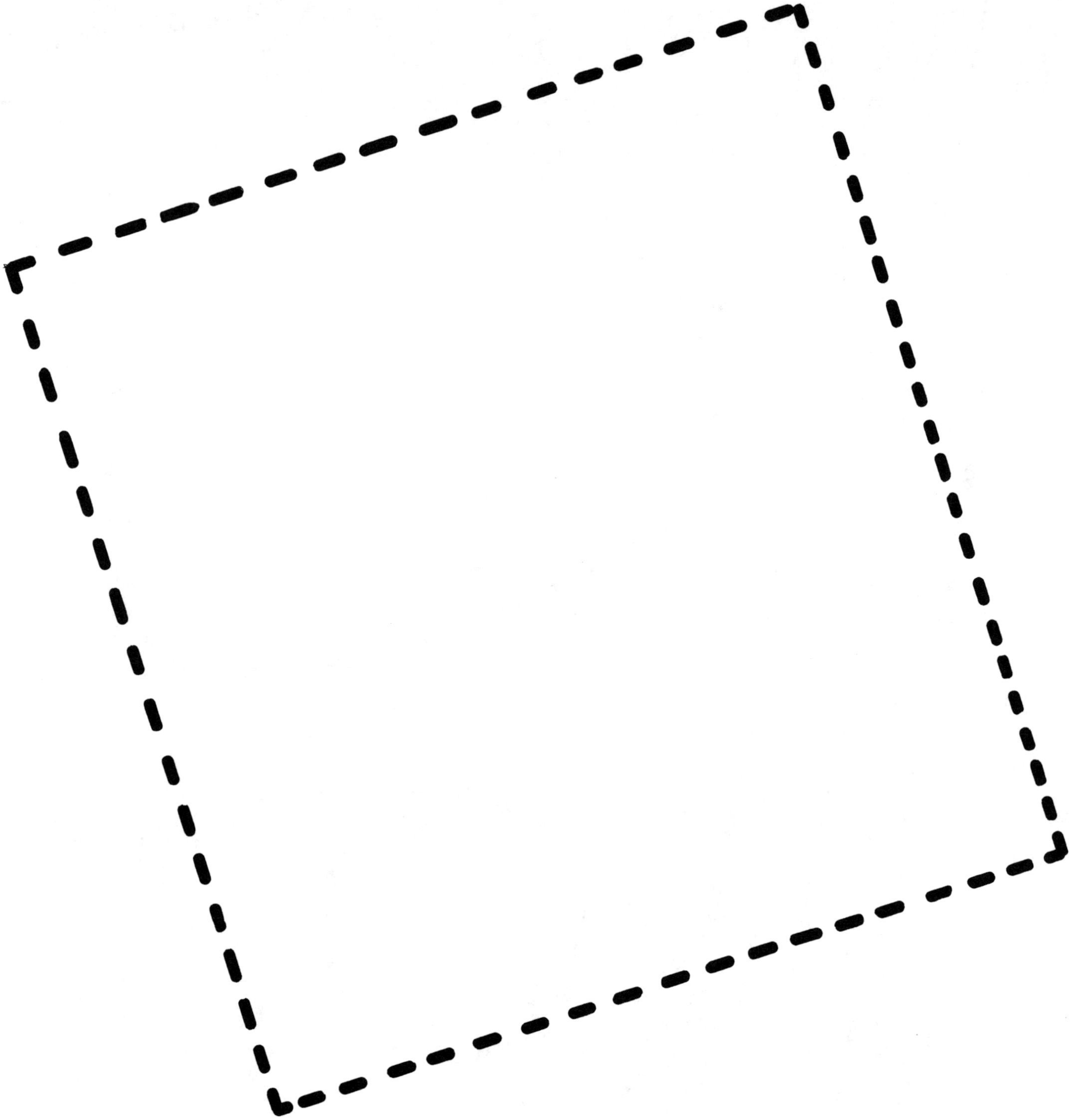

Truck

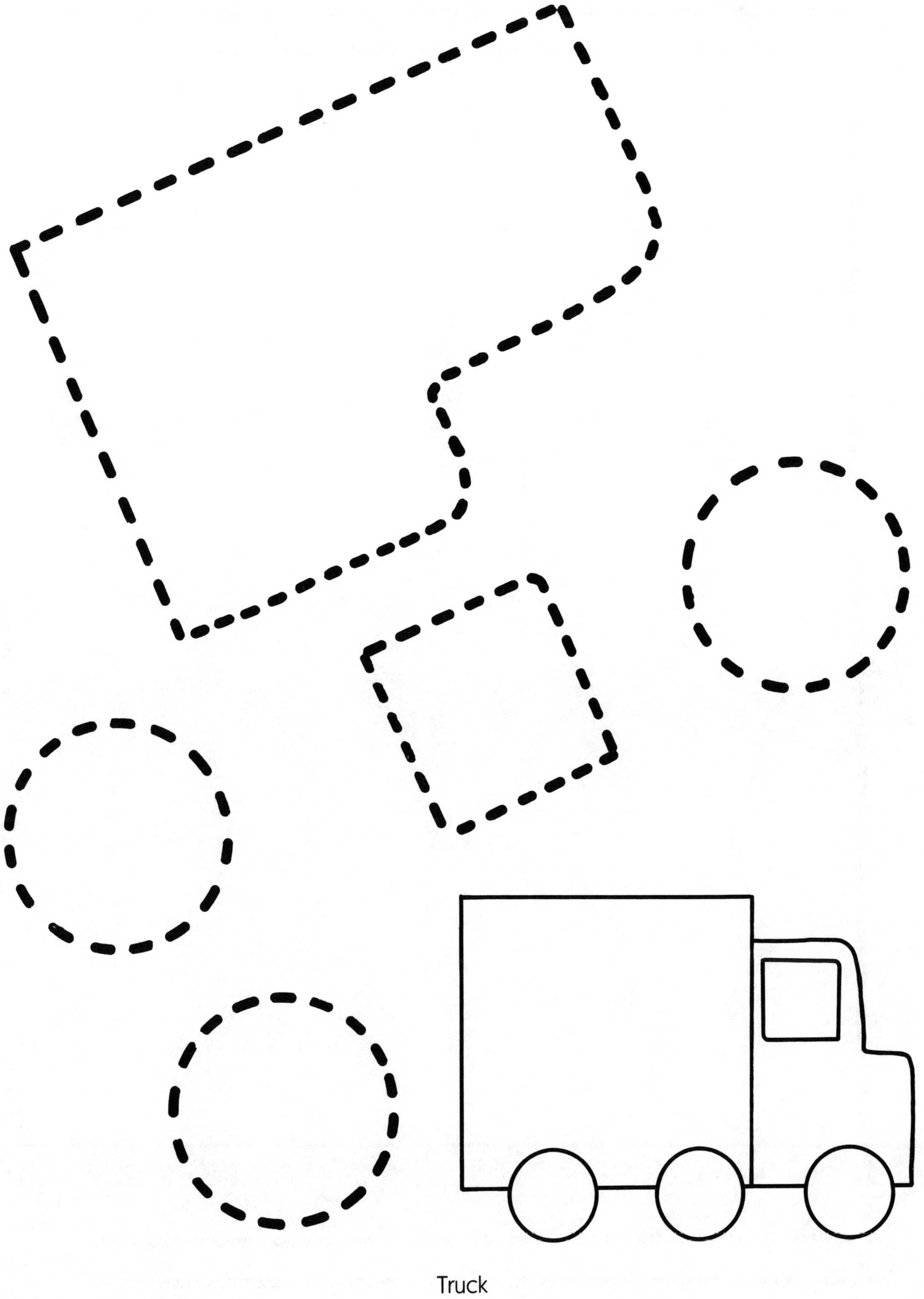

Truck

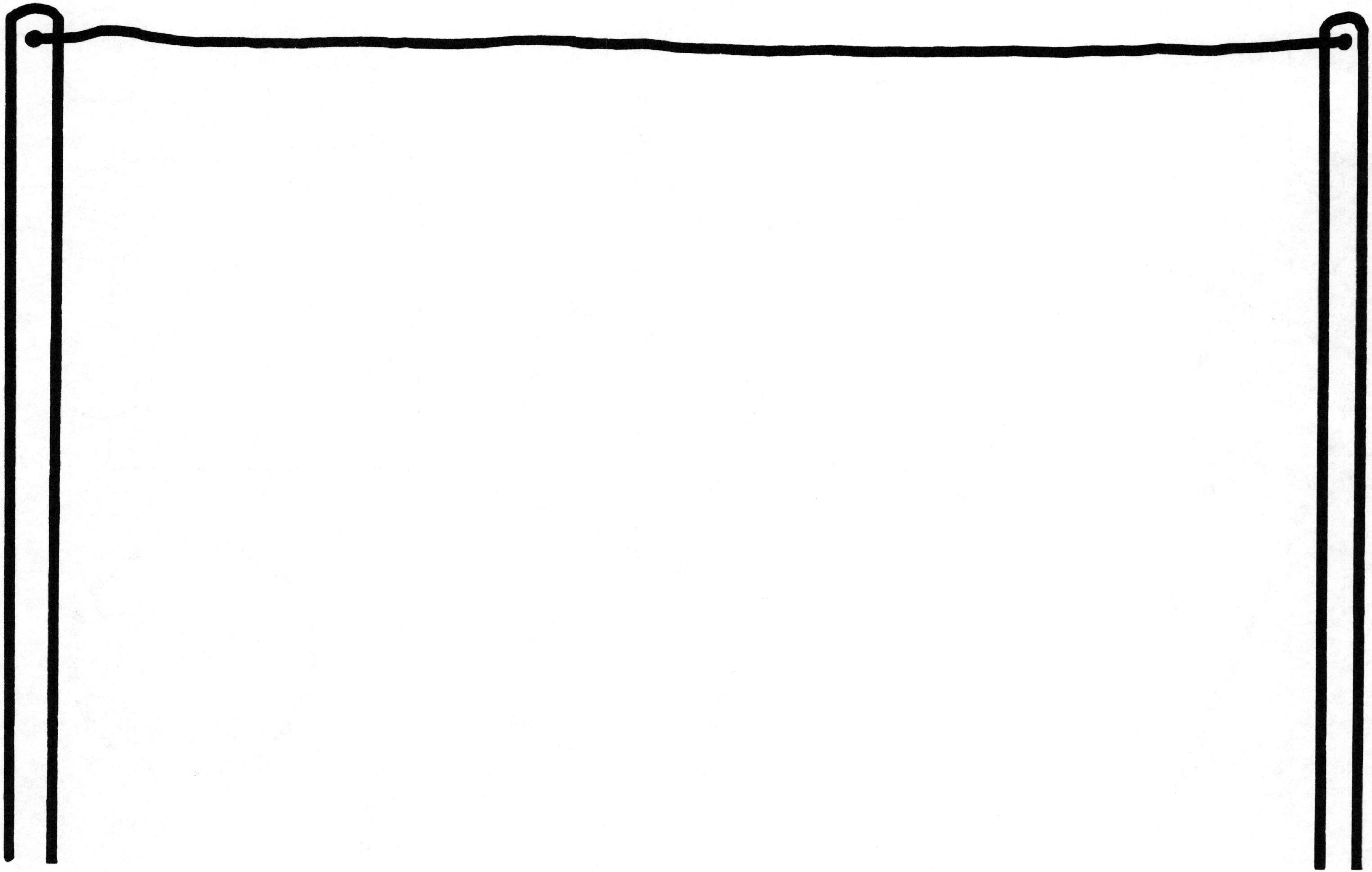

Clothesline

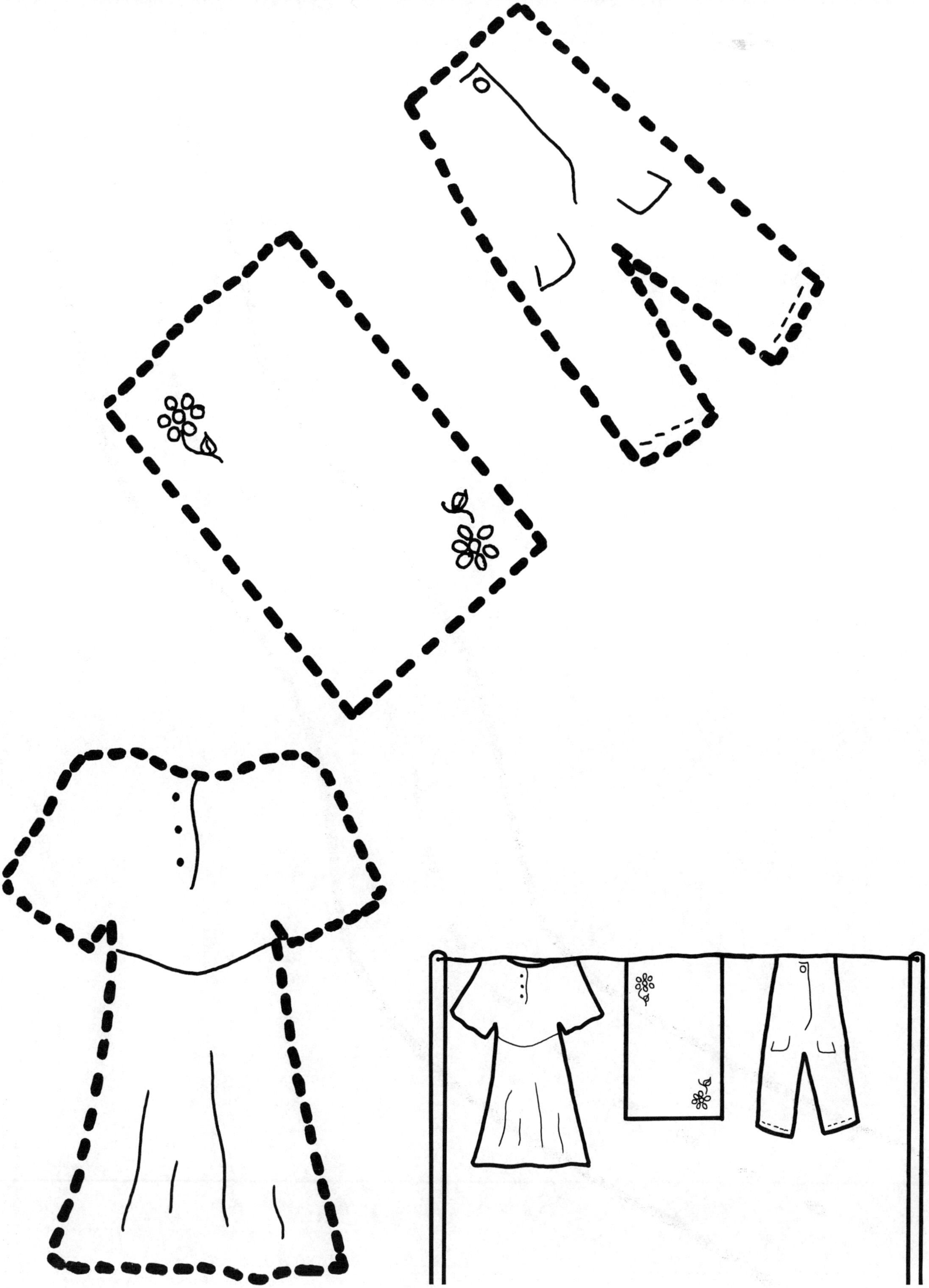

Clothesline

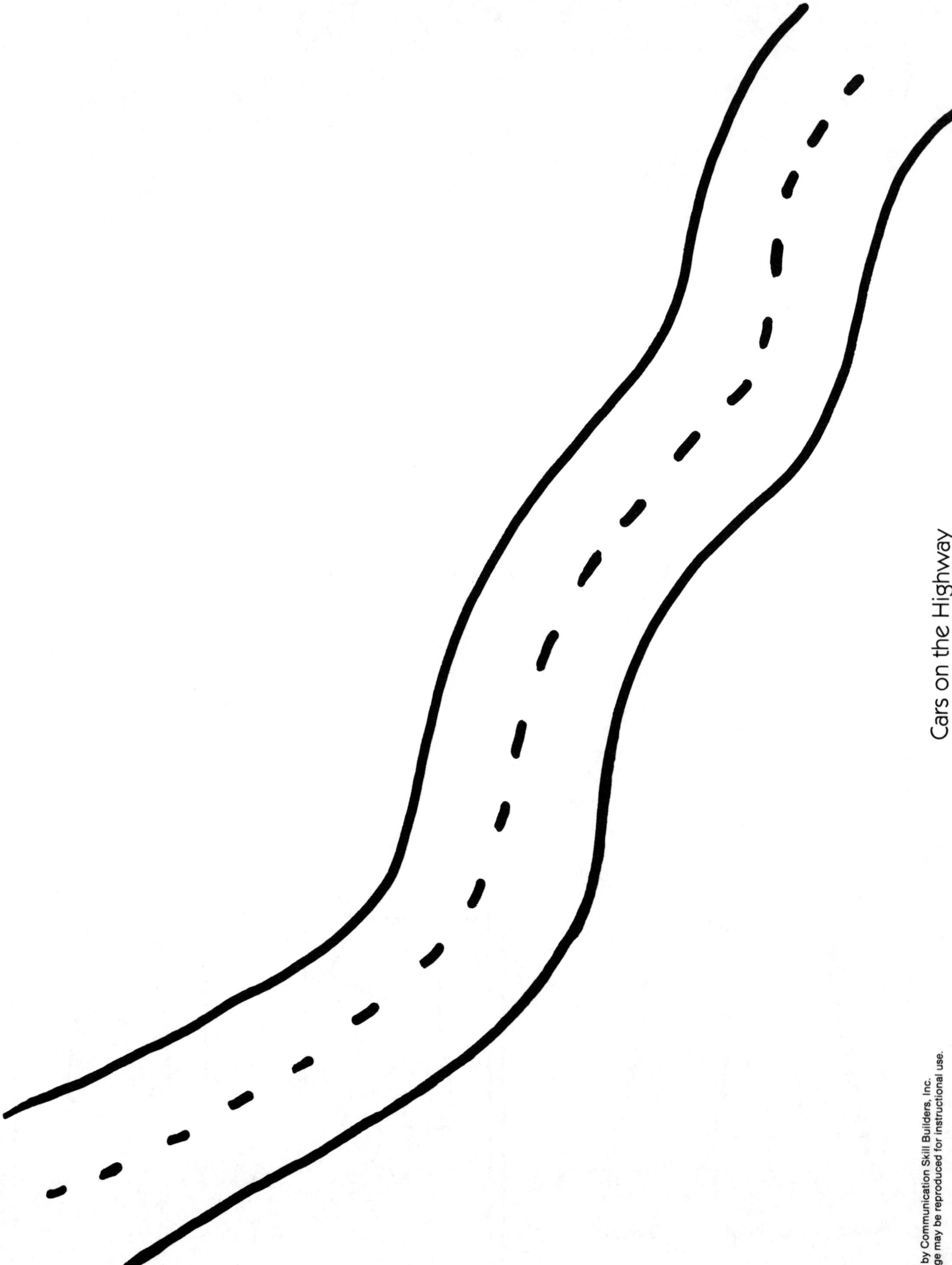

Cars on the Highway

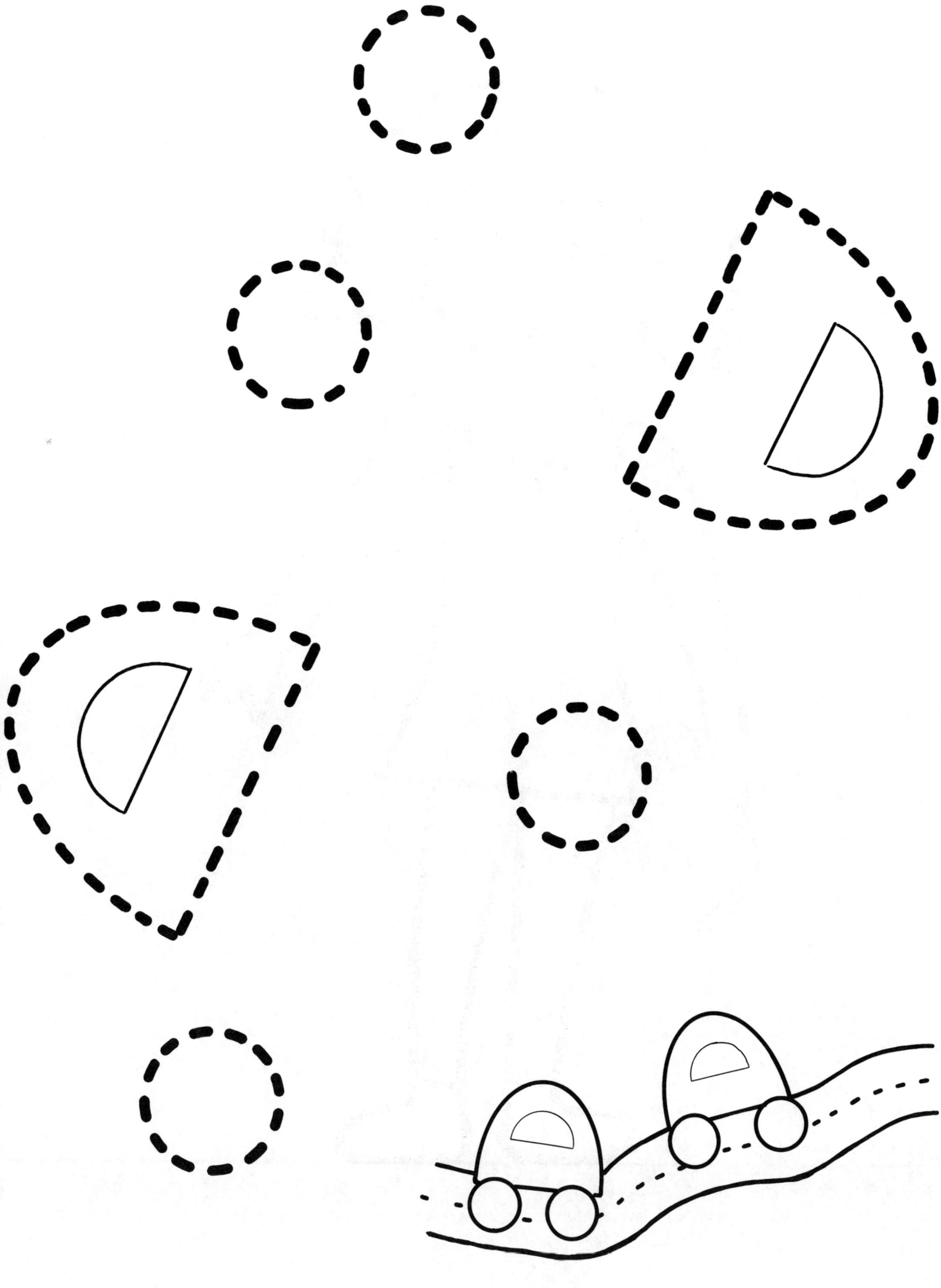

Cars on the Highway

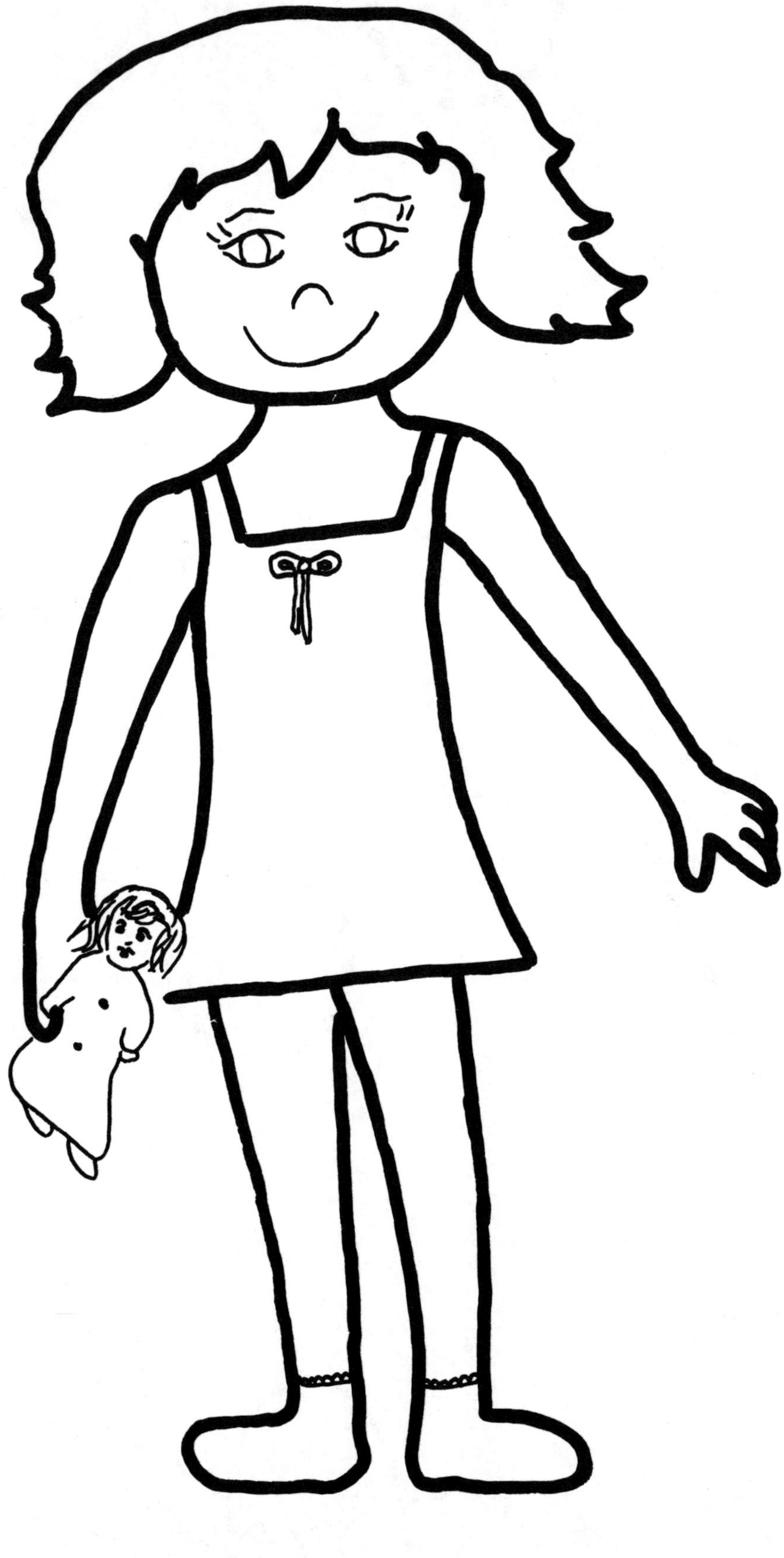

Dress the Girl

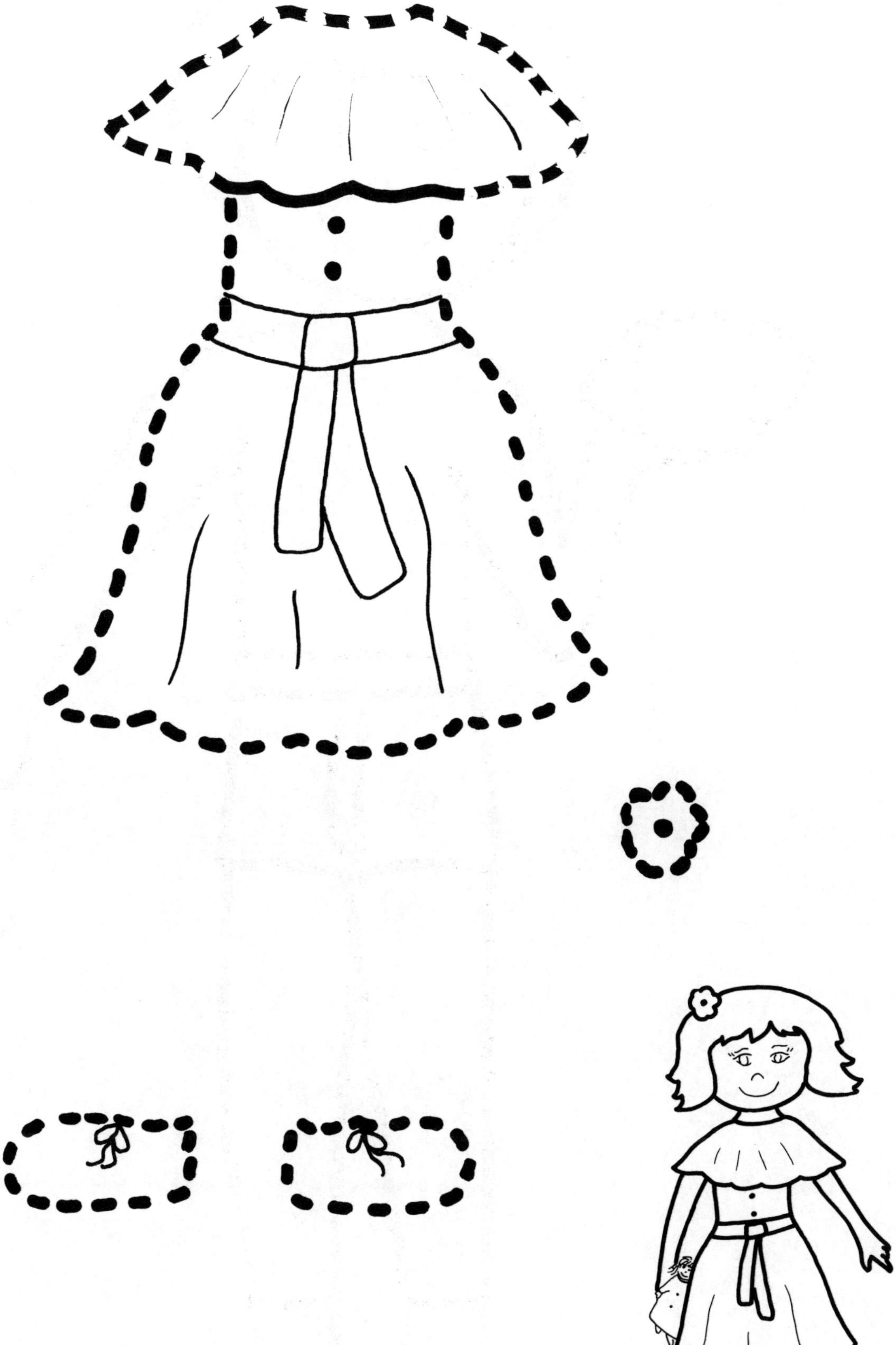

Dress the Girl

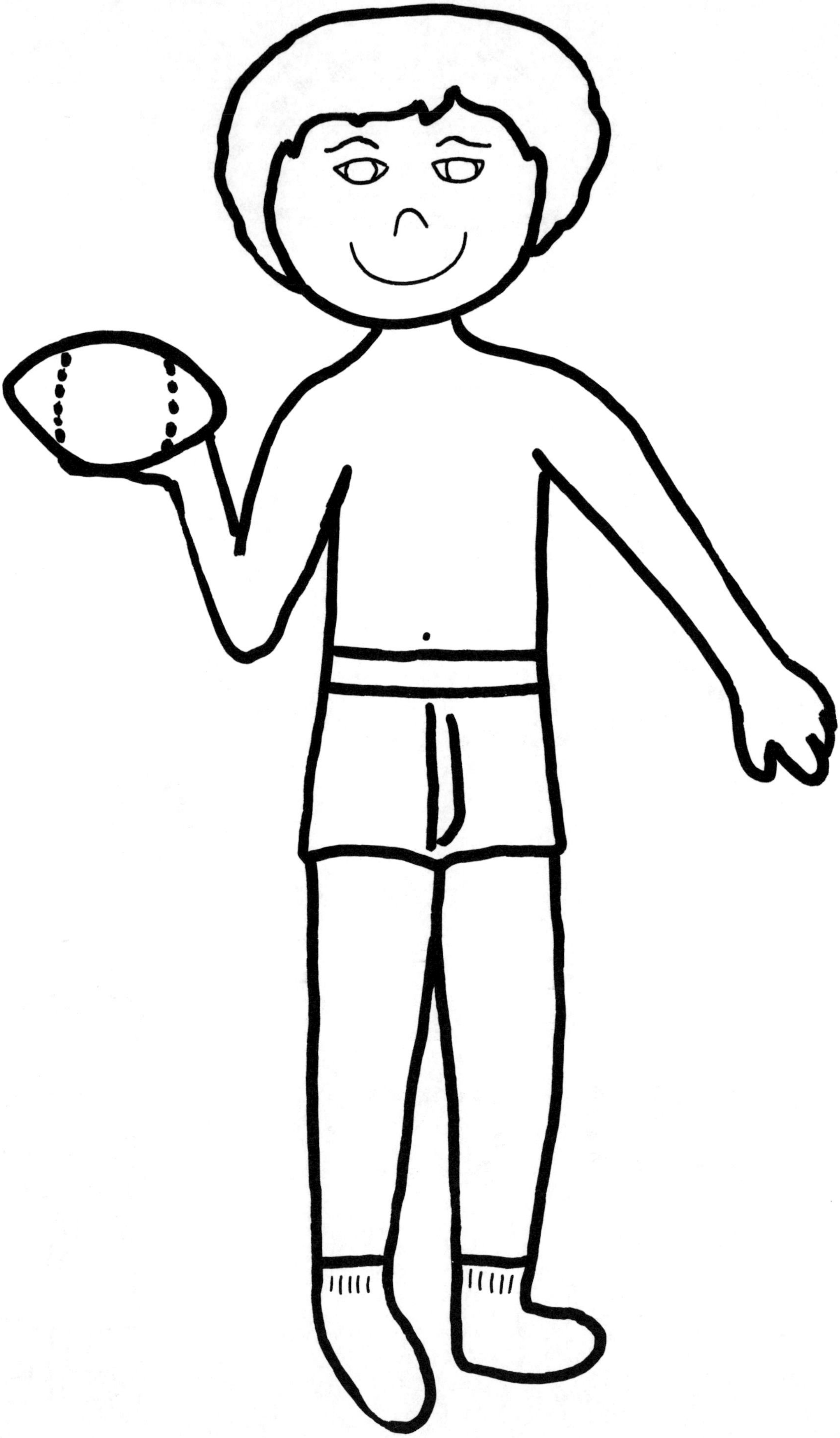

Dress the Boy

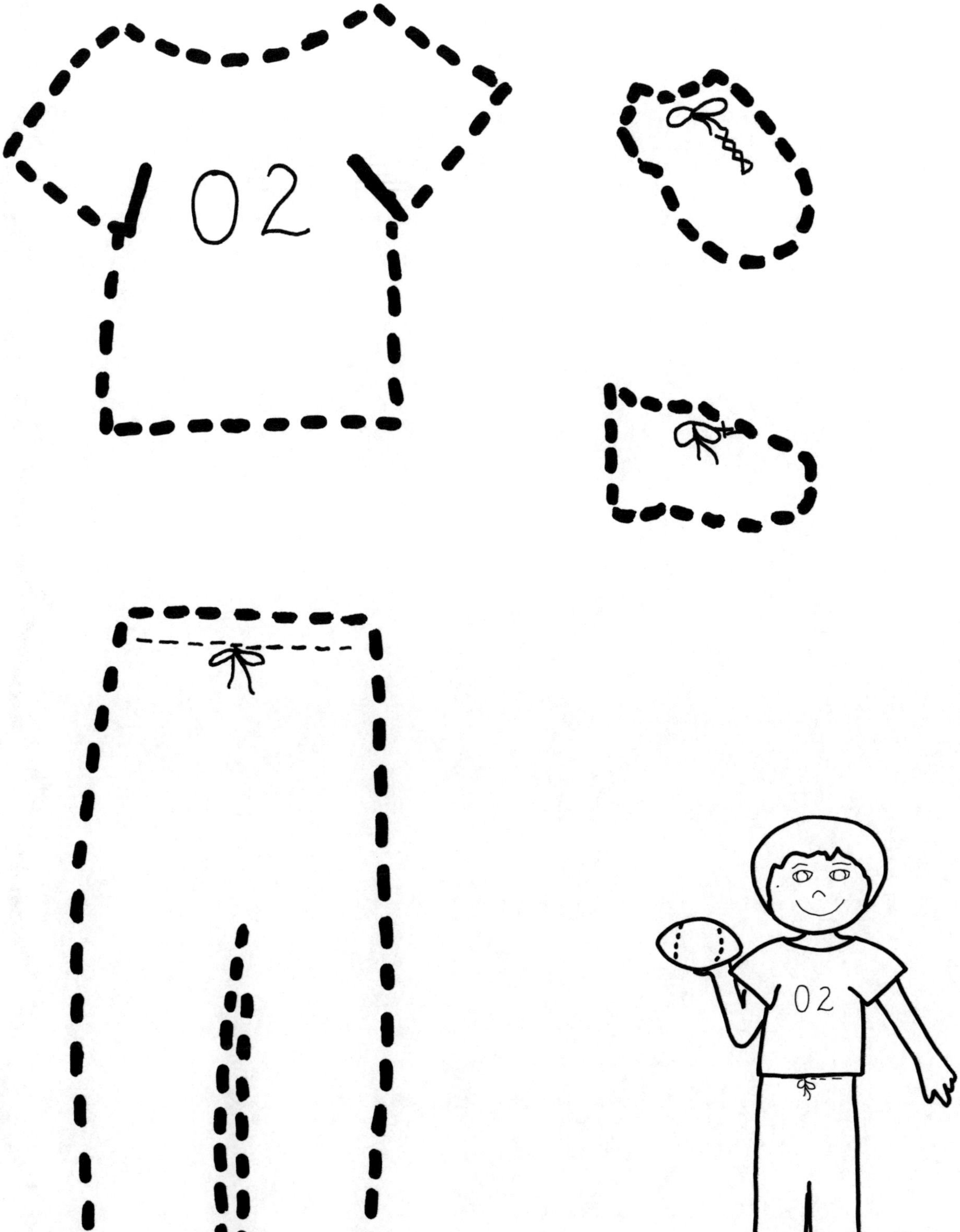

Dress the Boy

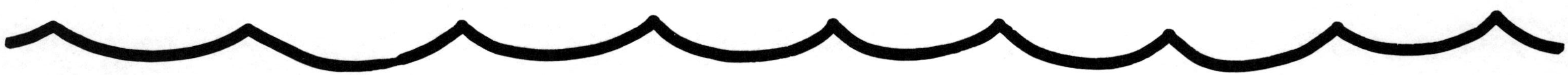

Sailboat on the Lake

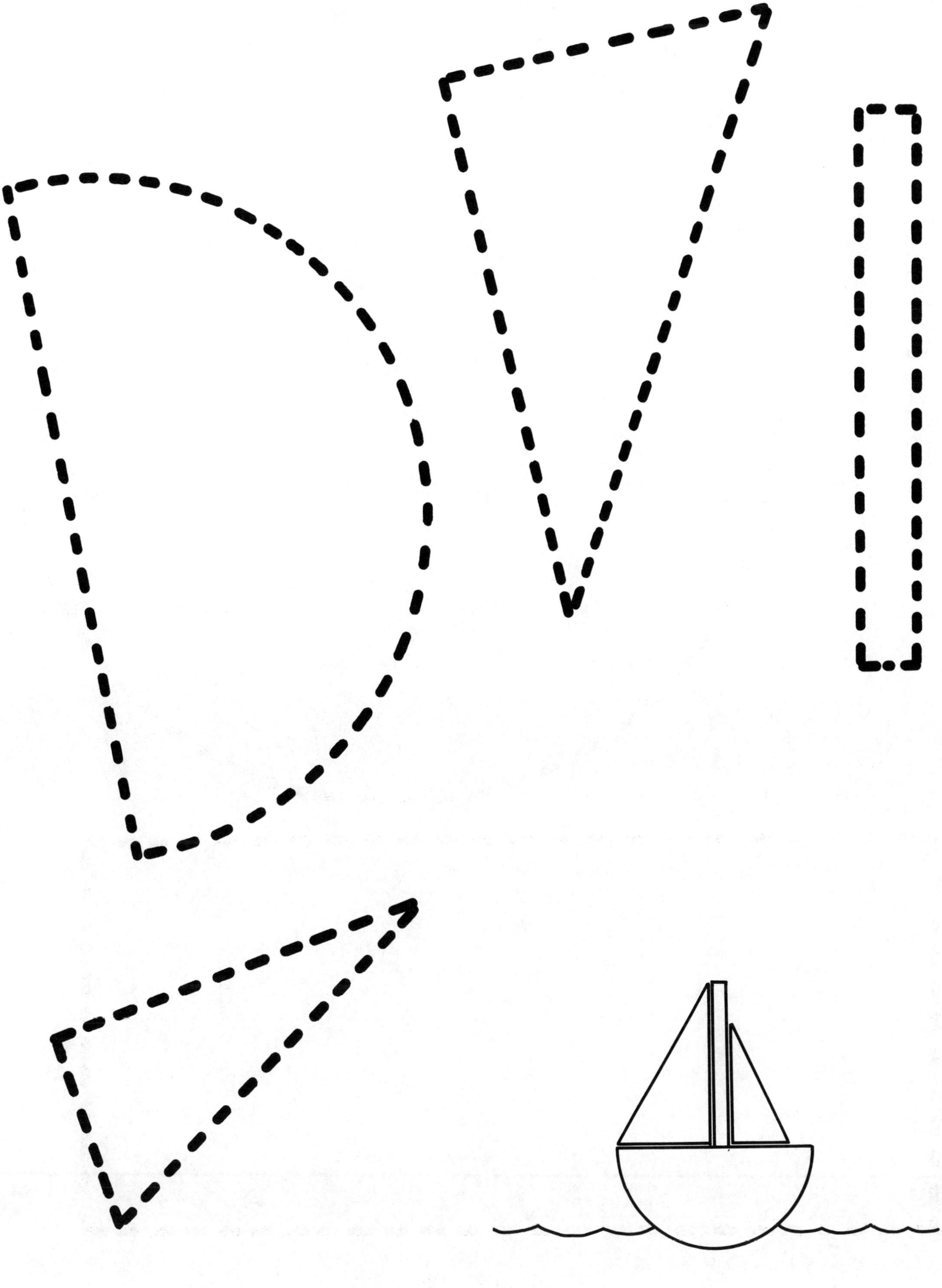

Sailboat on the Lake

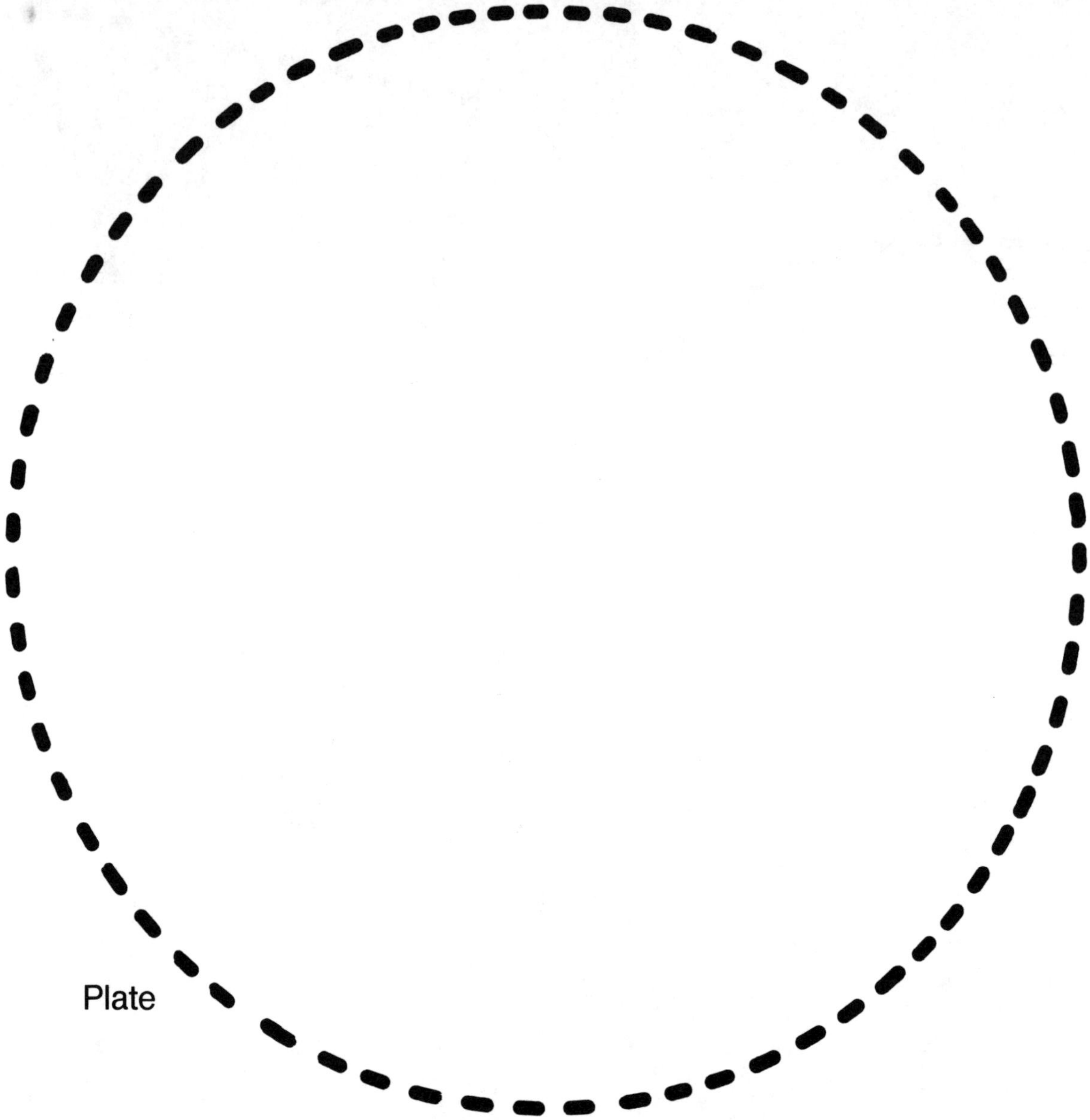

Plate

Napkin

Set the Table

Set the table on a placemat. (See instructions and patterns on pages 316-321.)

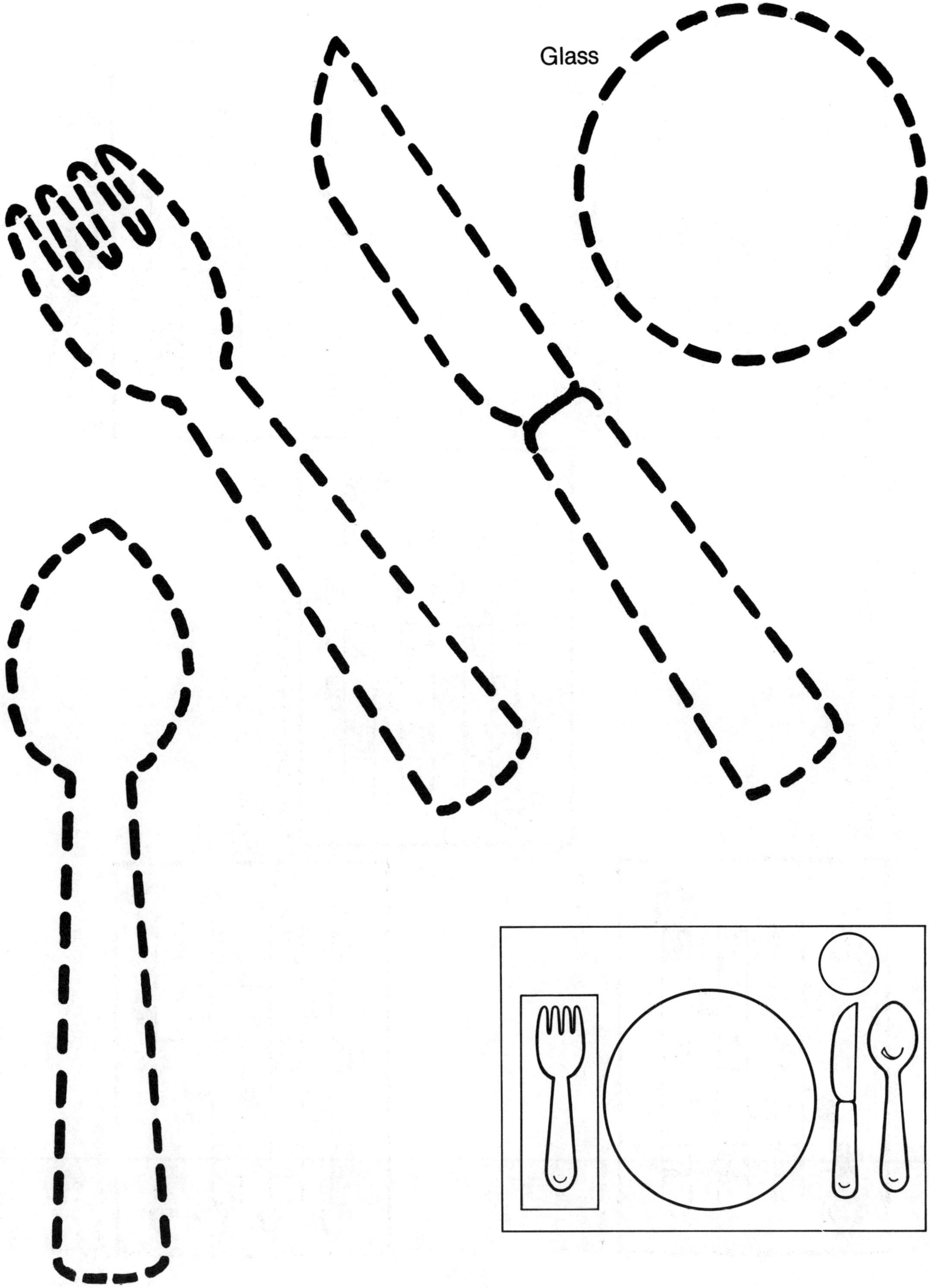

Set the Table

Seasonal Placemats

Placemats can be used for lunchtime, parties, or to take home as gifts. They may be laminated for durability.

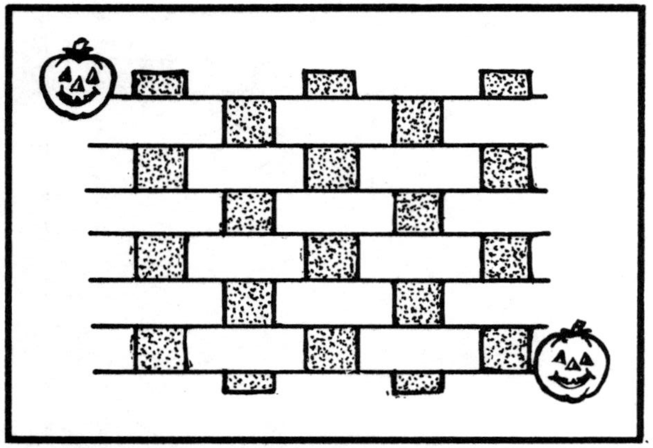

Halloween Placemat (page 317)
Weave orange strips through black construction paper.

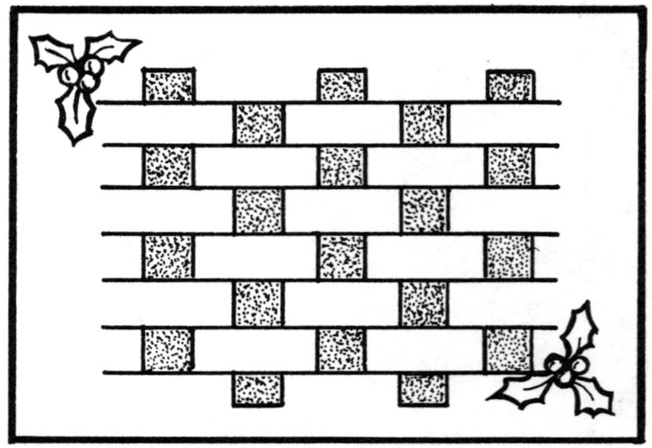

Christmas Placemat (page 318)
Weave white strips through red or green construction paper.

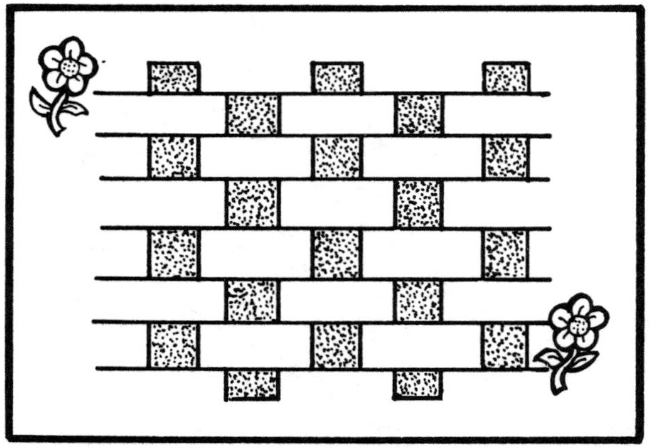

Springtime Placemat (page 321)
Weave yellow strips through light green construction paper.

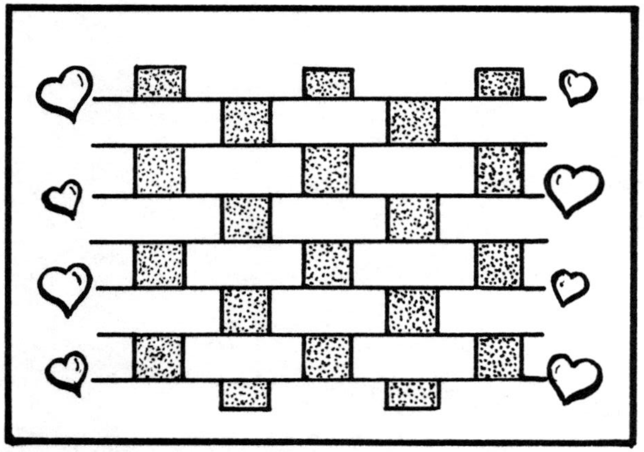

Valentine Placemat (page 319)
Weave pink strips through red construction paper.

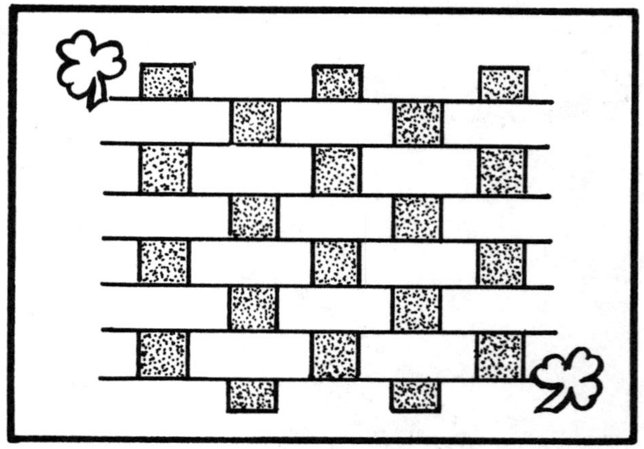

St. Patrick's Day Placemat (page 320)
Weave light green strips through dark green construction paper.

See pattern on page 337 for strips for weaving.

Halloween Placemat

Christmas Placemat

Valentine Placemat

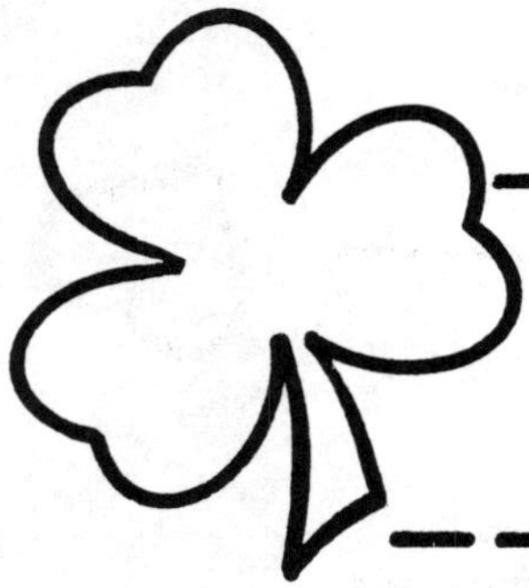

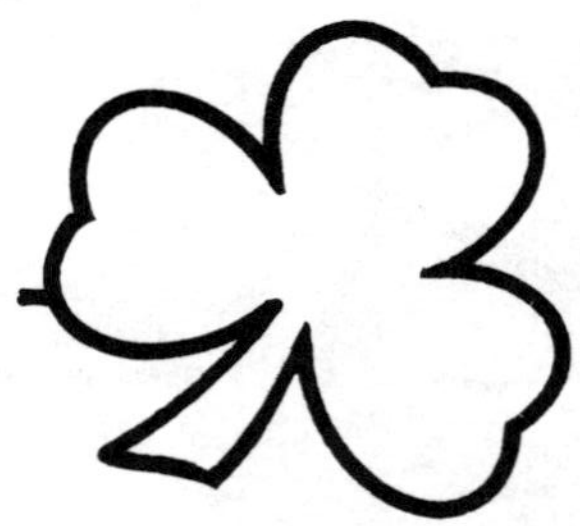

St. Patrick's Day Placemat

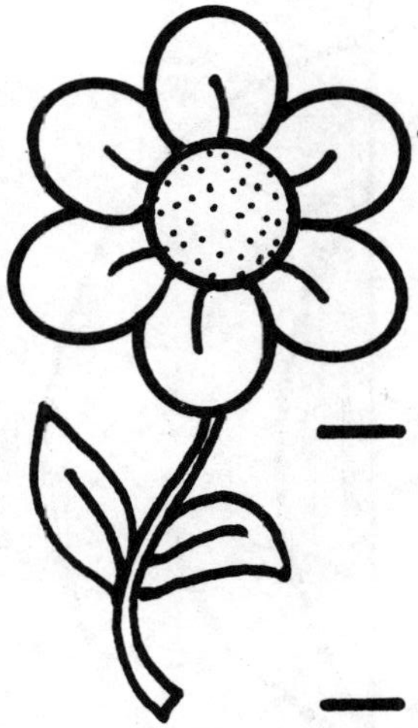

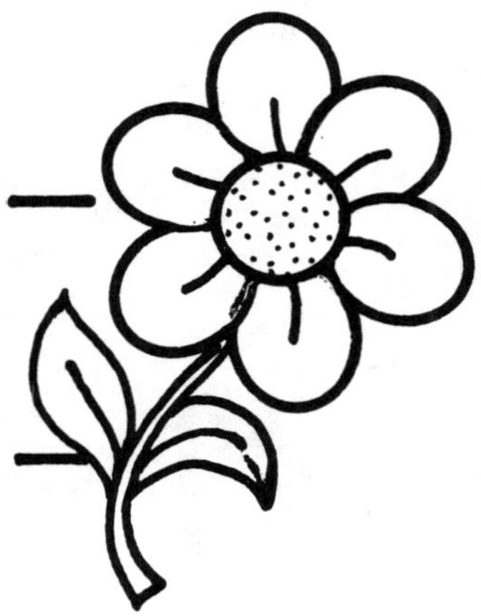

Springtime Placemat

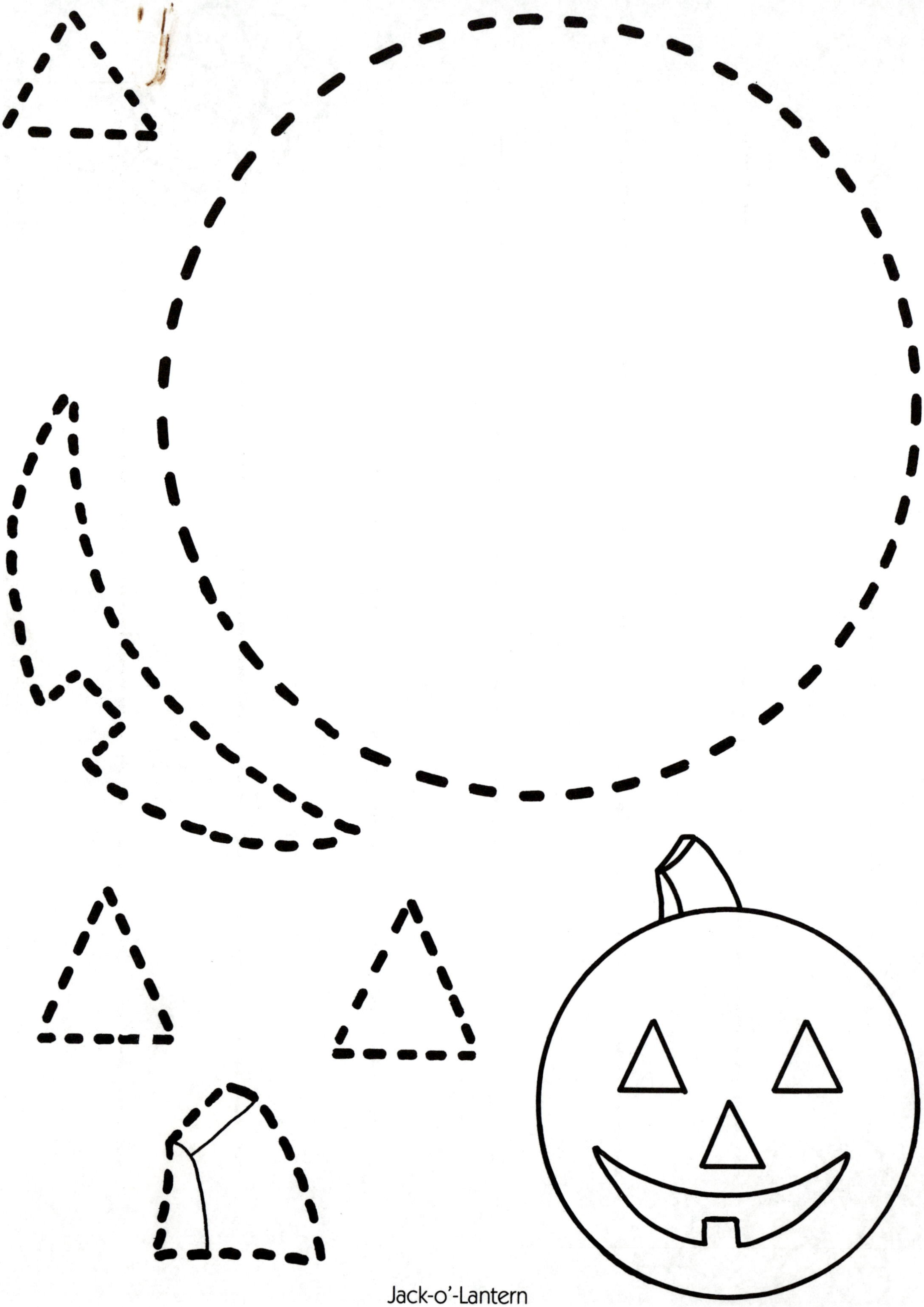

Jack-o'-Lantern

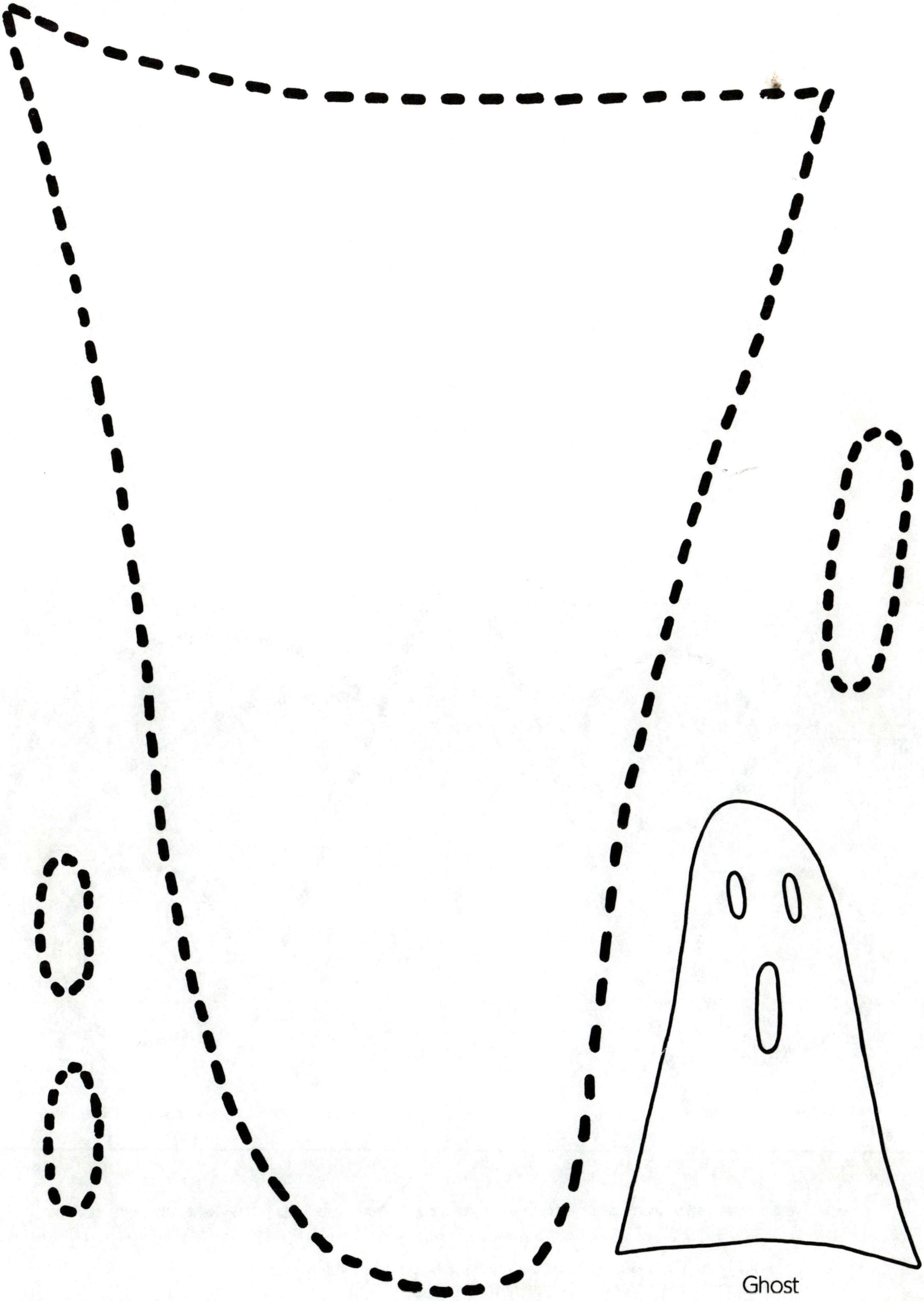

Ghost

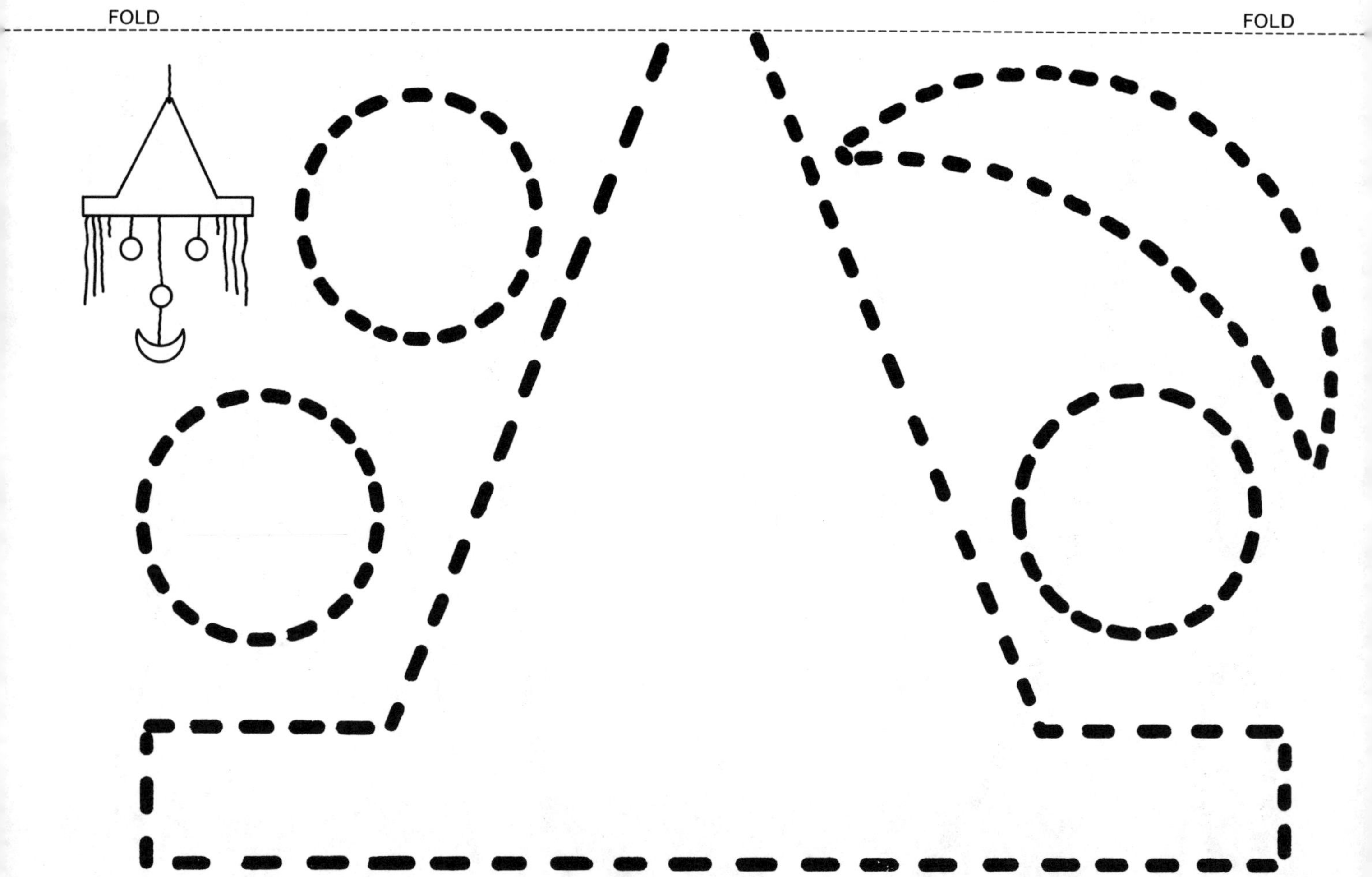

Witch Mobile

Fold in half; cut out pieces. Use yarn for hair and to hang mobile. Put yarn between the two pieces and glue them together.

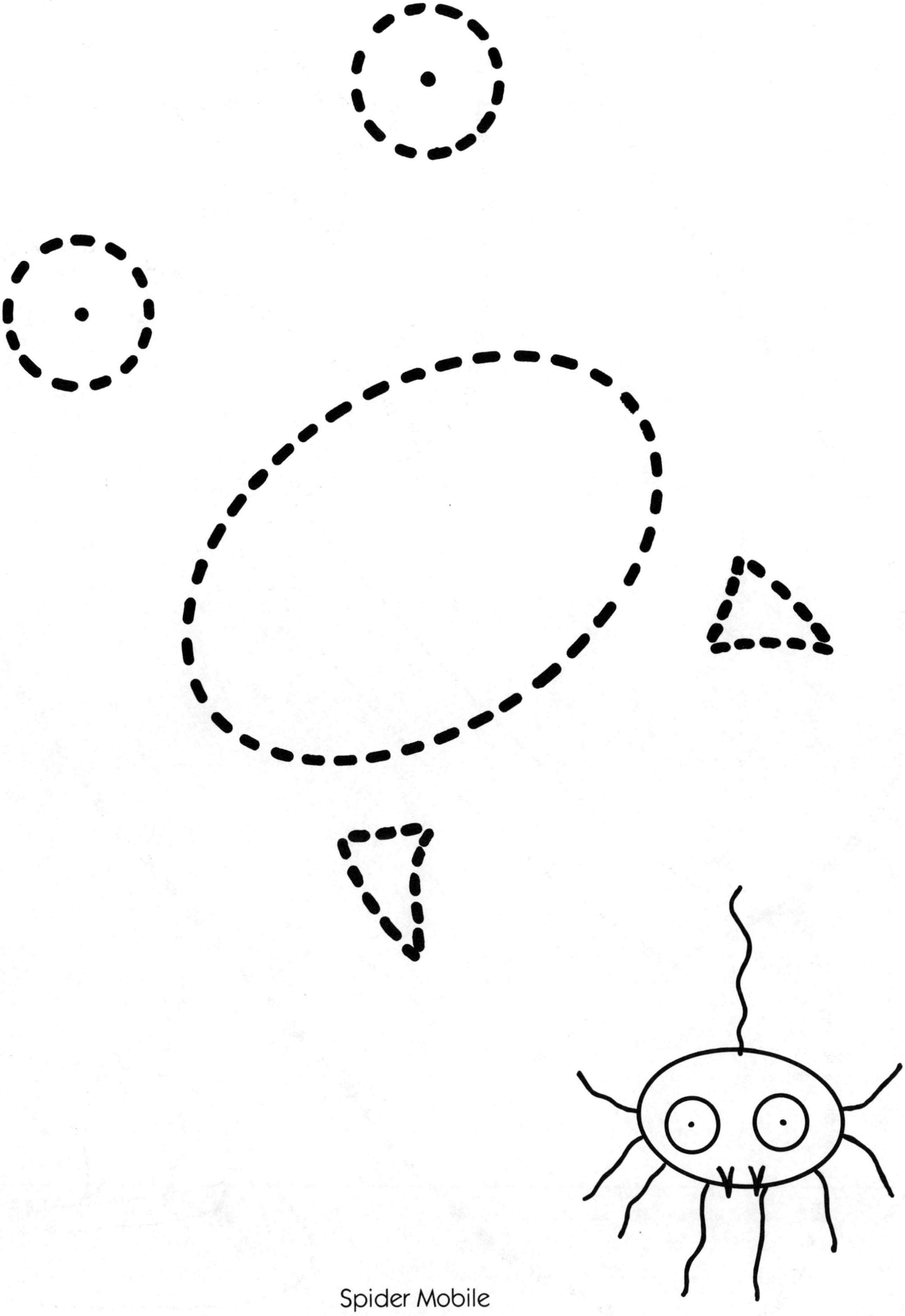

Spider Mobile

Cut rubber bands to use in making the spider.

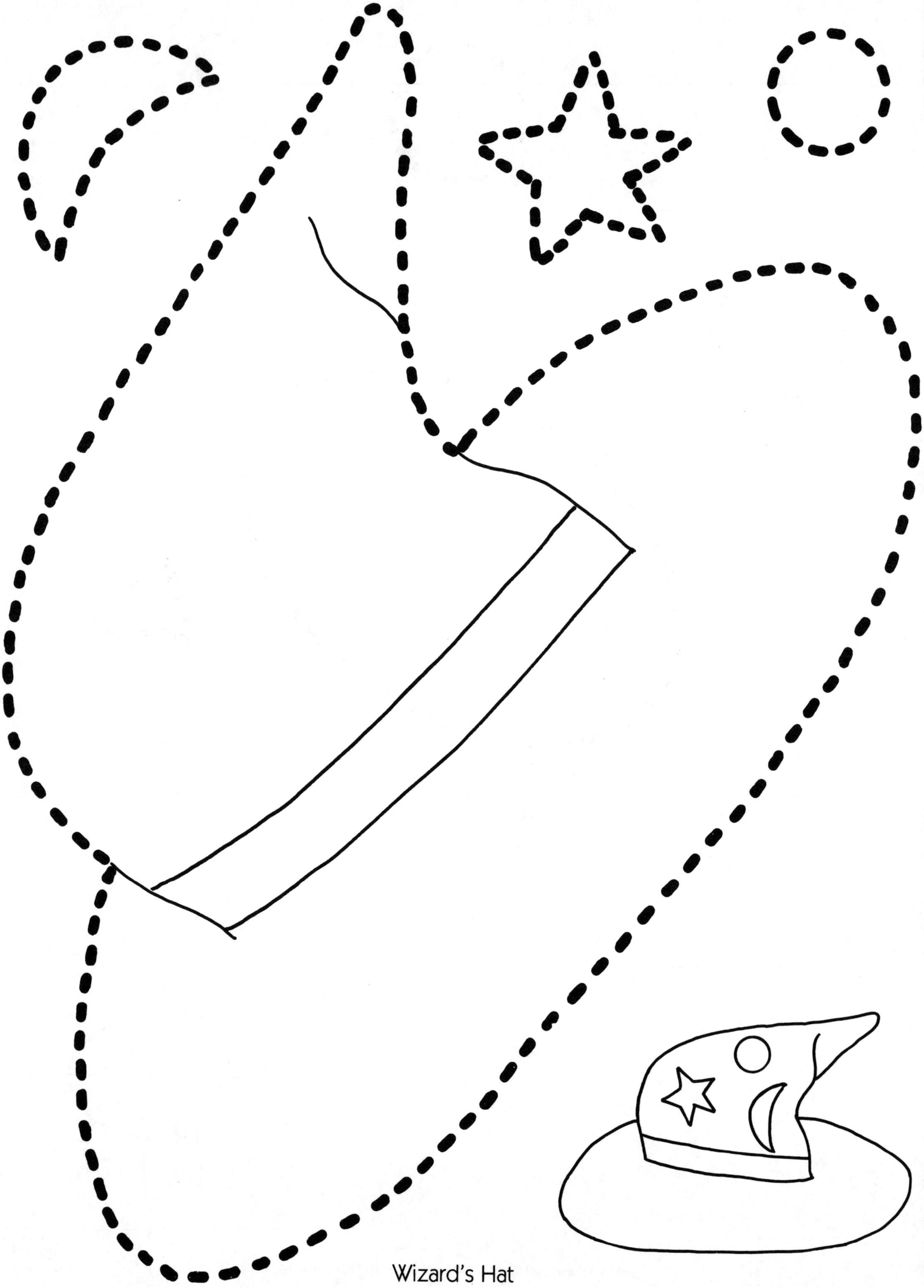

Wizard's Hat

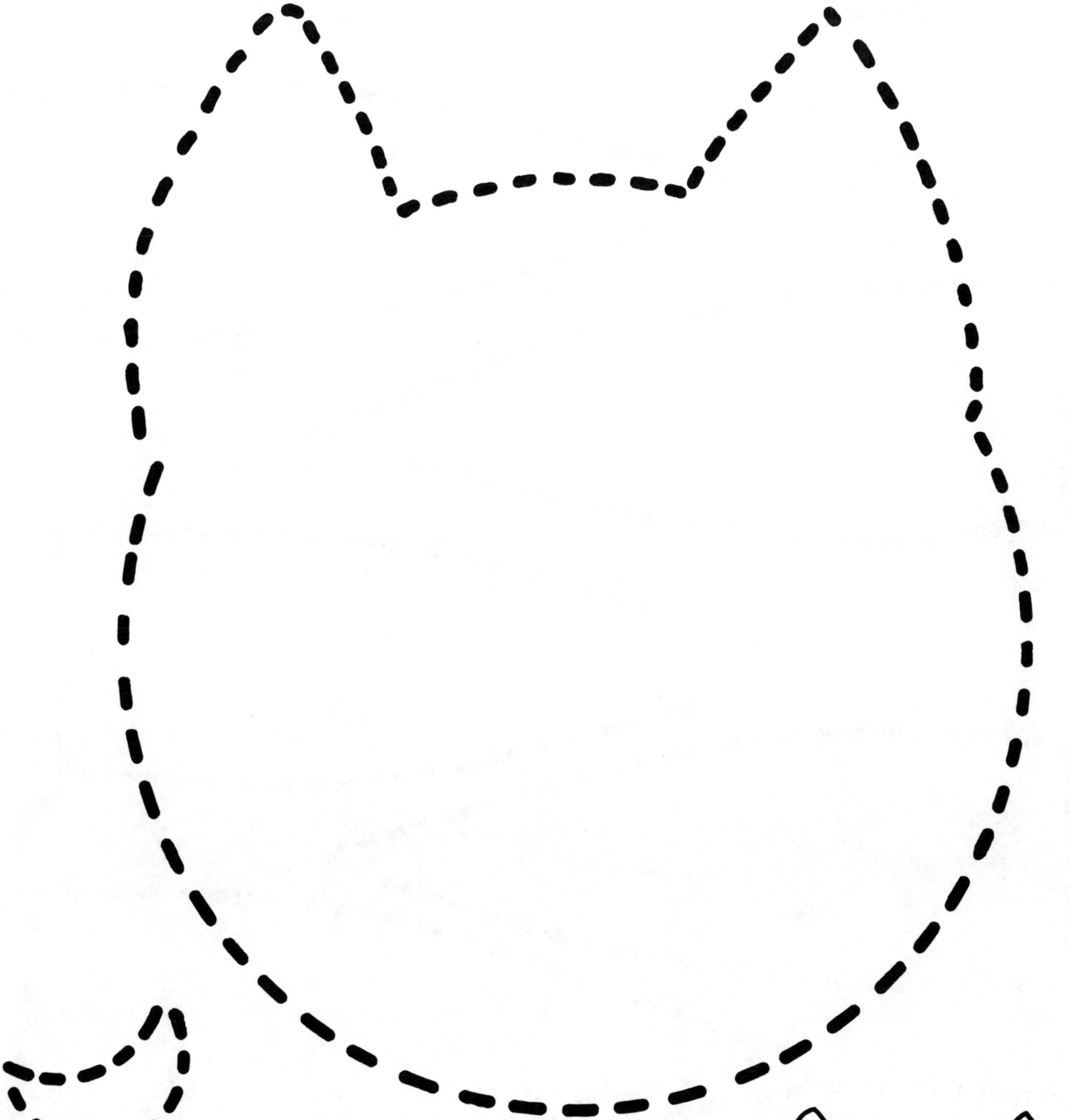

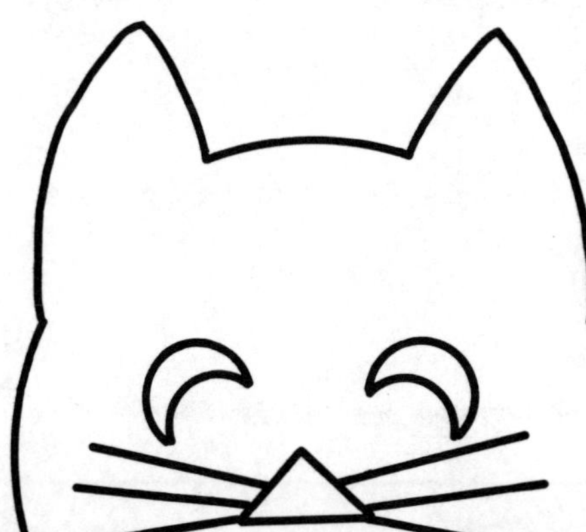

Black Cat

For whiskers: Draw on with a felt-tip marker, paste on pieces of black yarn, cut strips out of paper, or paste on broom straws.

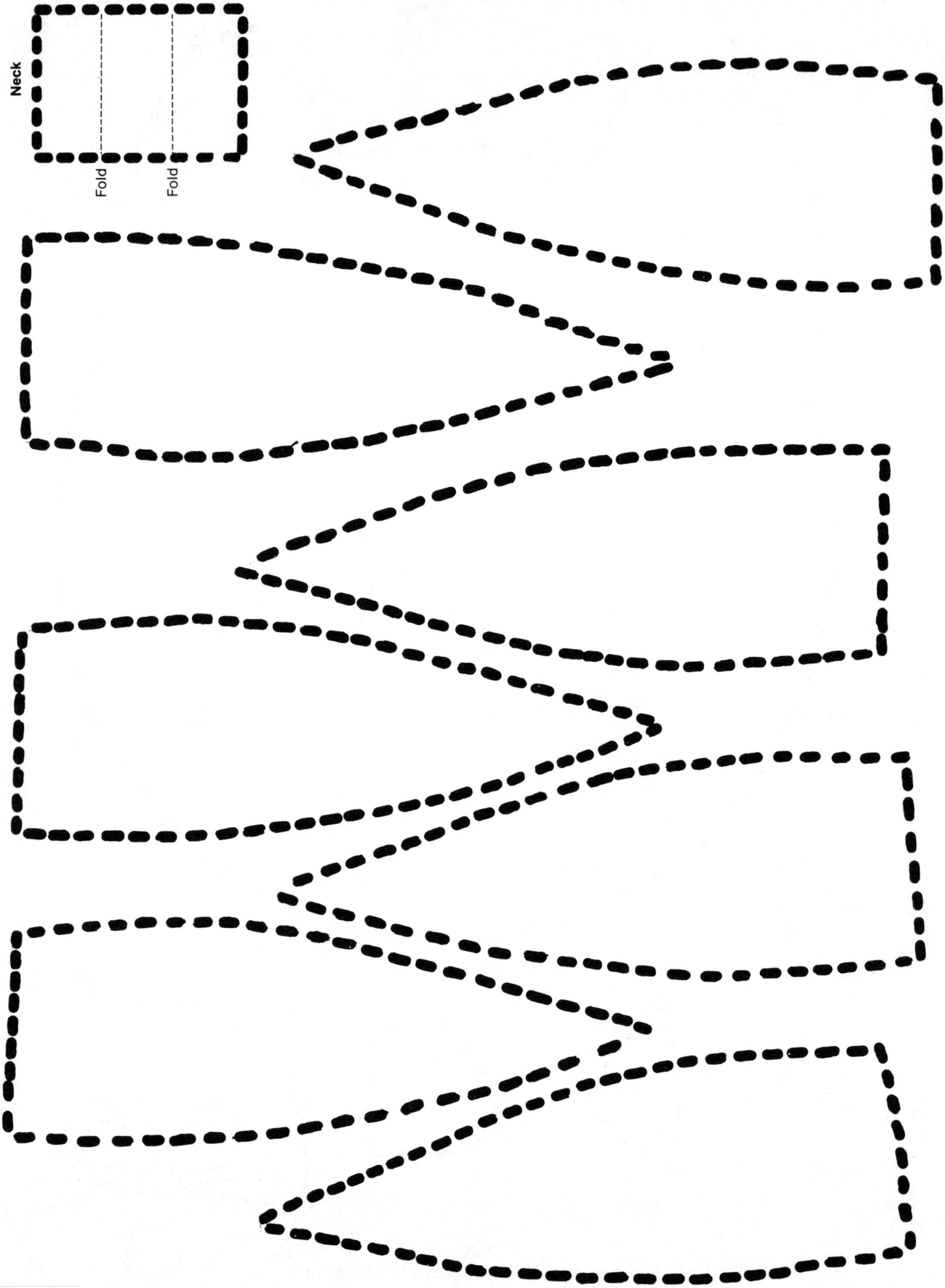

Turkey

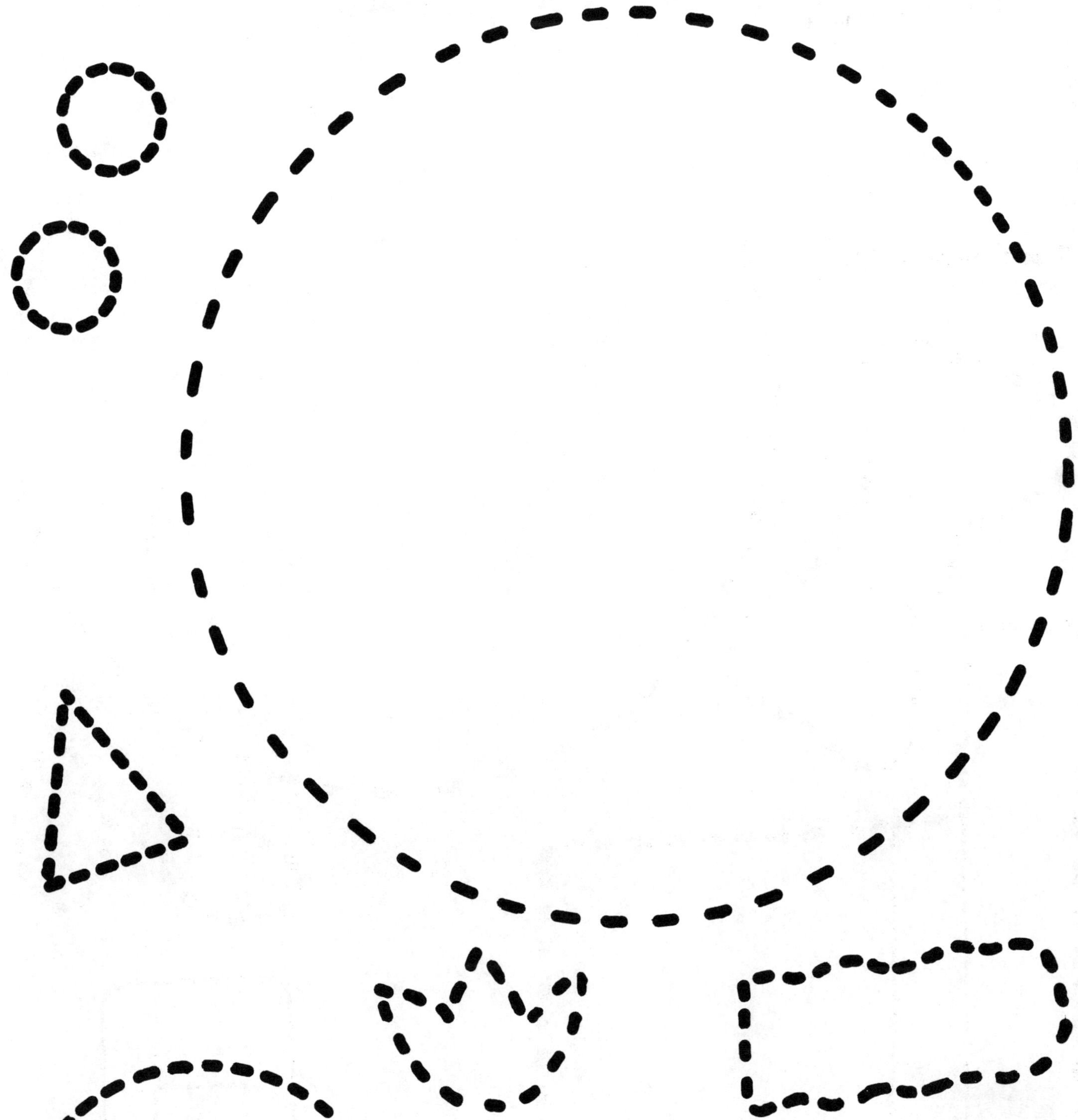

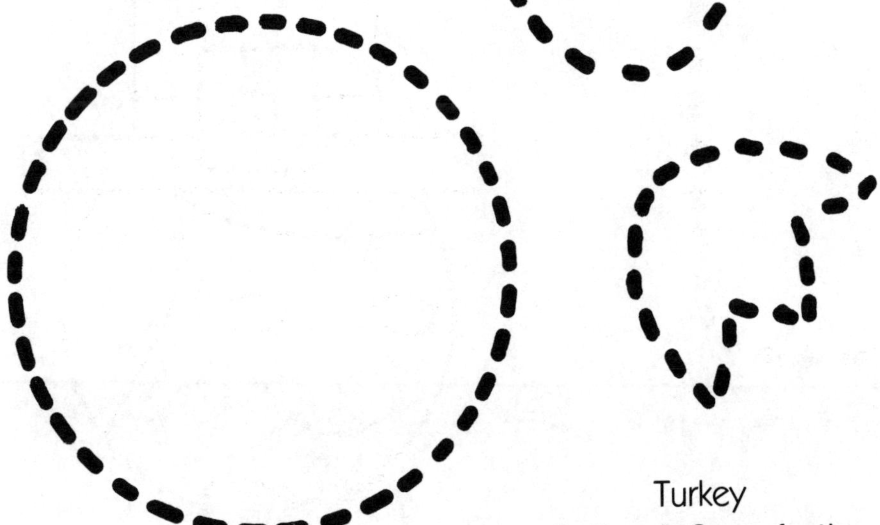

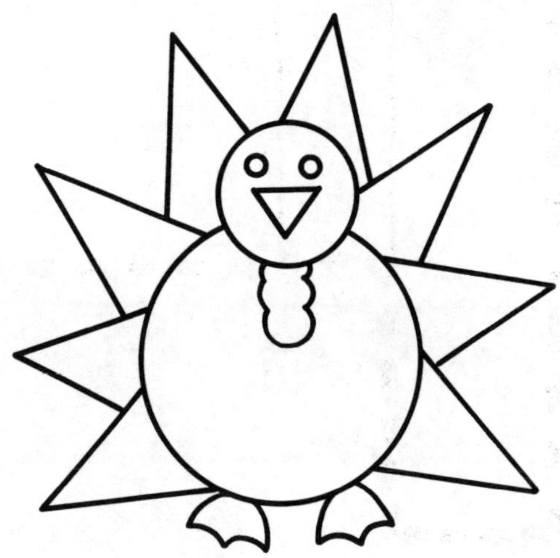

Turkey

Optional: Copy feathers on different colors of paper.

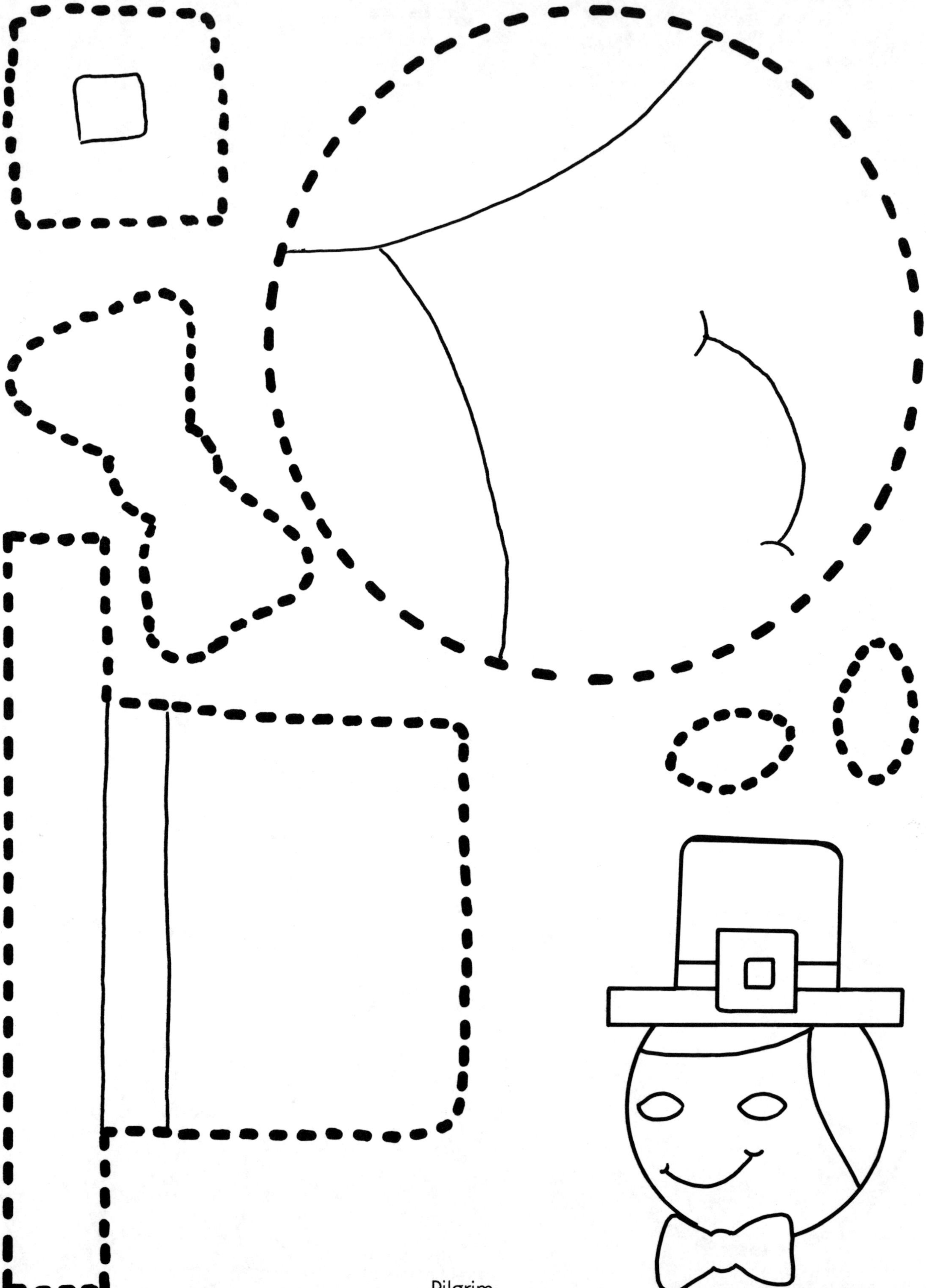

Pilgrim

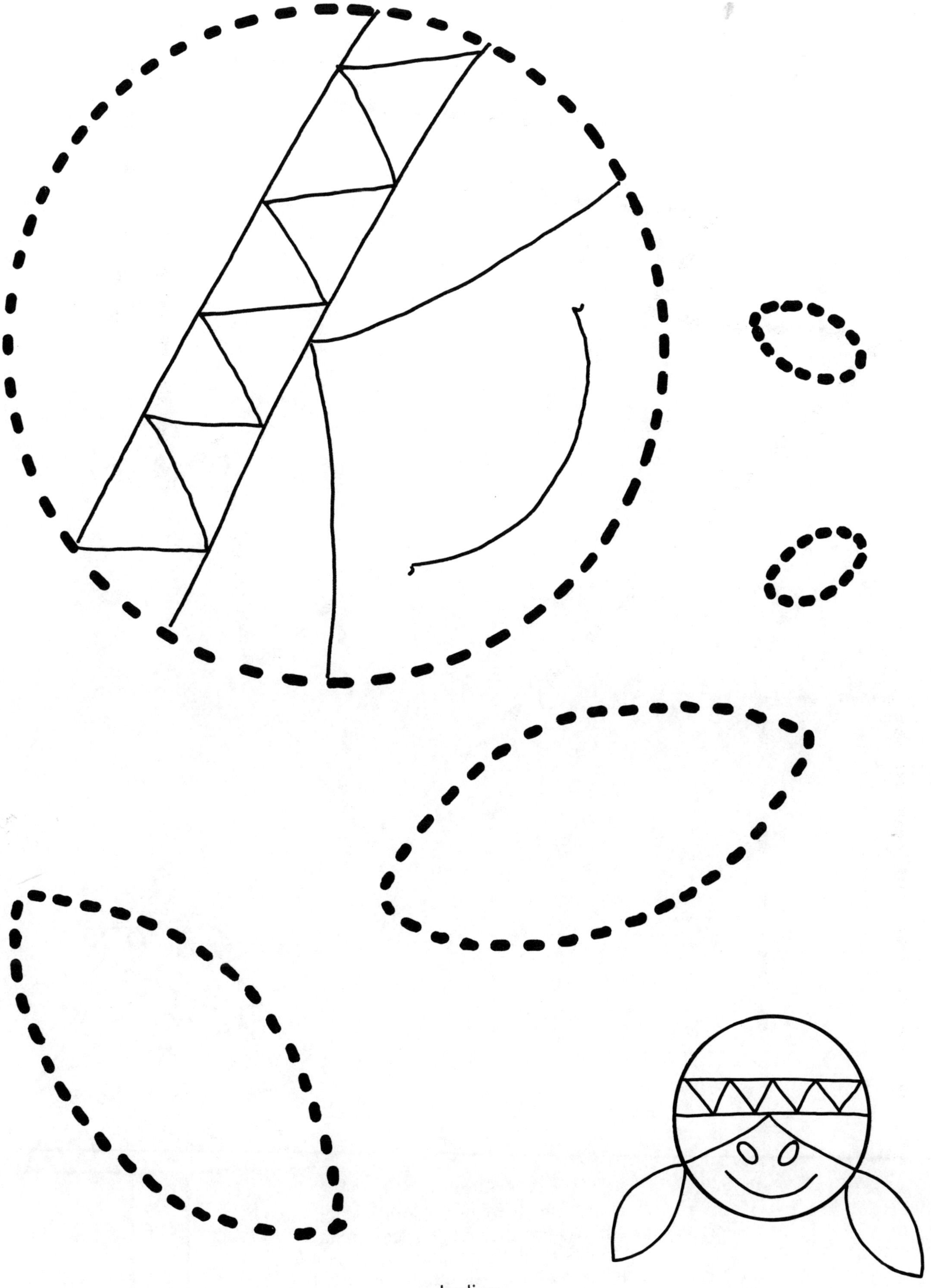

Indian

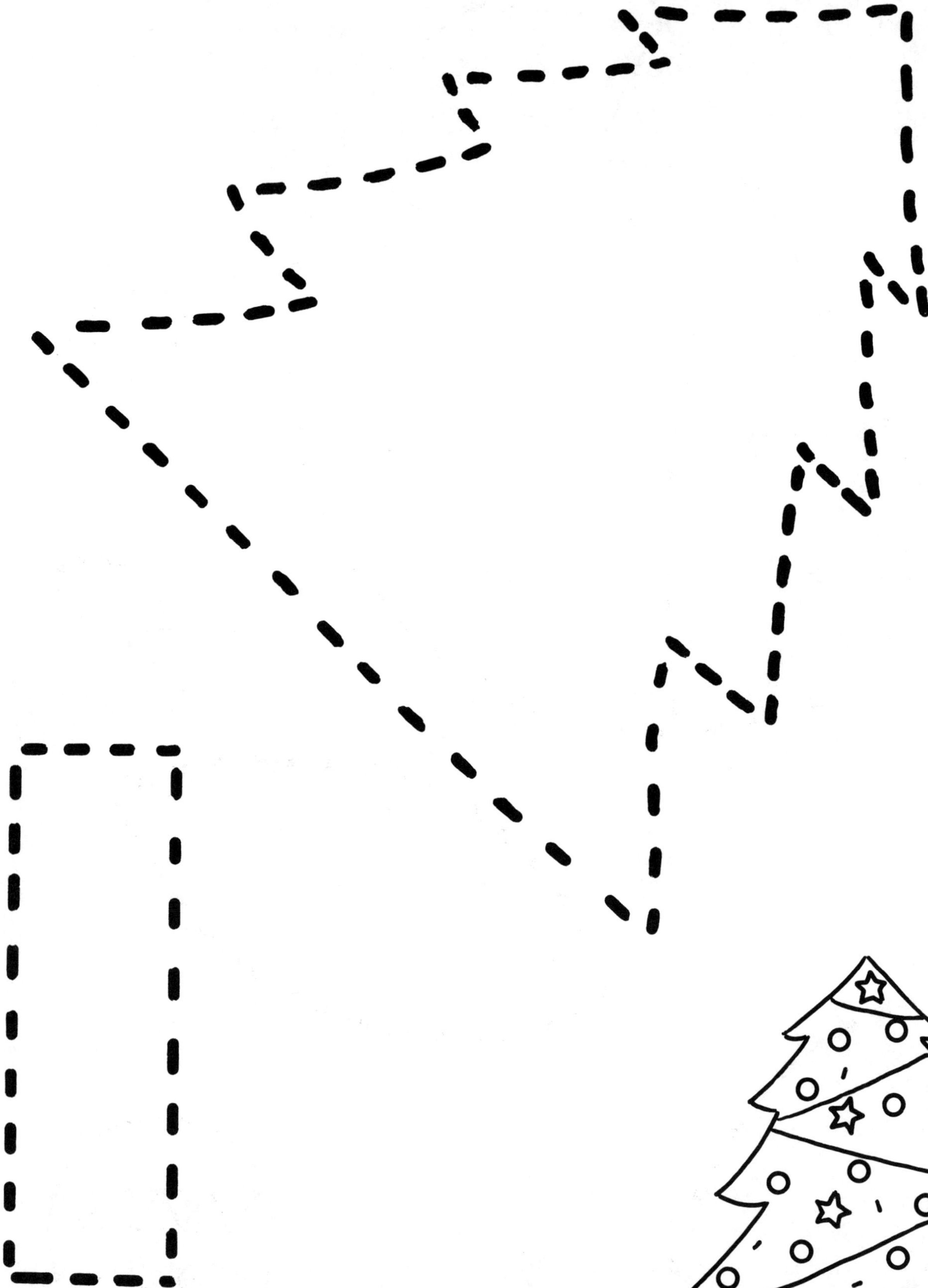

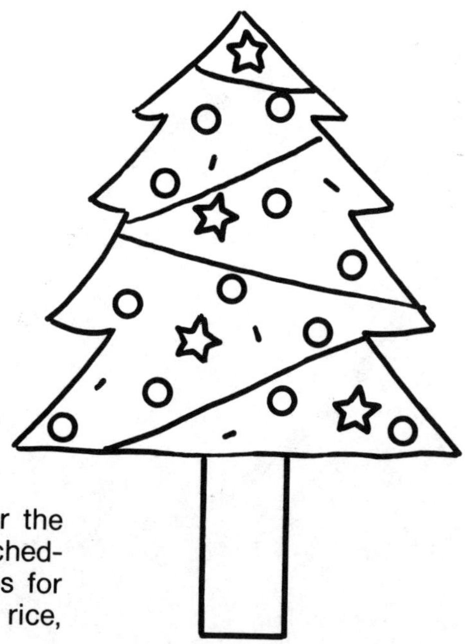

Christmas Tree

Optional: Use a tongue depressor for the tree trunk. For decorations, use punched-out colored circles or gummed circles for balls, pieces of tinsel, gummed stars, rice, popcorn.

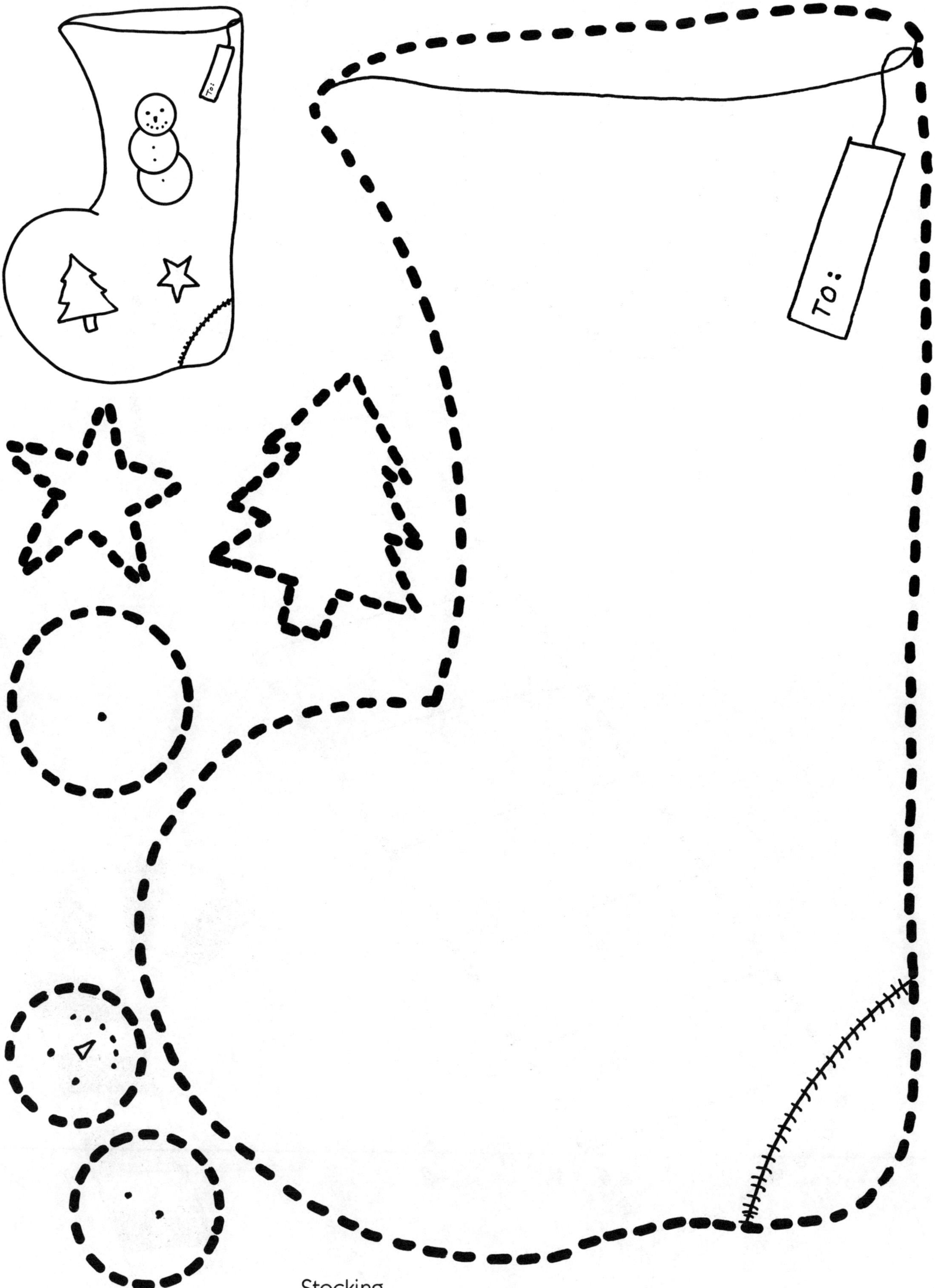

Stocking

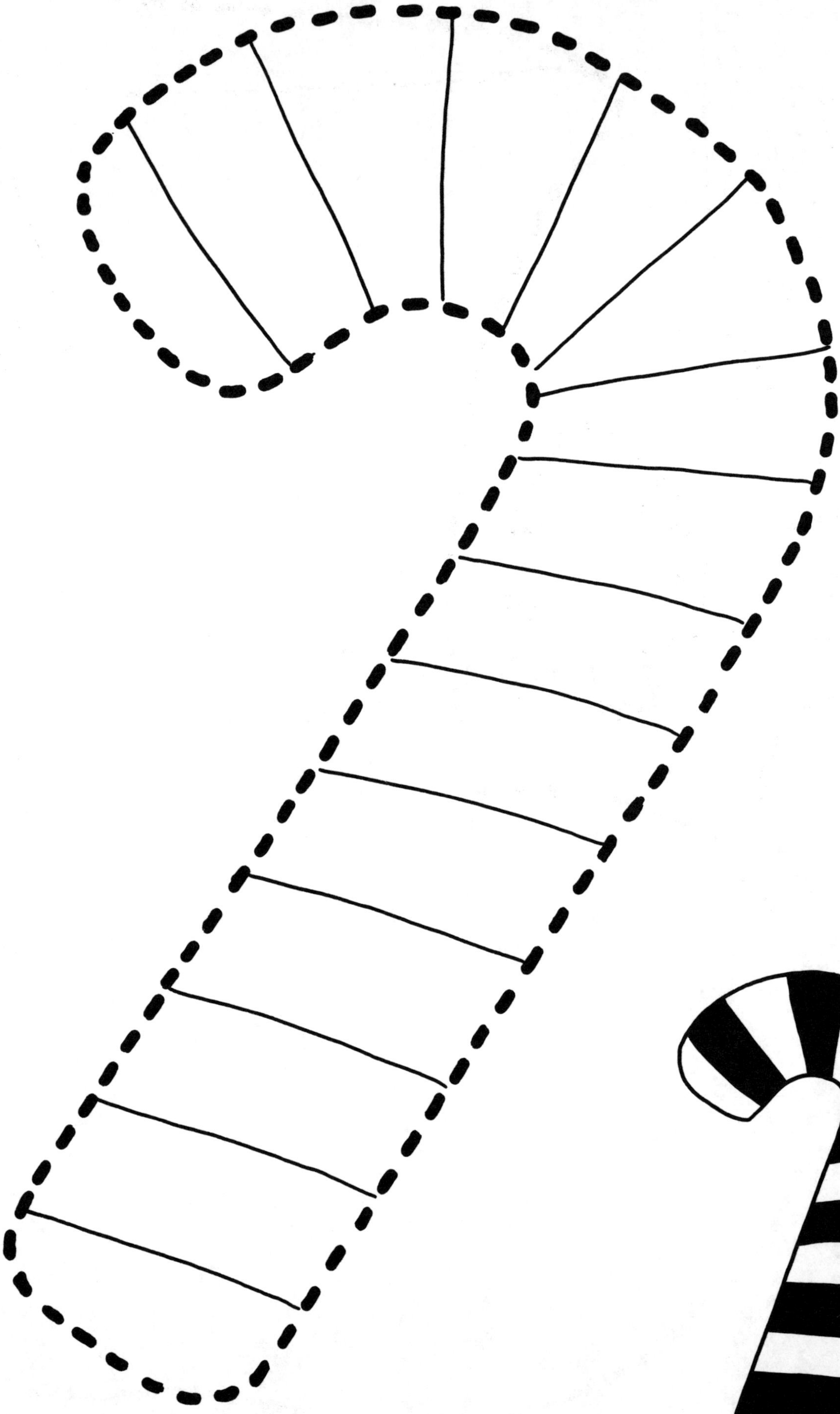

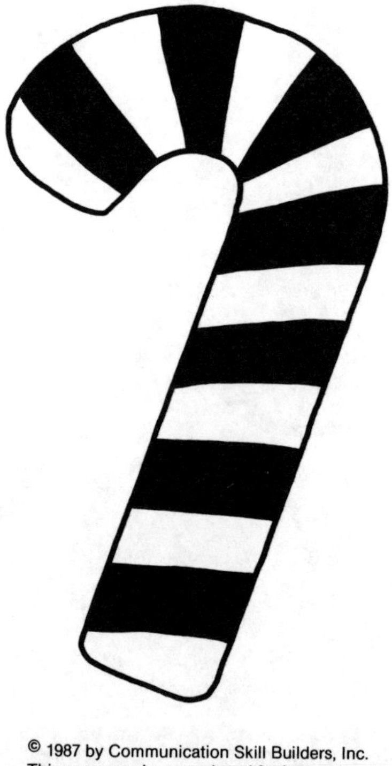

Candy Cane

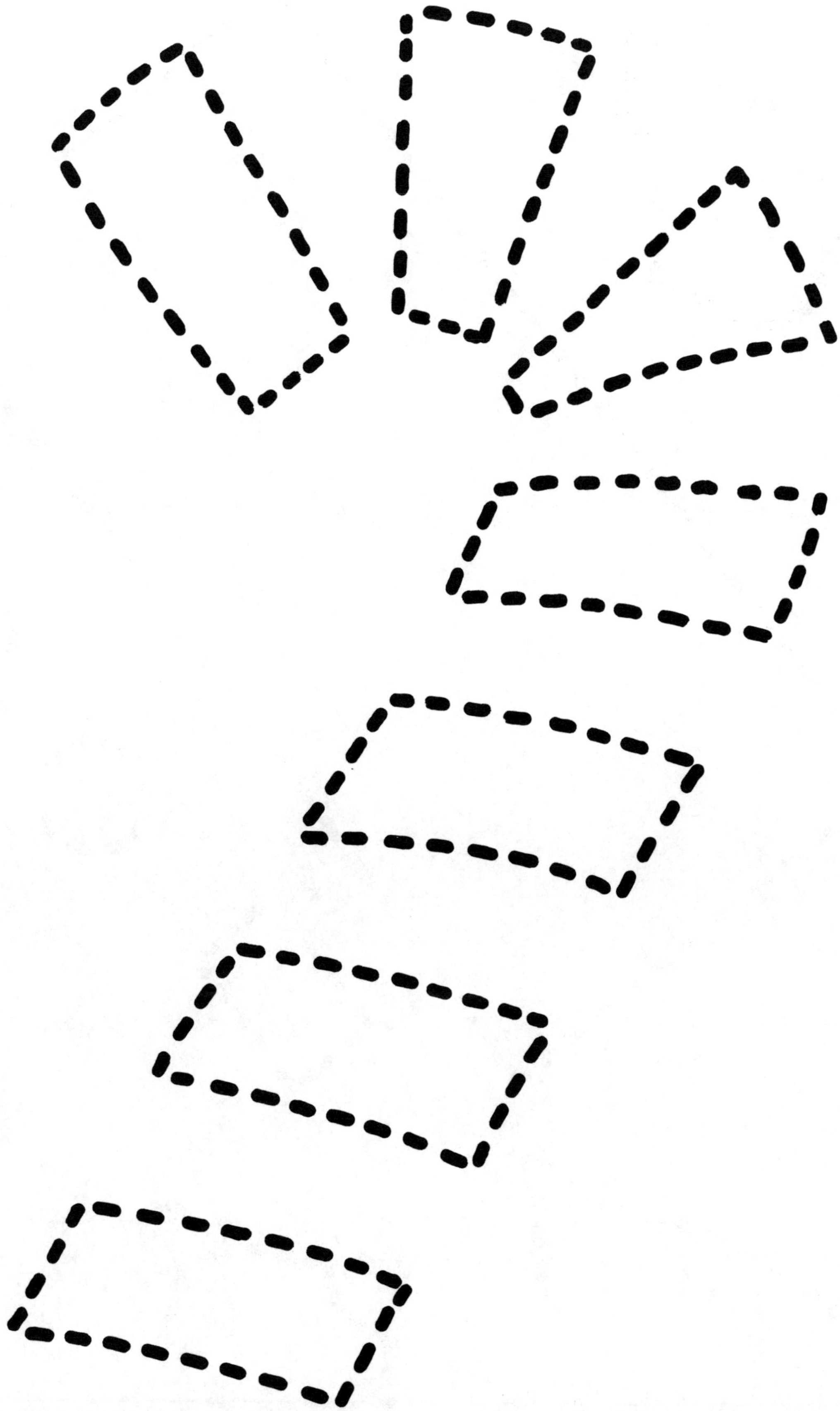

Candy Cane

Copy on red construction paper.

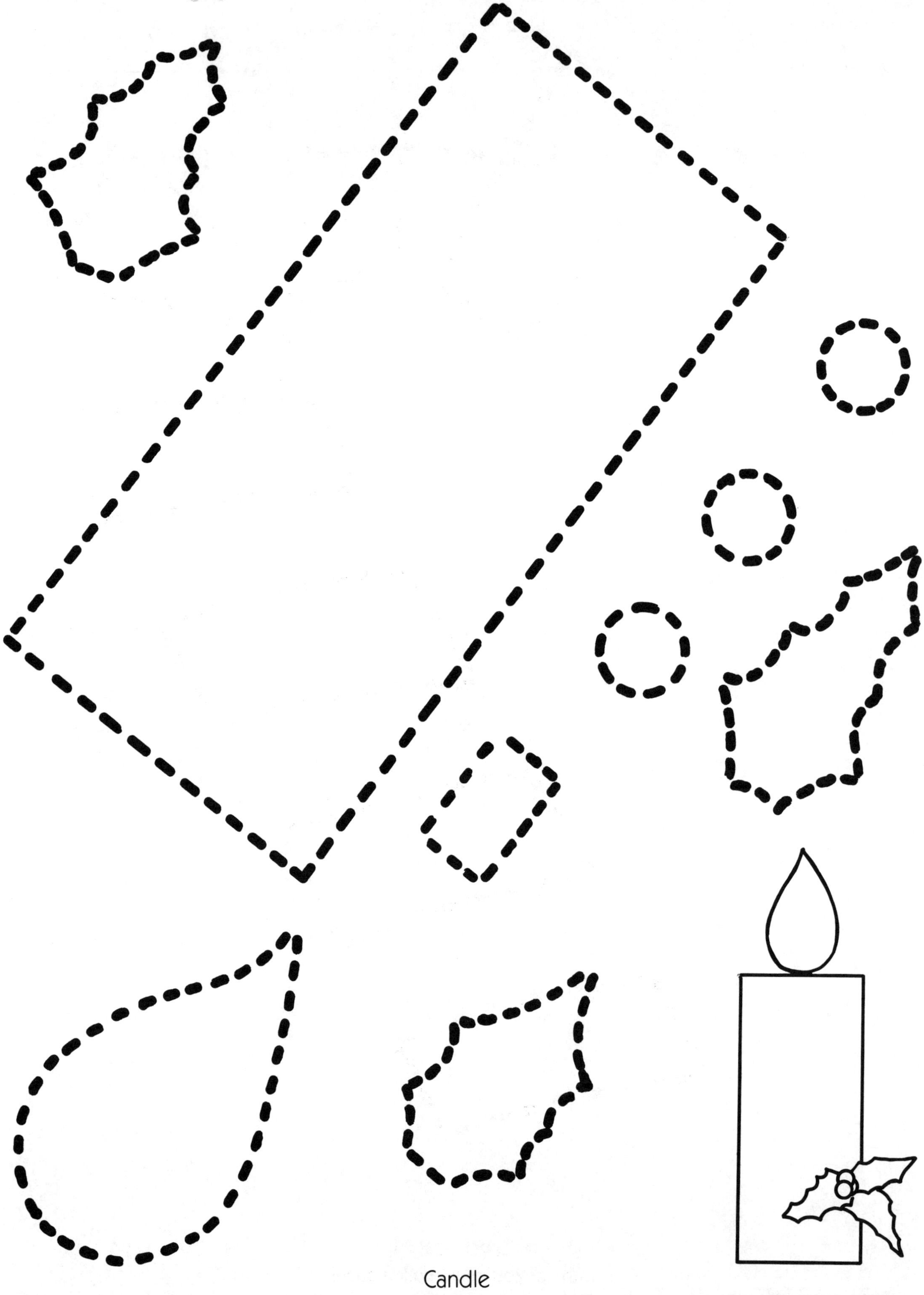

Candle

Paper Chains

Use these strips for Paper Chains and for Placemats (see pages 316-321).

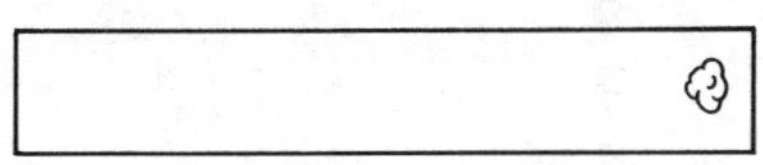

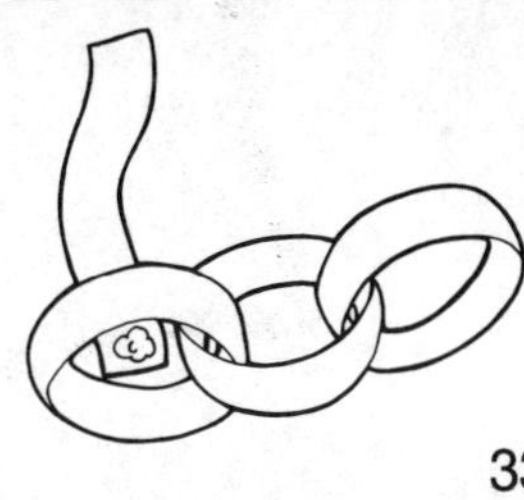

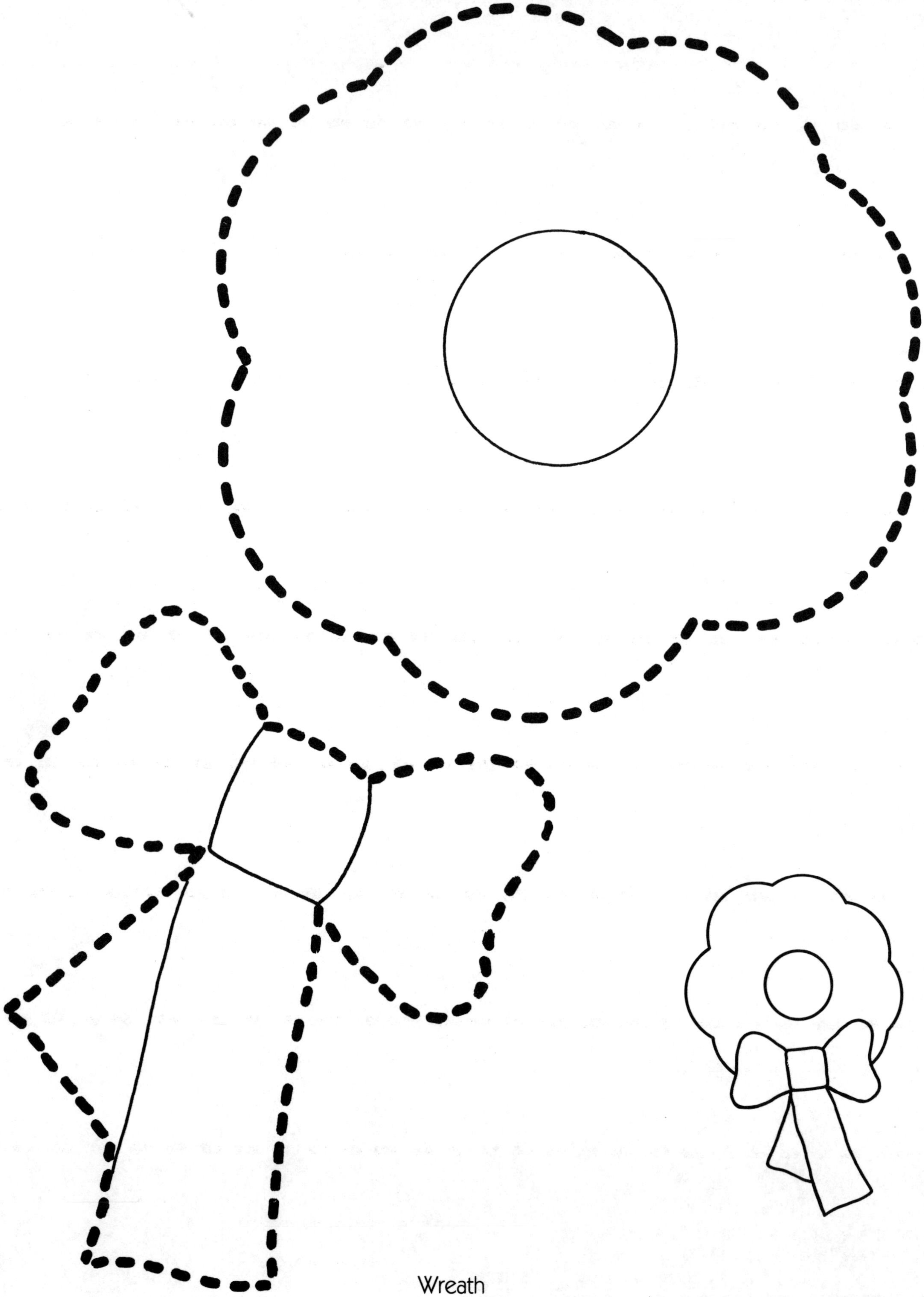

Wreath

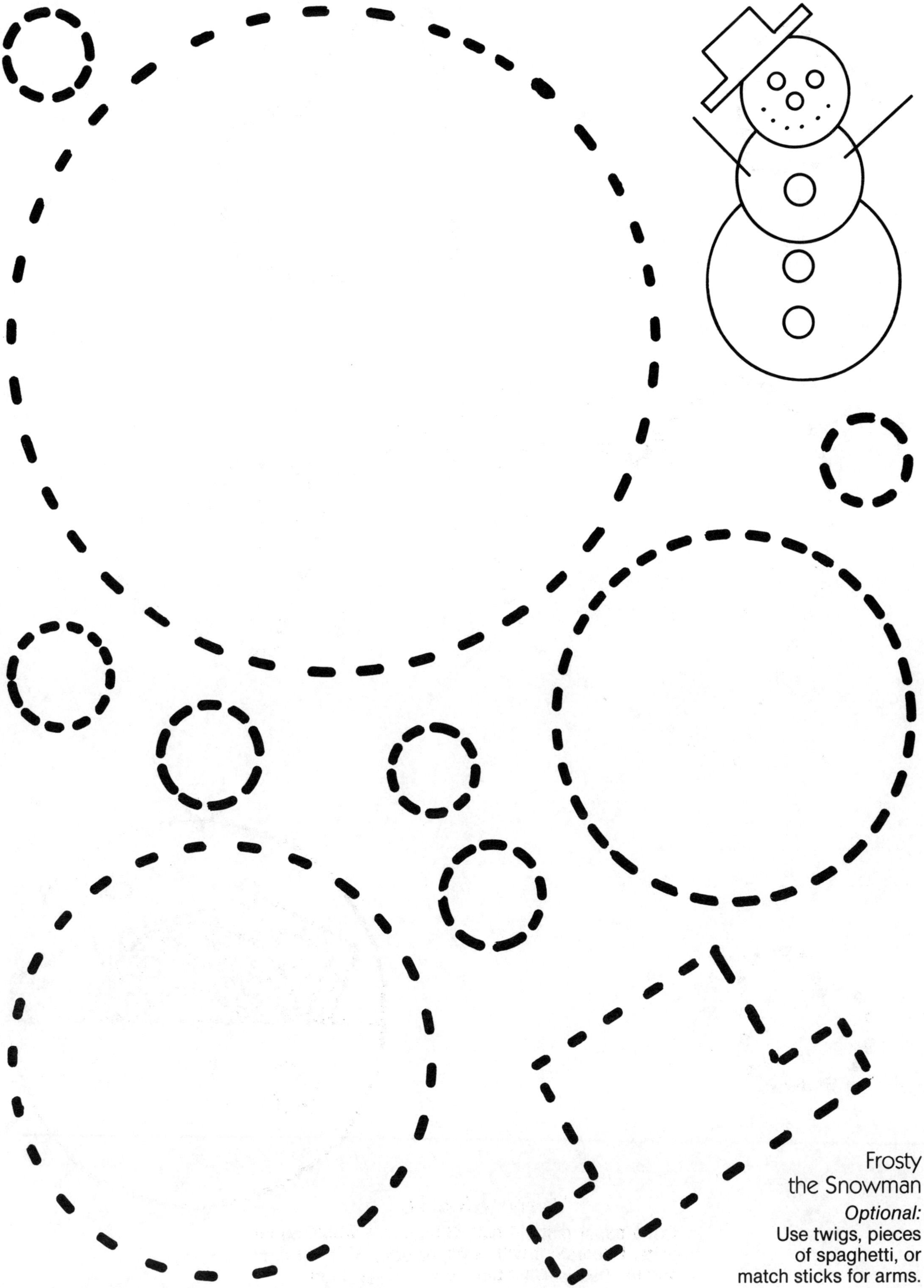

Frosty
the Snowman

Optional:
Use twigs, pieces
of spaghetti, or
match sticks for arms.

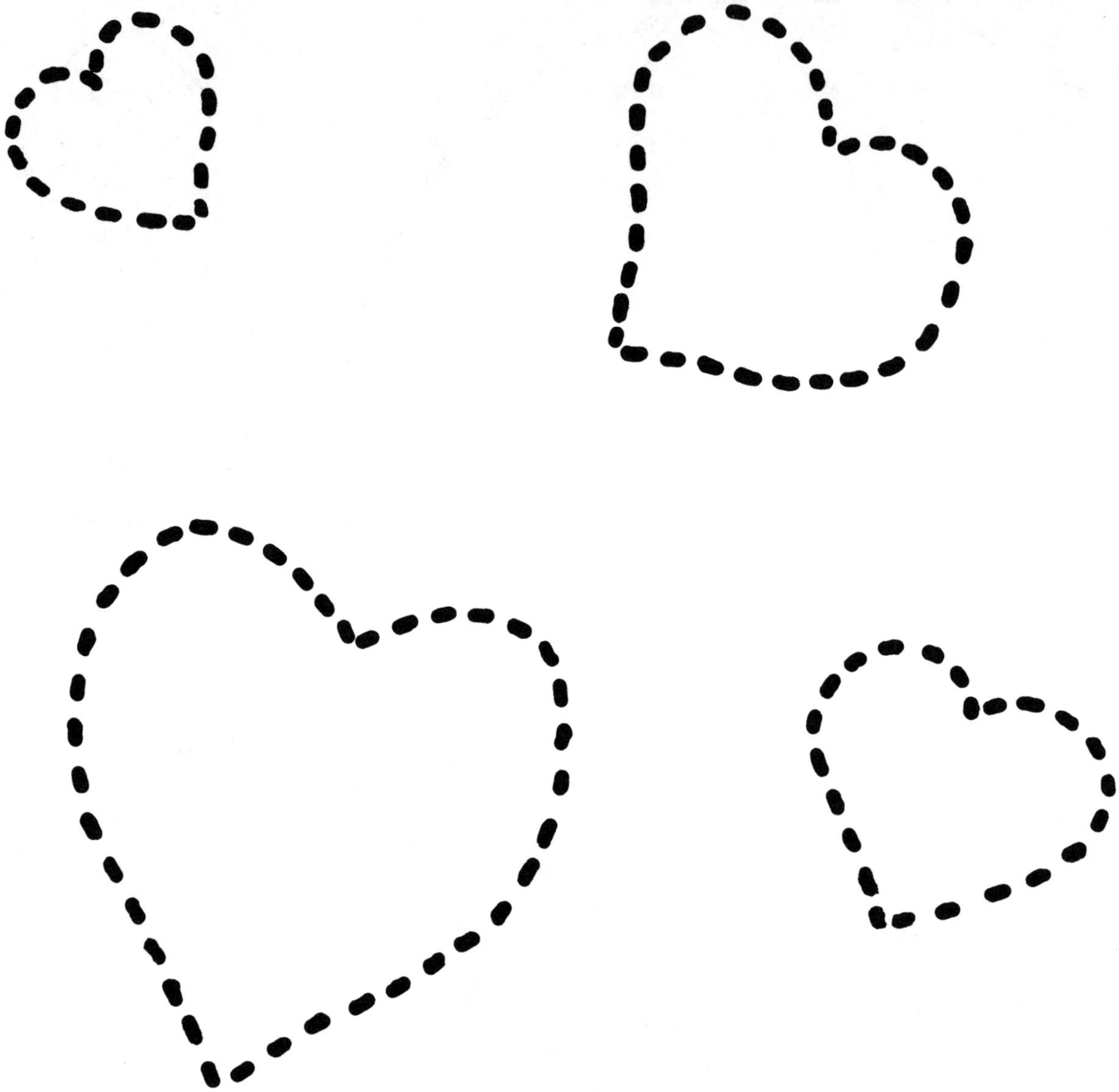

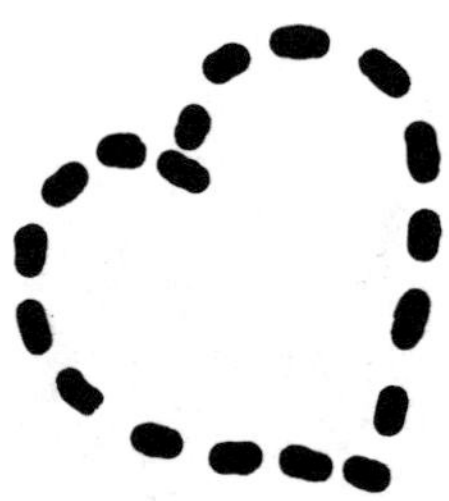

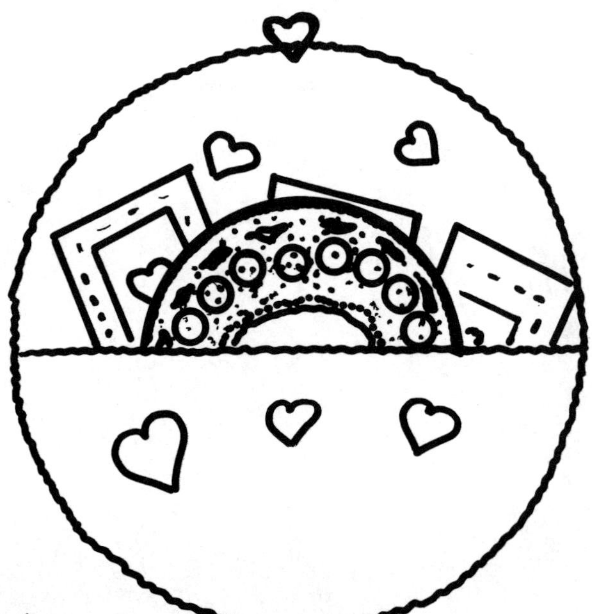

Valentine Mail Pouch

Cut a paper plate in half. Glue it to a whole paper plate. Decorate it with a paper doily. Cut out pink and red hearts. Glue them on for decoration.

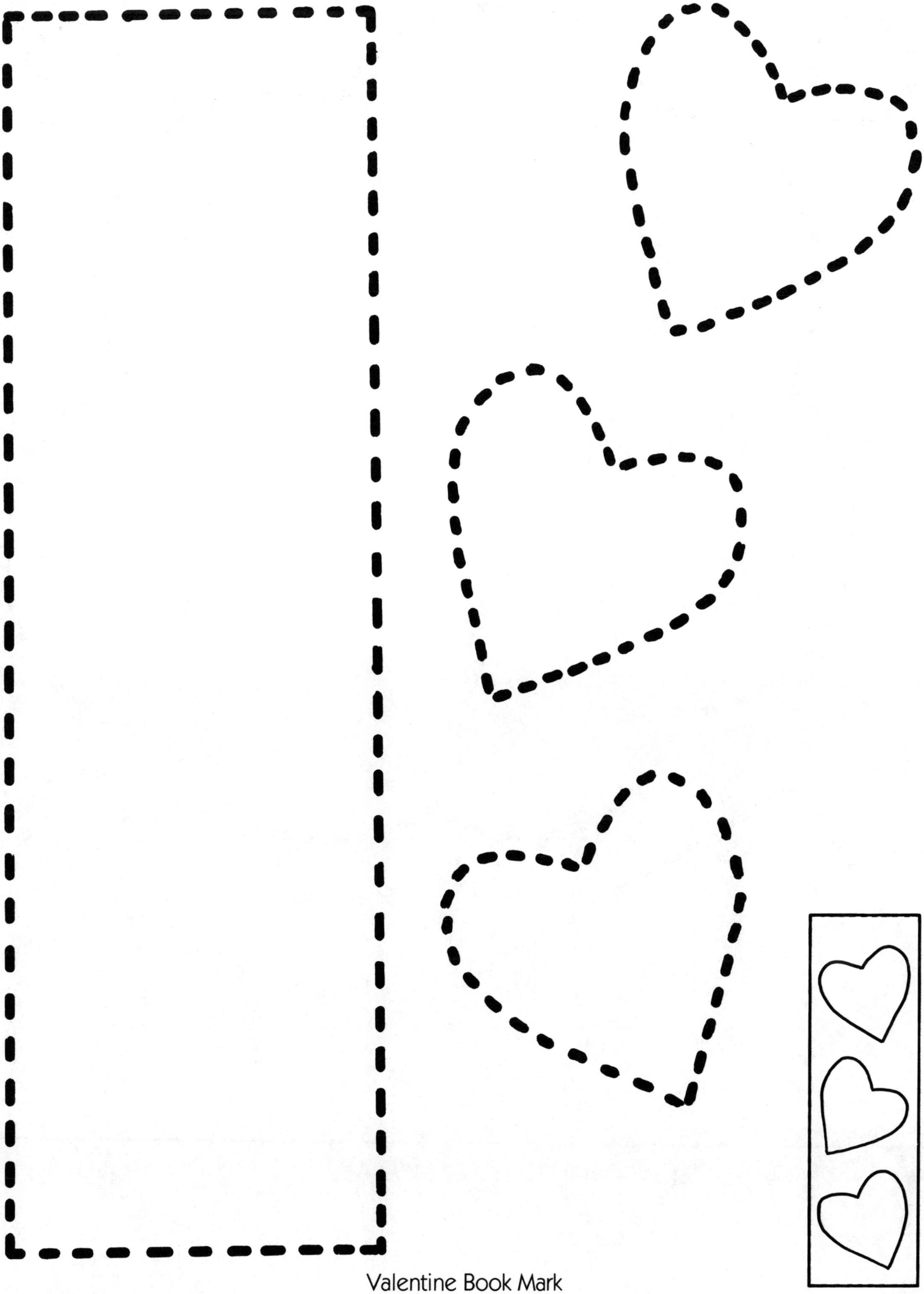

Valentine Book Mark

2 copies for Monday

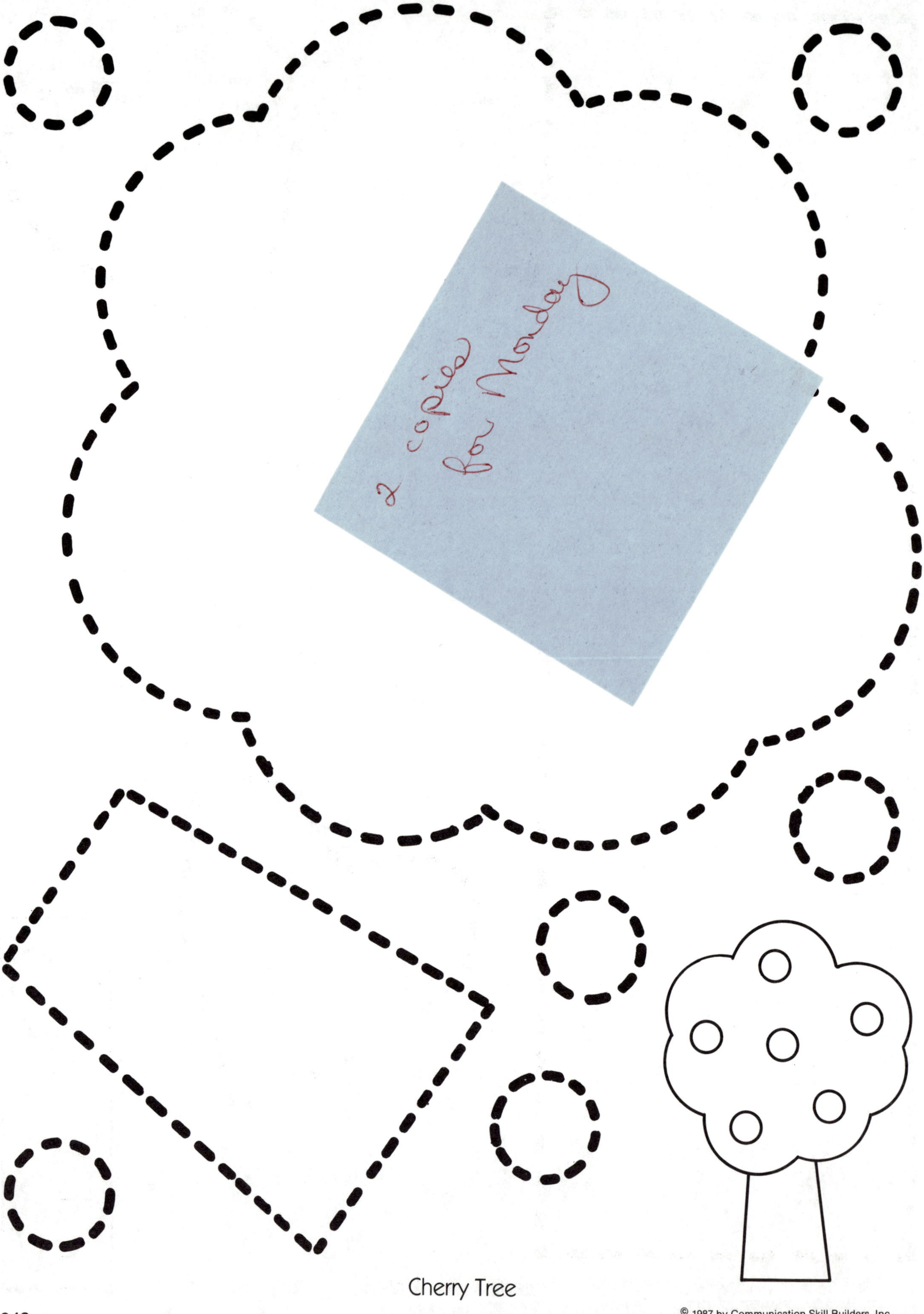

Cherry Tree

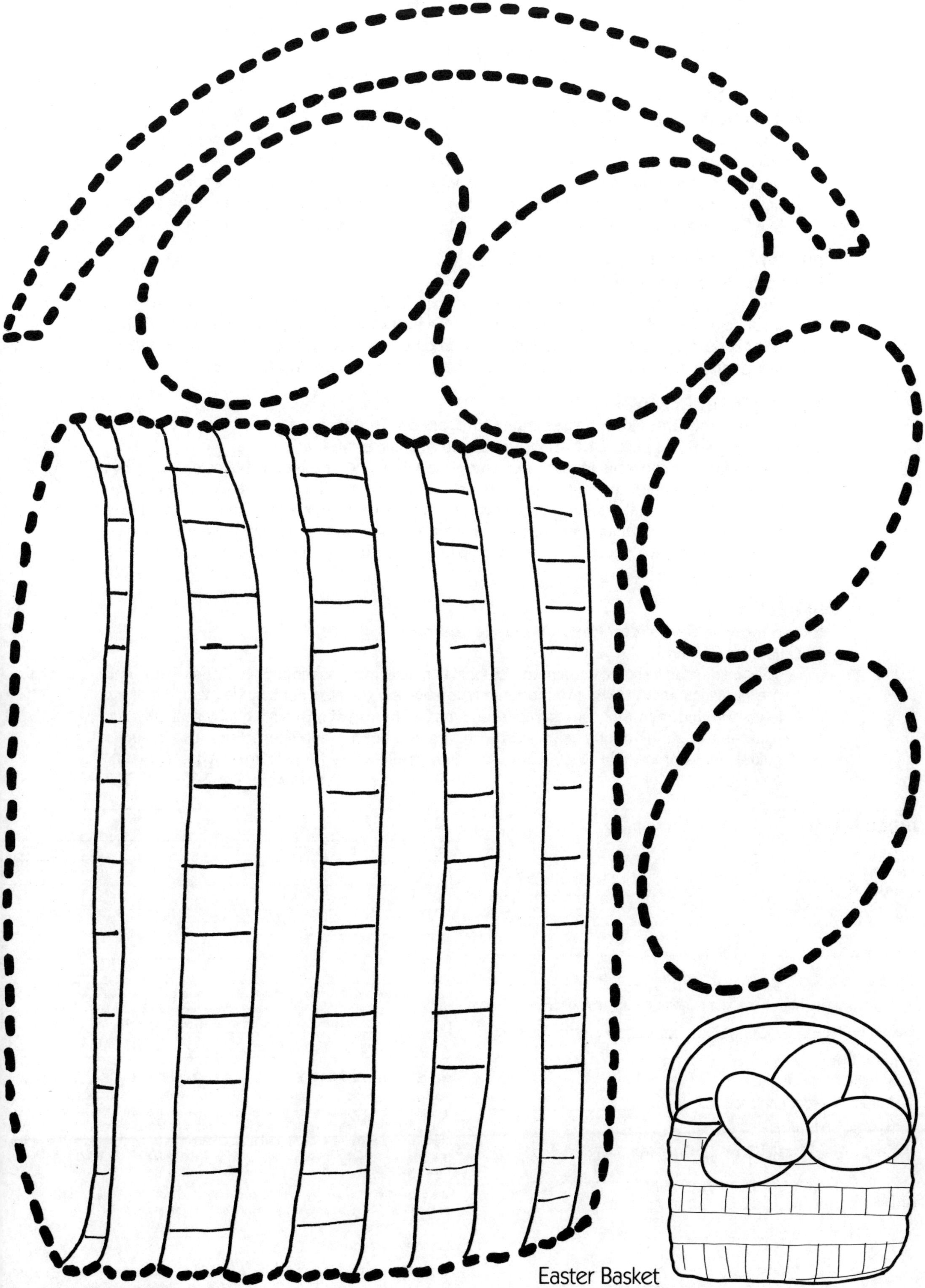

Easter Basket